D1784447

# LIVING WITH FEAR

## REFLECTIONS ON COVID-19

# LIVING WITH FEAR

## REFLECTIONS ON COVID-19

Copyright © 2020 Prince Ade Odunlade

All rights reserved.

No part of this book can be reproduced in any form or by written, electronic or mechanical, including photocopying, recording, or by any information retrieval system without written permission in writing by the author(s).

Printed in Great Britain

Although every precaution has been taken in the preparation of this book, the publisher and author assume no responsibility for errors or omissions. Neither is any liability assumed for damages resulting from the use of information contained herein.

A catalogue record for this book is available from the British Library

ISBN 978-1-8385360-39

Cover design by Japh Addico Ohatey at Onetouch Design Studio
Published by WritershouseConsultancy

# CONTENTS PAGE

## PART 3 – Conquering Fear

## PART 4 – Life after Fear

# Acknowledgements

This book is dedicated to every key worker, to their families and to their friends. Millions have worked tirelessly and courageously during the time of COVID-19. The original idea for the book was to honour the hard work and commitment you have shown, and to strive to help you make sense of the complex issues of fear and hope that have arisen during this incredibly challenging period.

The book was put together in a record time of two months, an astonishing achievement which would not have been possible without the passion and focus of more than twenty contributors and a committed editorial team: a diverse group of professionals working within healthcare and academia, nursing students, and people with lived experience of the virus. We hope the perspectives here offer you something that can help you come to terms with your own experiences.

*"The Authors have agreed that the profits from the sale of this book are to be donated to the CNWL NHS Foundation Trust Charitable Fund, a charity registered with the Charity Commission for England and Wales (Reg Nos: 1082989)"*

# Preface

## *Claire Murdoch CBE*
National Director for Mental Health
Chief Executive of Central North West London NHS Foundation Trust

I am very happy to introduce this book and its contribution to the thinking around the experience of COVID-19 in the NHS. I also thank the contributors for kindly donating profits to our Charitable Funds. It is far from definitive, and by no means a full commentary on the pandemic; it is more valuable than that.

It collects together the thoughts and experiences of many clinicians, therapists, nurses, student nurses, doctors, people with lived experience and academics; reflecting on what they expected, what they saw, and what they found from their point of view. It is eclectic, it reflects many professional outlooks and the experiences of individuals who played their part. Its value comes from 'being there' and bringing many aspects of the pandemic to the surface.

CNWL was proud to be part of a system response; our services were changed, staff were redeployed, we opened new wards and services. We had many staff who responded to the call, who worked and cared for patients who were often worried and fearful, despite their own worries and fears.

I cannot stress enough how proud I am of them all and how thankful so many people are to have been cared for by these wonderful people. One way of sharing our experiences is to start learning and that starts in these covers, with such rich opinion and experience.

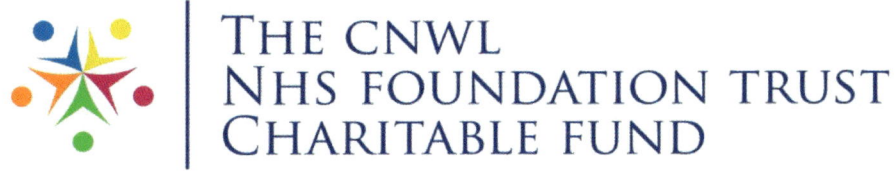

# THE CNWL
# NHS FOUNDATION TRUST
# CHARITABLE FUND

The CNWL NHS Foundation Trust Charitable Fund is a Registered Charity (Reg Nos 1082989), which enhances NHS services provided by Central and North West London NHS Foundation Trust, and Camden and Islington NHS Foundation Trust, through the receipt of donations and the payment of grants which benefit the patients, service users and carers of its services.

Our vision is 'to create a world where ordinary people are empowered to do extraordinary things and achieve outstanding outcomes, for the benefit of all regardless of whether they have, or care for someone, with a physical or mental illness.'

The Charity seeks to build resilient communities which allows the clinical work of the NHS to be sustainable, and enables patients, carers and staff the opportunity to lead lives which, as much as possible, fulfil their personal and professional aspirations.

If you would like to support our work by making a donation, you can do so using either:

1. Virgin Money Giving Donation Page:
https://uk.virginmoneygiving.com/donation-web/charity?charityId=1001865&stop_mobi=yes

Or

2. Pay Pal:
paypal.com/gb/fundraiser/charity/3160433
or searching for: **CNWL NHS Foundation Trust Charitable Fund**

**To get find out more, or to get involved, please contact Andrew Machin our Associate Director for Charity Development at**
**andrew.machin@nhs.net**

# Forward

## *Robyn Doran*

When I was asked by my colleague Ade to write the foreword to this book it made me reflect on my own experiences and earliest memories of fear, which was as a young child growing up in Napier, New Zealand. At the time, Napier was a town that frequently experienced earthquakes. Whenever there was an earthquake, I remember the haunted look on my Dad's face. I never fully understood that look. It was a look of utmost fear. Crippled by the event, we were not able to move him to the places of safety that we had been taught to move into in earthquake drills at school. I realised now that the fear I saw in my Dads eyes was probably as a result of Post-Traumatic Stress Disorder, which can often be associated with traumatic events. As a child he was at school in Napier in 1931, when a major earthquake ripped through the town and destroyed it, and many lost their lives. He witnessed this first-hand and never had any chance for treatment or help over the years as the town rebuilt itself (both the bricks and mortar and the community).

Some years later I had the privilege of working with the community of North Kensington and survivors and bereaved of the Grenfell Tower. I have heard and watched survivors tell the story of escaping from the tower on the night of the fire and how it impacted them. Members of the community watching people jump from the tower trying to survive or shouting out the windows for help from their neighbours and friends; many of them suffered from PTSD following their horrific experiences.

This book is about trying to make sense of fear that millions are experiencing today. It is written in the midst of the biggest pandemic the world has ever seen for many generations. Each chapter is written by individuals who have different perspectives and reflections to share. A number of the authors are health professionals who come from a range of backgrounds. Many have been delivering frontline services in the midst of this pandemic and have a first-hand experience of fear. The book has both very experienced clinicians at the top of their career giving us their insights, and student nurses who came into work carrying out their daily shifts, and then found themselves working on a ward with a number of fragile COVID positive patients. They will share their experiences of taking a break in the middle of a shift and an hour later when they returned to the ward, 5 of the 12 patients had died. Some of the authors are academics and some train our clinicians of the future. Their perspective is different again, as they are also able to reflect on their own fear and suffering that individuals and families have experienced during this unprecedented time.

You will find insight into how some people have managed during this period. You will also find some social comment from a political perspective, and one of the authors gives us a psychodynamic viewpoint about those in power in this country, questioning whether their "collective omnipotent delusion" made a situation that was bad even worse. Unlike other countries that took a pragmatic lockdown approach early on, the British "keep calm and carry on" approach probably did not help us. A large group of older adults travelled to Berlin to see an orchestral concert; the Prime Minister was proud to be shaking hands with people who had the virus; a quarter of a million people went to the races at Cheltenham.

Many health care workers will be suffering from Moral Distress and or Moral Injury from their experiences over the last 10 weeks since the pandemic began. Where at times they did not feel that they had the right equipment and protection to keep themselves and their patients safe. I will never forget the recent conversation I had with nurses on one of the learning disabilities wards within the Trust where I work. The nurses were fearful for themselves, their families and their patients. Despite the guidance around social distancing, what do you do when the patients you are committed to working with do not understand or adhere to social distancing? Even with full PPE they were still experiencing fear.

Where are we now? At the time of writing this foreword, the UK had a death total of 38,489 and was just starting to come out of lockdown. The fear is still real and prevalent in my own Trust. I still have regular conversations with staff at all levels that fear for themselves, their patients and their loved ones. We do not know what will happen next.

# Introduction

*Professor David Sines*

## Living with Uncertainty – The Challenge of Rediscovery

I regard it as both a pleasure and a privilege to have been invited to produce the introductory chapter of this reflective and insightful book that takes us on a journey to enlighten our understanding of the experiences, effects and lessons to be learned from the 2020 global COVID-19 pandemic. During the past four decades, I have been personally associated with the lives of people whose autonomy has been challenged for a range of reasons and with their families and their professional supporters. A unifying factor that I have witnessed in my professional journey relates to the need to learn to live with uncertainty when our autonomy is compromised or challenged. Such compromise to our autonomy correlates directly with the imposition of enforced change that might have occurred as the direct result of the imposition of restrictions on our personal freedom or the removal of the rights, status and societal position of members of our local and national communities.

However, as this insightful text will bear witness one thing is certain, we can never assume constancy in our lives. Rather, we are all engaged in a lifetime journey of uncertainty. This requires us to build personal resilience to enable us to adapt meaningfully. To enable us to acquire the capacity, confidence and capability to respond effectively to the imposition of unexpected life events and externally imposed sanctions that demand us to recalibrate the ways in which we construct our normative 'lived reality' and engagement with society.

This book takes us on a journey that combines personal insight and narrative with an evidence-based exposition of human behaviour and an underpinning exploration of how members of society prepare, respond to, and recover from the effects of sudden change and imposed threats to their personal health and wellbeing. The book reflects a rich tapestry against which to explore and understand the key stages of transition that occur as individuals journey through personal and professional uncertainly. Through reliance on narrative witness accounts and theoretical elucidation, the chapter authors synthesise the characteristics of the life challenges shared by a myriad of people and in so doing provide a sense of global, corporate memory to inform future generations of ways in which to build greater personal resilience in the face of unexpected and perceptibly uncontrollable adversity. The book penetrates the key challenges faced by members of society during the COVID-19 pandemic and explores their reactions to the same. The cost to our collective emotional and mental health is hard to gauge, but estimates suggest perhaps half the population are feeling more anxious or depressed than normal. In some ways, we all need to learn to cope and offer an explanation for how individuals can build and face a new reality, whilst retaining a sense of courage, hope and recovery.

Having read this book, I was reminded of a previous text that I read during my mental health degree nursing training whilst studying at the Maudsley Hospital in 1974 ('The Fear of Freedom'), published by Erich Fromm in 1941, which explored 'man's' relationship with freedom and adversity. Fromm was writing at the time about the rise of Nazi Germany in the early 1930s' and notes that in our quest for freedom and human rights that we are increasingly reliant upon 'the realisation of the individual self'. Fromm argues that although 'freedom' has brought us independence and the right to rationality, it has resulted also in members of society becoming susceptible to imposed and unexpected isolation, anxiety and powerlessness.

During times when isolation is imposed, Fromm advised that 'isolation can be unbearable. The alternatives man is confronted with are either to escape from the burden of this freedom into new dependencies and submission, or to advance to the full realisation of positive freedom which is based on the uniqueness and individuality of man'. Fromm postulates that we all have a need for sensuality and emotional security and the need for co-operation and socialisation. He argues also that we have a need not to be alone in order to manage our inter-dependencies and also to enable us to avoid becoming overwhelmed by our own 'insignificance'. In my opinion, there are parallels with Fromm's thesis and the experiences that we all are sharing and experiencing during current COVID-19 pandemic situation. As such, this book is an analysis of the physical, psychological and emotional character structure of humankind, which provides us also with a salutary reminder that we cannot take life for granted and that we are all the subject of the need to evolve and adapt to meet the urgent needs of the times in our quest for stasis, hope and survival.

A further parallel to the current book is the fact that Fromm recognises that human nature, whilst not being without its 'omnipotence', can adapt significantly to social change. He argues also that humankind strives to seek security by forging ties with the local and national community but does so at the potential cost to personal freedom and the integrity of the individual self. Fromm advises that this is a dialectical process that involves increasing inner strength and resilience, but states also that this is limited by society, which can determine just how far individuality, freedom and autonomy can be expressed. The paradox is however that the sense of separation of 'individual self' from society may be experienced as anxiety and fear. When this occurs, the world can be experienced as threatening and overpowering. Under these circumstances, I would argue that such a challenge to one's autonomy and right to seek socialisation can result in one feeling that one's sense of integrity and self-worth is debased, compromised and threatened. At such times we can become vulnerable when we are exposed to external pressure to conform to unfamiliar sanction and threat to our personally constructed concept of normality and security.

This book advises in *Part 1, Section 5 – (Anna Maratos)* that we develop '*a psychological defence to protect its proponents from feeling afraid of an uncontrollable, invisible threat which requires a degree of unity, inter-dependence and collaboration to be defeated. Cultural forces in the west and perhaps particularly in Britain, promote independence and invulnerability over openness and leaning on others; stoicism is seen as resilience while being in touch with one's vulnerability and inter-dependence on others, may be more likely to be associated with weakness'.* In the same way the building and maintenance of sustainable communities and neighbourhoods is one of the most powerful and visible expressions of today's society. This fact remains a precept since it relates to a concern that wherever possible local communities should be permitted to reinforce their own lawful norms, rules and sanctions in order to maintain a sense of communal order and personal protection. This has become an expected and unifying ideal across nations, and down the generations.

This is a characteristic of a social system that belongs to us and which we have come to take for granted as members of a 'free and open society'. Such sustainable communities that we have all come to take for granted in recent decades are characterised by members of the population assuming that our habitat provides an impenetrably safe and secure place to live. One where people can receive the protection they require, to live their lives to the full without fear of harm, threat, intimidation or restriction or compromise to their health status or to their right to freedom of expression and lifestyle. This has become the practical expression of a shared commitment by our nation which can be regarded as a commitment to 'shared governance'.

Any approach to shared governance involves a fundamental shift in mind set. From one that is perceived as imposing sanctions and restrictions on others, to one that is founded on the cornerstone principles of partnership, equity, accountability, and personal ownership that form a culturally sensitive and empowering framework; enabling sustainable and evidence-based decisions to determine how we can conduct our lives safely in accordance with our personal values, drive and determination to self-actualise and protect others. Shared governance requires us to promote and foster a facilitative, rather than directive approach to how we encourage the emergence, the co-design, re-setting and implementation of adaptive behaviours that enable us to regain psychological stability and purpose in our lives.

So, in its simplest form, shared governance is shared decision-making based on the principles of partnership, equity, accountability, and ownership at the point of service. This process model, whilst being empowering, requires all members of our local communities to have a voice in decision-making, thus encouraging diverse and creative input that will help advance the common cause of social and moral justice. In essence, we need to encourage and empower every citizen to have a personal stake in the future governance of their local community and plead to the principle of common purpose and alignment to locally held values of moral purpose, justice and fairness and above all public protection and health security. Such approaches are reported to lead to increased citizen satisfaction, safety and welfare, and encourage local people to take greater ownership of their decisions and of the consequences of their actions and are more vested in community focused outcomes. In our quest to regain control over our lives, and to construct a 'new normal', following the current global pandemic, we will all be required to assume a new sense of moral purpose and responsibility. Such then is the principle of participative management, collegiality and shared governance.

There is no doubt that the current challenge will undoubtedly result in the creation of a new paradigm with goals and objectives that are encompassed within an organisational learning environment. Leaders, administrators, local citizens and front-line employees are constantly learning and implementing new ways of responding to the pandemic. They seek to secure public confidence, compliance, encouraging society to 'keep people safe' and engaging in new ways of thinking and working. In the process, we are recognising increasingly that the delivery of 'the new normal' at the point of personal and community engagement is key to organisational success. We are preparing for new ways of working, new ways of engaging with society, and new ways of participating with others. Shared governance is about moving from a traditional hierarchical model to a relational partnership model of engagement with the public accompanied by a strategic change in organisational culture and leadership. It involves a significant realignment in how local citizens, system leaders, front line employees, and public health and social care systems transition into new relationships and responsibilities. At its best, it results in a triad of shared responsibility – the health and social care services, adherence to local community norms and individual internalised accountability, underpinned by shared governance and external scrutiny.

So, what is that we should strive to achieve? A safe, reliable and trusted service that is there whenever we need it, often at the most profound moments in our lives. Also, during times when we are confronted by some of the excesses that manifest as the result of some of the most fundamental elements of the human spirit that exist with our local neighbourhoods. These are the times when as local citizens we experience the public health and social care system in an intensely vivid and personal way. For the main part, our local citizens stand alongside our public health services, and continue to give thanks for the service; for the skill, and for the understanding and assurance that the front-line guardians of our health security, societal values and norms so capably display.

Despite these challenges, the recent pandemic has reaffirmed that our health and social care systems (and those who work within them), continue to act as guardians of our societal norms and health protection systems, and continue to defy any attempt to compromise the veritable standards of professional health care practice that underpin our national health and welfare systems. In this way, we owe a debt of gratitude to all of our health and social care practitioners for their determination, resilience and commitment to sustaining the provision of responsive, effective, non-compromised and safe healthcare services to members of our population.

However, to be proud of our health care system is not to be blind to its imperfections. It's to be honest about its achievements, while holding ourselves to aspire to an even higher standard. An analogy exists here with the NHS when Aneurin Bevan predicted that the Health Service, "must always be changing, growing and evolving" so that "it must always appear to be inadequate". So here's the paradox: To continue to succeed in the future, our health and social care system must always be impatient with the present and look forward with hope for a sustained positive future. Within which we all seek to build trust, confidence, competence, capability and effective collaboration in order to protect the public and to promote a renewed sense of purposeful engagement, as we build and engage with a new safe and enduring future. This will be a connective journey, informed by both an internal and external experience of reflection and "making sense of" our lived experiences.

This book confirms that creative service responses can be designed by health care professionals to ensure that people who present emotional and psychological trauma are afforded the opportunities to re-connect purposefully with themselves, others and their social world. These opportunities could occur through the medium of caring communication and exploration of life realities, as identified by those who have experienced trauma, fear and anxiety. Our health care professionals have provided authentic knowledge-based support to persons whose autonomy is temporarily compromised or challenged 'through the delivery of receptive and people-centred qualities and skills to validate people's lived realities, reawaken personal aspirations and care for expressed human needs' (Feely, 2007).

In delivering effective and responsive support during times of personal and global crisis evidenced based care, it is important that the voice of true experts [service users] are heard. Through sharing a range of respondents' narratives, this book offers a first-step contribution to understanding how we can work together to build a positive future. This book confirms that our service response is not powerless, even if we are sometimes challenged by extreme circumstances and internal and externally imposed conflict. One thing is sure – we as a global society and economy are determined to win the battle to re-establish a sense of personal and societal control and to manage our expectations as we confront a new 'normal' and seek to 'reset the dials' to direct the way in which we behave, interact and commune in the future. We must seek to reach a new understanding with each other, with government and with the wider public about how we can further adapt and become even more resilient as individuals and as society as a whole with the aim of overcoming unexpected adversity and learning to live purposefully and effectively with uncertainly.

# The Diary of an Accident and Emergency Consultant

*Dr Ian Ewing*

As a medical consultant mid-way through my career in the NHS, I have gradually reached the stage of feeling competent to deal with whatever comes through the door. I don't worry about being on call for emergency admissions: experience tells me that I can cope. Thursday night feels different though and I struggle to sleep. I am about to cover my first weekend of the COVID-19 crisis and will be the senior medical opinion for all patients admitted to hospital from Friday to Sunday.

In the last few days, I have heard of vastly experienced Consultant colleagues breaking down during on calls, overcome by the volume of patients with respiratory failure, fatigued by difficult conversations and decisions, and struggling with the uncertainty of trying to determine likelihood of benefit from critical care interventions, such as mechanical ventilation.

What really has me worried though is the hospital engineers' concern about the oxygen delivery system. We know that our tank will not run dry, but nobody is sure if the network of pipes can deliver oxygen in sufficient volume to cope with the demand of so many ports turned up to the maximum flow rate. In addition, we are trying an intervention, continuous positive airway pressure (CPAP), to try and stave off ventilation in selected patients. CPAP is even more oxygen hungry than a high flow reservoir mask: perhaps 25 litres of oxygen per patient per minute. I may have to ration the use of oxygen. I find the possibility terrifying and cannot understand how I will run the on call without this most basic resource. This is the fear that keeps me awake.

Under usual circumstances our hospital admits 25-30 medical patients with emergency problems every 24 hours, comprising of conditions such as, minor heart attacks, exacerbations of chronic lung disease, pneumonia, diabetic emergencies, and drug overdoses. I begin to accumulate patients under my care on Friday night and head in early on Saturday morning to start seeing them. There are 17 admissions, not an unusual number, but the list is remarkable: next to 15 names it simply says '?COVID'; only two patients have come with regular medical problems.

Two things worry me. Firstly, the volume of patients suspected to have COVID-19 (all of those on the admission list currently require oxygen). Secondly, what has happened to patients with regular medical problems; are they suffering at home fearful to come to hospital during the pandemic?

I take the junior doctors around to see the first few cases. At the severe end of the spectrum, COVID-19 seems to be quite a homogeneous illness, blood test and chest X-Ray results for the patients we see are similar. The most striking feature is the very low level of oxygen in the blood and correspondingly high oxygen flow rates needed to correct this. My anxiety about the hospital's oxygen circuit resurfaces, but I try to put this aside and move on.

Mid-way through the admissions round we encounter an extremely unwell man in his 80s. He is visibly short of breath from across the ward, but is trying to stand up and pulling at his intravenous lines and electrocardiogram (ECG) heart monitor. I go to his bedside with a nurse and though he is delirious and confused, we are able to settle him and reattach the monitor.

The admitting junior doctor had suspected COVID-19 and started treatment with oxygen and antibiotics to cover any additional infection. The patient is unable to tell me much about his illness due to confusion. He has a fever and some X-Ray changes of COVID-19, but ECG tracings are abnormal, and the heart muscle marker in the blood is elevated to more than 50 times normal. I suspect that he has suffered a big heart attack some days ago, but tried to remain at home despite this. His carer called the ambulance on finding him febrile and breathless during an evening visit last night, probably due to COVID-19 infection exacerbating acute heart failure, but unfortunately his transfer to hospital is too late.

He will not survive this illness and would not benefit from admission to intensive care or mechanical ventilation. Indeed, the chances of causing a cardiac arrest by placing him under anaesthesia to receive ventilation would be extremely high. Instead I start treatment to address his symptoms with intravenous diuretics and a small dose of morphine to relieve breathlessness. I urgently call his daughter to explain the gravity of the situation and why treatments such as ventilation or cardiopulmonary resuscitation would not help. His daughter makes it in to hospital in time to see him; he goes on to die peacefully late on Saturday evening.

I finish the admissions round and head to our CPAP ward, where a group of patients are grouped together in a bay behind a sliding glass door. An orange light on the oxygen control panel is illuminated and a buzzer sounds continuously. The nurse in charge tells me that this has been the case for a few days, and she has been reassured by the engineers this morning that oxygen flow is currently 'adequate'.

The personal protective equipment (PPE) needed to see patients with COVID-19 receiving basic interventions, such as oxygen by reservoir mask, is simple: surgical mask, apron and gloves. This equipment has been in good supply on the wards we have visited. The situation is different for CPAP, which forces oxygen into the airway under pressure and is classed as an aerosol-generating procedure: potentially a much greater risk to staff in terms of exposure to quantity of virus in the immediate atmosphere. To enter the CPAP area enhanced PPE is required: full surgical gown, face shield, filtering face mask, hair cover, and gloves.

The on-call registrar has just seen all of the patients behind the glass and emerges having already removed her enhanced PPE. We discuss the situation and decide that I will not enter the area myself in order to conserve PPE equipment. We review the patients' monitors through the glass. Of the six patients one is clearly dying and has already been deemed unfit for ventilation. We find a bed on one of the regular COVID-19 wards and transfer him for palliative care. More encouragingly, a younger patient has improved significantly with CPAP, and avoided the need for ventilation. He also returns to the regular ward. I am relieved that we have managed to get two patients off CPAP but slightly disheartened to note that the orange light and buzzer continue unabated.

The remainder of the weekend follows a similar pattern. Each morning and evening I have about 15 new patients with suspected or confirmed COVID-19, and an ongoing oxygen requirement to accommodate, and a handful of others with conventional problems who we try to keep out of hospital. I make it to Sunday evening, and find that with support from medical and nursing colleagues from emergency medicine and intensive care, we have coped and somehow accommodated everyone who came through the doors.

I spend Monday and Tuesday helping to organise training for doctors from other specialities who will be redeployed to help treat patients with COVID-19. These doctors, of all grades and experience, are universally apprehensive. I explain to them that I have just come through an on-call weekend, that things were alright and that the hospital is coping. I show them some X-Rays and blood results to familiarise them with what they will be seeing, and we discuss some of their anxieties around covering unfamiliar roles.

Elective work in my usual speciality has almost completely ceased due to the pandemic, but we are still conducting a handful of telephone consultations to try and sort out those with the most urgent problems. Almost nobody is being called to the hospital for a face-to-face consultation due to the risks of infection, but I am approached by our cancer specialist nurse on Wednesday to ask if I could make two exceptions. An elderly man with an established cancer has phoned in with troublesome new symptoms, and may require an urgent invasive procedure, and a young father who has completed aggressive surgery and chemotherapy needs to be seen to explain that scans now show widespread recurrence of cancer, which has become incurable.

I arrange to see both patients in my otherwise empty clinic on Thursday. I am relieved to find the elderly patient better than expected. A simple prescription should alleviate his symptoms. Thankfully we do not to have to undertake an urgent procedure, with all of the associated risks of hospital admission at this time.

The consultation with the young father is much more difficult. He has attended alone and has worn his own PPE, a mask covering most of his face and latex gloves. A baseball cap pulled down low conspires to obscure much of the rest of his face, but his eyes convey the fear of being called up to hospital at such an extraordinary time. We sit two metres apart on opposite sides of the consulting room and I wonder how to establish the trust and rapport delivering this devastating news requires. I go through his scans, explain the prognosis, and try to outline what lies ahead in the final months of life. His words are calm, but I can make out his tears from behind the mask. The consultation draws to a close and our specialist nurse takes him aside and gently talks him through the services and support available in the community.

I return to my office to dictate the letters. I had felt mildly unwell prior to the clinic, and now I begin to cough. A colleague walks in and declares that I look ill. I try to brush this off but as I continue to cough, it is clear that I am developing suggestive symptoms and must no longer remain in the hospital. I hastily pack up my things, call occupational health and email my departmental manager.

Unlike many NHS workers I can access COVID-19 testing, which I complete on my way out. Sitting in an isolation room I am approached by a nurse in PPE. I am suddenly struck by the reality that medical staff now require protection from me, which is hard to swallow after a weekend of endless hand-washing, mask, glove and apron changes. The nurse takes a swab from deep in my pharynx and both nostrils, looks at my suffused eyes and speculates that it will be positive. I withdraw to isolation at home and wait for the result.

On Friday morning my muscles ache and I am sweaty, but I still feel well enough to work remotely. As I check some patient results on my laptop my phone rings from a withheld number. It is the Consultant Virologist. The swab is positive. I am infected with COVID-19. My first reaction is indignation. This is inconvenient. I don't want an enforced week off work at a time when the health service is so stretched. I exchange texts with a colleague. She tells me to stop working, to rest, to recover. She is right. The first wave of minor concern washes over me. I look online for survival data for otherwise fit patients under 50 with COVID-19 infection. Somewhat reassured I retreat to bed and reflect on an extraordinary working week on the frontline of a pandemic.

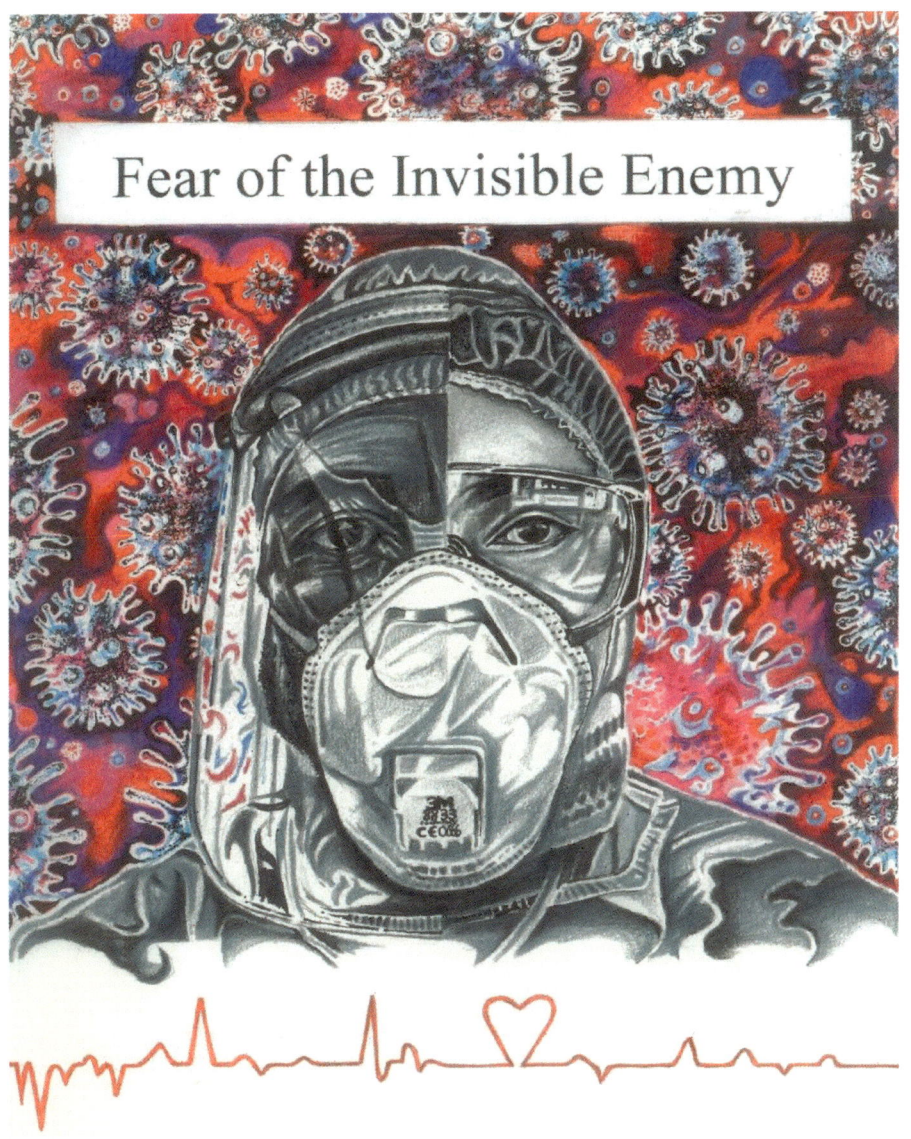

Fear of the Invisible Enemy

Artist: Neil Gardner

# Part 1

## The Manifestation of Fear

# Observing the Leadership and the Surrounding World in the COVID Landscape

## *Ade Odunlade*

It's 2:45am, and I wake up sweating. I sit up in bed and wonder what's going on. Getting to my feet, I start pacing up and down the room. The whole house is dead quiet, my family sleeping. I start ruminating on the events of the day: losing three staff in my Division and five within the National Health Service Trust where I work. As I pace across the room, I picture each of these staff members and what it would feel like for their family, friends, and colleagues. Sweating and fearful in the dead of the night, wondering where the world is going with this coronavirus outbreak. I speculate what could happen to the services if we lose more staff. It's difficult to imagine what somebody high up would be going through; I'm far below the rank of people like my chief executive officer (CEO) and the national director.

Now it's 4:30am. I can see my suit and shirt hanging, ready for me to slip on and become the general; to go from being this frightened leader to being someone who can give hope, calm, and encouragement to the team. Can I still get some sleep? I need to get going in an hour. Duty calls.

Suddenly, I remember that I'm not alone. The evening prior, my chief executive had called to talk things through with me and gave me lots of acknowledgements and praise. I recall my divisional director colleagues, along with the texts and emails from the entire executive team. Confidence starts to emerge. Time to go back to bed and catch an hour sleep, before getting into the well-pressed suit and shirt and setting off for another day of frantic battle. I mutter to myself, and remember the words of Nelson Mandela:

"I learned that courage was not the absence of fear, but the triumph over it. The brave man is not he who does not feel afraid, but he who conquers that fear."

In our Trust, the leadership has been exemplary, beginning with the tier of operation established by our chief nurse. She threw herself into the work, blending compassion and focus in a way that's marvellous to watch. She continues to tirelessly bring much-needed knowledge, honesty, openness, and visibility in managing the new terrain in which we all find ourselves.

The entire leadership became more visible, available, and supportive. The pace of decision-making is fast, thus making the delivery equally fast. Working with the chief nurse, the central hub became a command centre, manned by an energetic, passionate, and excellent staff. They worked tirelessly, often ignoring their need to take a break until reminded to take one. It was not unusual to see members of the executive and senior leadership asking staff to go home, then waiting around to ensure that they actually leave the building. A very caring leadership was a beautiful thing to watch.

"Leaders establish trust with candor, transparency, and credit."
— **Jack Welch, former CEO of General Electric** (Welch, 2020)

At the height of the pandemic, I received a phone call from one of my borough directors. Several patients in one of our units had tested positive for coronavirus, and this had caused heightened anxiety among the staff. Her response was to go to that location with one of her senior managers and work alongside the nursing staff for the day. This started a spate of daily leadership presence in the unit. The divisional director of nursing also moved in to work with the staff, and all anxiety suddenly started to diminish. What was most significant, however, was that most of the patients who are categorised as being in the 'at risk' category survived the virus.

I visited a unit during the outbreak, because they had just had a number of positive patients. I was met by the ward manager who was new in post. I was a bit worried about how he would cope, but had been told that he is a good man and a good leader. I had a brief chat with his director about my anxiety but was astonished by the response I got from her: She said that she believed in his ability to lead the team, and that she would be offering support in the background. Almost a month afterward, we all heard the story of how the ward manager had successfully led his team to ensure that all the patients survived and were cared for. He told us a story about going to the supermarket to buy some groceries and suddenly realising that shopping with strangers presents more risk than patients who are on the ward. He used this example to encourage the staff to work on the ward, explaining that at work they have personal protection equipment which they wouldn't have when shopping with strangers. He spent time working alongside his staff and led the team that worked in the Red Zone. A new leader was born, proving that champions are born out of challenges.

> "Leadership is about making others better as a result of your presence and making sure that impact lasts in your absence."
> — **Sheryl Sanberg, COO of Facebook** (Sanberg, 2020)

> "Do what you feel in your heart to be right – for you'll be criticized anyway."
> — **Eleanor Roosevelt, former First Lady of the United States** (Roosevelt, 2020)

Moving away from our local leadership observations and turning attention to national and international leadership observations, this unprecedented COVID-19 outbreak has challenged the leadership everywhere. The Queen, Winston Churchill, Nelson Mandela, Mahatma Ghandi, Dalai Lama – these people are part of a long list of world leaders who have led others through trials and challenges. However, it is important to understand that the COVID-19 challenge changed leadership interaction. It has been very interesting watching the countries around the world, along with the huge variations in their leadership approaches. New Zealand Prime Minister, Jacinda Ardern, has become the symbol of a leader that speaks to touch the heart of the nation and provide authenticity in interaction with her people. Her messages and quick proactive decisions seem to have had a positive outcome, and resulted with very few cases of coronavirus. The United States, in contrast, has seen a huge number of cases, with Donald Trump constantly speaking what comes to his mind.

The lack of synchronised messages has undoubtedly led to inconsistency in the approach of dealing with this pandemic. China adopted a containment approach - not only to the disease but its communication as well, with a managed flow of information. This has allowed people to cast doubt on the integrity of the information coming out of China. A long list of countries - namely Brazil, Mexico, Italy, Spain, Iran and even our own Great Britain - underplayed and were slow in grasping the severity and level of dangerousness of COVID-19. This no doubt affected the responses of each of these countries to the pandemic, resulting in many of them being caught unprepared.

> 'Leaders have the courage to make unpopular decisions and gut calls.'
> — **Jack Welch, former CEO of General Electric** (Welch, 2020)

> '"Because fear kills everything," Mo had once told her. "Your mind, your heart, your imagination."'
> — **Cornelia Funke, *Inkheart*** (Funke, 2020)

However, it is important to explore the power of science and the NHS in this pandemic in the United Kingdom. As a result of being caught off guard by the pandemic, the politicians soon realised the only way to get the public to understand the magnitude of the situation was to turn to science and the NHS. It is also worth mentioning that both science and the NHS have been a political football for politicians, and world politicians have been very disparaging about science. Especially when you consider the whole debate about climate change. The apathy to the science of climate change has frustrated many who believe we should acknowledge and use science and its evidence in managing the future of the planet. However, COVID-19 has changed this viewpoint, as politicians have no solution other than to turn to the NHS and science.

People trust their NHS, as it has remained a reliable organisation since its establishment. The UK appears to have adopted a strategy of using science and the NHS as the cornerstone of decision making. The visual presentation of daily briefings was an attempt to manage the messaging, by ensuring that what is presented to the people is the voice of science. This approach has helped the government manage the continuity, even when Prime Minster Boris Johnson was unfortunately hit by the virus.

> "I must say a word about fear. It is life's only true opponent. Only fear can defeat life. It is a clever, treacherous adversary, how well I know. It has no decency, respects no law or convention, shows no mercy. It goes for your weakest spot, which it finds with unnerving ease. It begins in your mind, always…so you must fight hard to express it. You must fight hard to shine the light of words upon it. Because if you don't, if your fear becomes a wordless darkness that you avoid, perhaps even manage to forget, you open yourself to further attacks of fear because you never truly fought the opponent who defeated you."
> — **Yann Martel, Life of Pi** (Martel, 2001)

The positioning of scientists and the NHS in the messages to the public has been measured and focused on the task at hand, moving away from any self-adulation or societal praise. The leadership of Simon Steven, CEO of the NHS, has been interesting. It was as if a general went into a massive battle plan and quietly implemented it. The NHS has seen an unprecedented change to its system, with tremendous staff and leadership response. The development of Nightingale Hospitals, the establishment of new services, and increase in digital offerings- all within a few short weeks- is no mean feat! While there have been various issues ranging from personal protection equipment (PPE) to testing, the NHS has remained focused on doing what it does best.

London was the most impacted area in the UK, and NHS London has been integral to wrestling with the biggest challenge in century. The partnership, along with a range of stakeholders like the army, has been tremendous in ways that will possibly lay the foundation for future cooperation and service delivery. Consequently, we now know that we can make change happen quickly, and that cooperation and collaboration is better than solo service. We now perceive that we are better as a whole and collective system, rather than the disjointed and fragmented system that the Commissioning and Provider split forces upon us. We now know that the focus of our efforts can be on the needs of the population, instead of the drive for Commissioners Key Performance Indicators (KPIs). The future now belongs to outcomes for the population, involvement of the community in care delivery, and the expansion of the community services. Additionally, we have become increasingly aware that there is no dichotomy between health and social care. All that has been hidden in our population is now out for open scrutiny by the public. We have come to realise the stark evidence of inequalities in health through the mortality rates of COVID-19, and that the healthcare of the rich is better than that of the poor, and that our Black and Asian Minority Ethnic (BAME) population needs to be better cared for.

I have been using the phase 'we now know.' What this means is that we do not have to sweep all these issues under the carpet, and use the words 'investigation,' 'inquiry,' 'research,' and other ways in which we placate people and drive these things underground. COVID-19 has brought all this out into the open for us to see, so that we may reconsider the type of society we want, the type of service model that we want, and the type of relationship we need to develop as a society.

What is even more revealing with COVID-19 is the type of employers people have. The pandemic has brought out the best and the worst in people. Society now has a choice going forward. However, I am a student of history and not under any illusion that human beings have a way of putting things behind them, forgetting, and gradually migrating back to the old ways. Whatever happens, COVID-19 has made a significant change in our world view.

Several NHS soldiers have fallen, and my heart goes out to their family, friends and colleagues. It is heart wrenching, and I have no doubt that we will forever remember them and their invaluable contributions to the NHS. One of the interesting observations is the lack of openness by a number of areas, in terms of how COVID-19 was being discussed at the early stages. Another observation was the attempt for people to explain the calamitous events away, rather than acknowledging them and mourning the loss. In future years we will know more, but right now it is just important to feel the loss, and to strengthen the family, friends and colleagues of those who are here no more.

> "Remember, feedback is meant to address the problem, not the person."
> — **Travis Bradberry, author of *Emotional Intelligence 2.0***
> (Bradberry & Patrick, 2009)

> "We are not interested in the possibilities of defeat; they do not exist."
> — **Queen Victoria** (Inspirational Quotes, 2020)

BAME staff across the country have experienced a strange feeling, considering the overrepresentation in the mortality rates for COVID-19. The NHS is a mirror of the society, and what happens in the wider society is reflected within the system. There is a lot to learn, despite the quick intervention of leaders in the NHS. Despite the praises that I have lavished on the NHS- of which I am equally part of and culpable too- it is now vitally important that staff well-being, happiness, hope, and aspirations should now take the centre stage.

The NHS cannot function without its staff, its most precious asset. Staffs need investment in order to be developed towards reaching their maximum potential. For a number of years, Workforce and Race Equality Standard (WRES) and Equality and Diversity (ED) have become an optional extra, and something that is done at the mercy and interest of leaders, rather than as a requirement. We praise ourselves by increasing small percentage each year, with London having the worst picture in the country. In spite of research telling us that we get more productivity and better services for people, we have not paid as much attention as we should in looking after our staff across the NHS.

A pandemic like COVID-19 has galvanised the society and business organisational response with a lot of freebies, and appreciation of NHS staff demonstrated through national weekly clapping on Thursday nights. It is quite overwhelming, and impressive to see how individuals and organisations are supporting NHS staff. What a wonderful way to encourage the staff who continue to put themselves on the line for people. I hope that this act of generosity will not cease with the end of the pandemic, and that companies will see this as part of their social responsibility and individuals will support their local NHS Trust through volunteering. Collaboration between companies and individuals with the local NHS Trusts can bring so much more to the local population.

> "As we express our gratitude, we must never forget that the highest appreciation is not to utter words, but to live by them."
> – **John F. Kennedy** (Kennedy, 2020)

> "Appreciation is a wonderful thing: it makes what is excellent in others belong to us as well."
> – **Voltaire** (STANDS4, 2020)

> "The roots of all goodness lie in the soil of appreciation for goodness."
> – **Dalai Lama** (Lama, n.d.)

Prior to COVID-19, the NHS was overwhelmed, and services were unable to cope. During the pandemic, there was a huge reduction in the demand for a number of services- possibly out of fear of catching infection or attempting not to overwhelm the NHS. This is an interesting phenomenon worthy of further research. It is worth finding out where the resilience and self-management has emerged. We have always wanted to see our General Practitioners, but we now know that consultation via a digital platform could be equally effective. A new dawn has arrived in terms of access to healthcare and how we experience the delivery. The future of patient participation in care and self-management is another road to watch as it emerges in the years ahead. As we drive into this future, productivity and outcomes start to emerge as the lingo for future investment in the NHS.

Our attitude about how we use the NHS will no doubt have to change, as we need to preserve it and not misuse it. It is even more important to note that the cost of COVID-19 will have an impact on future spending, showing that we are going to have to reduce bureaucracy and increase access to health. The need for integrated services as well as a focus on the health of the population paints a portrait of the future where NHS will not be the only solution to people's health, but rather each key establishment will have to play their own part.

> "I must not fear. Fear is the mind-killer. Fear is the little-death that brings total obliteration. I will face my fear. I will permit it to pass over me and through me. And when it has gone past, I will turn the inner eye to see its path. Where the fear has gone there will be nothing. Only I will remain."
> — **Frank Herbert, *Dune*** (Herbert, 2005)

The definition of key workers during the COVID-19 outbreak brings an interesting dynamic into what is necessary for a basic society to function. The interplay between the NHS and the delivery of services by these key workers has provided us with an interesting piece to study. I am in admiration of the supermarkets. Their leadership has been exemplary and have managed challenging and complex problems. They have kept the supply going, despite our attempt at buying up everything in the supermarkets. The pictures of empty supermarket shelves evoked a feeling of fear and loss of control, and pandemonium ensued. The ample global reserves have helped in a way that health organizations and other sectors should emulate. What we also need to learn is the diet and food consumption of people who are stuck at home. Are people eating healthier than they have managed to do in the past? What impact will this have on the population health, and how much people will be returning to the old ways?

The biggest impact of this pandemic is going to be on mental health. The effects of people dying alone- without their loved ones being able to say goodbye or be present at either the passing or the burial- will linger. The need for bereavement support for individuals and families will dominate our attention in months and years post-outbreak. The significant impact of the resultant fear and anxiety that this has generated will no doubt increase, with people seeking much-needed support and calling for expansion to our Improving Access to Psychological Therapies (IAPT). The Mental Health Long Term Plan has provided us with a template for the future, and adding the lessons of COVID-19 will no doubt be the template by which we can map out the future of mental health services. We will begin to see the need for mental health services. The effect of the virus on the brain and impact on mental health has yet to fully unravel. It is not known if a COVID-19 infection may cause mental health disorders or have an impact on neurodegenerative disorders months or years after the pandemic.

"Fear cuts deeper than swords."
— **George R.R. Martin, *A Game of Thrones*** (Martin, 2011)

"The moments when the United Kingdom has come together to applaud its care and essential workers will be remembered as an expression of our national spirit, and its symbol will be the rainbows drawn by children."
— **Queen Elizabeth** (Queen Elizabeth coronavirus transcript, 2020)

Another impact on mental health may also lie in the effect of social distancing, and the emergence and expansion of communication via digital platforms. This could also impact on our social norms, expression of empathy, communication of compassion, and how we show that we care. Gestures such as touching, hugging, and shaking hands are some ways in which human beings maintain and express connection. It begs the question: what is the new norm, and how do people react and respond without a feeling of rejection and abandonment? The impending challenge of paying back the cost of COVID-19 and the massive change to various organisations with poor social care will no doubt be a source of many problems for mental health. Prior to COVID-19, there have been arguments around the implication of austerity for mental health. Should mental health services start to get worried about the economic challenge and the COVID-19 aftermath?

COVID-19 has changed our world in unprecedented ways. The leadership of politicians across the globe has been challenged, demonstrated by mixed messages and inconsistency. UK politicians rose up to the challenge with a reliance on science and the NHS to deal with this pandemic. The operations of the NHS at macro and micro levels have been impacted, with access to GPs and other NHS services being delivered through digital consultations. Inequalities in health between the rich and poor and within the NHS – which is a microcosm of society – has been exposed, depicted by the high mortality rates for COVID-19. The post COVID-19 era calls for centrality of staff well-being and development in the NHS, and for staff being perceived as the most precious asset of the NHS. Collaboration, integration, seamless care delivery across health and social services, expansion of community services, focus on the needs of the population, and lessons from the pandemic could be the driving forces to shape the NHS in the post-outbreak landscape.

> *"Things done well and with care exempt themselves from fear"*
> — **William Shakespeare**

> "This is the time for facts, not fear. This is the time for science, not rumours. This is the time for solidarity, not stigma. We are all in this together; we can only stop it together"
> — **Dr Tedros Adhanom Ghebreyesus, Director General of the World Health Organization** (WHO, 2020)

# Fears on the Frontline of COVID-19

*Harvey Wells & Nikki Yun*

Fear is the dominant emotion during the COVID-19 pandemic: people are scared of being infected; relatives are worried for their loved ones; there is fear about the impact of COVID-19 on employment, society, and the economy; and the patients who are infected are fearful for their lives. Despite the shared experience of fear, it is rarely disclosed or acknowledged by those working to treat patients with COVID-19. This chapter explores the experience of working in Intensive Care with patients who have COVID-19, having fear as a constant companion, the impact that fear can have on clinicians, and how talking about fear may help to lessen its impact.

## I Wonder, What are You Feeling?

We have a briefing at the start of each shift in the Intensive Care Unit (ICU). In this morning's meeting, a team of intensive care nurses, ward nurses, specialist nurses, healthcare assistants and medical students have been brought together to care for the COVID-19 patients for the next 12 hours. Our Matron starts his briefing by sharing how proud he is of the team and how well everyone has adapted to the current circumstances. He expresses his awareness of the psychological impact coronavirus is having on us all. He paused and asked, "I wonder, what are you feeling?" We all sit there, staring at each other or looking away at the wall. A colleague finally broke the silence and said the word that each of us were feeling: *"fear."*

This book was written during the coronavirus pandemic. It is a difficult time for many people, and most of the things that were normal before the pandemic have been suspended or entirely changed. Our daily and weekly patterns have been radically altered by lockdown; many of us are working from home, or furloughed;

and the usual distinction between work and home has blurred. Social distancing protocols have separated us from our friends and families. All the things we know or expect in our daily lives are changing so quickly. We cannot predict what will happen in a few months. Many of the things that were certain are now uncertain.

In writing this chapter, we have cited evidence to support our arguments, as is to be expected. However, unlike most topics, so little is known about coronavirus; it is an unfolding situation that is still fairly new. Publications have yet to catch up with events. Therefore, we have used media that can respond much faster than traditional print formats. We have used websites, podcasts and news reports as evidence, as these are where people have captured their experiences.

## Coronavirus is Scary

COVID-19 is a scary virus. It is invisible, easily transmitted between humans, and potentially deadly. It affects the respiratory system, causing the worst-affected to struggle to breathe – a terrifying prospect. Patients who need ventilator support are treated in ICUs which have been adapted to treat COVID-19. At the time of writing, over 20,000 patients have died of coronavirus while in hospital care. Family members are not able to visit their loved ones in hospitals, which can be a cause of frustration, anxiety, and feelings of guilt at not being able to be with them at the end.

When someone develops a new illness or condition, they can often get an idea of the prognosis, or the course and duration of an illness, or a healthcare professional can provide that information for them. COVID-19 is so new that it is hard to predict its course – from being asymptomatic, to having mild symptoms, to the need to be ventilated. The illness is unpredictable and scary. Can we keep ourselves and our families safe from this virus?

Coronavirus is also new and largely unknown. The information available is incomplete and evolving. There is much that is uncertain, and this can lead to more anxiety and fear. The early stories in the media made it seem as though coronavirus only affected the elderly and people with underlying health conditions; the young and the fit had little to be concerned about. However, that story has changed; young people without underlying health conditions have fallen victim to coronavirus and become severely ill, and some have now died, sadly. No one is safe from coronavirus; people are right to be afraid of COVID-19.

**What is Fear?**

Fear is a key driver of human behaviour; we typically try to avoid situations where we are scared. Fear has evolved to protect us from threats by alerting us to the presence of danger. It was crucial in keeping our ancestors alive when the dangers were life-threatening. Today, many of the things we are anxious and scared of – such as public speaking, failing an exam, or losing our job – aren't life threatening, but we have the same fear response.

The fear response can be divided into two areas: biochemical and emotional. The biochemical part is what happens to all people, while the emotional aspect is individual. Fear starts in the amygdala. A perceived threat triggers a response in the amygdala, which triggers the release of hormones such as adrenaline, in preparation for us to be more efficient in the presence of danger. The brain becomes more alert and our mind focuses on the here and now. Our pupils dilate and our breathing rate increases. Heart rate and blood pressure rise, which increased blood flow and provides more glucose to the muscles. Organs that are not vital to short term survival, such as the digestive system, slow down. The body is prepared for us to "fight or flight" our way out of danger. However, it is our brains that process whether a threat is real or not.

Once the body has prepared for a threat, the hippocampus and prefrontal cortex help the brain interpret whether the perceived danger is genuine. If the threat is genuine, then our bodies have the resources to respond. Following the event, we can feel exhausted as those resources have been utilised and we are depleted. If we identify that a threat is not real – watching a scary movie, for example – then we overcome the initial "fight or flight" rush. We are often left feeling satisfied, reassured of our safety, and in control. However, the body has been primed to deal with a threat and has to process the hormones that have been released. This outlines the individual's response to fear; however, we are influenced by the fear of those around us.

Emotions can also be contagious. We are social animals and we recognise emotions in others, which can in turn influence our own emotions. You may see a friend looking relaxed in a stressful situation, and this can have a calming effect on you; the message is 'there is nothing to worry about' (you may also interpret their relaxedness in a myriad of other ways, such as "I wish I felt that confident," or "they don't see this as important"). However, if you see a colleague looking anxious and you too feel anxious, this confirms that there is something to be anxious about. In the short term, the fear response is useful. In the long term, being in a state of constant fear can cause problems.

## What are the Long-Term Effects of Prolonged Fear?

Fear is the human body's reaction to a threat, but it has evolved to be the reaction to a short-term threat. Once the threat has passed, we return to our normal state. What happens if the threat lasts days, weeks, or months? How does the body adapt to prolonged fear?

Chronic fear can have profound effects on our health. LeDoux (2015) explained that the potential long-term effects of fear on a person's health may include: disruption to sleep; dysregulation of the digestive system; and dysfunctions to the immune, endocrine, and autonomic nervous systems. Chronic fear can also impact on our emotional health and lead to the development of various problems, such as anxiety disorders, depression and mood swings, learned helplessness, dissociation, and difficulties with relationships. Fear can also have a profound effect on the way we make decisions. It forces us to focus our attention on the threat, primarily whether to fight or flight. This is incredibly helpful in the short term. In the long term, however, that focus may stop us from making more reasoned decisions. Fear also has profound effects on our memory. At times of stress, we can go blank and forget things that were previously easy to recall. Given that the coronavirus pandemic has (at the time of writing) lasted several months, and is predicted to last significantly longer, what will the long-term effect of coronavirus be on the health of the population?

On 15 April 2020, The Independent reported that the world is likely to face a mental health crisis after the coronavirus pandemic has passed (Lintern, 2020). It cited an article written in the Lancet and stated *"the scale of this problem is too serious to ignore, both in terms of every human life that may be affected, and in terms of the wider impact on society"* (Holmes, et al., 2020). It is truly scary to think about the repercussions of the coronavirus pandemic, as there is already so much of which to be frightened.

**Fear is the Emotional Backdrop**

Even prior to walking into an ICU, fear was the overriding emotion at the start of the coronavirus pandemic (Walker & Gerada, 2020). A report by the Office of National Statistics reported that the average anxiety rating in the UK in March 2020 was 5.18/10, which was an increase from an average of 3/10 in January 2020 (ONS, 2020). As the World Health Organisation declared the coronavirus a global pandemic, the immediate emotional response from the public was fear (Richards, 2020). People were panic-buying toilet roll, hand sanitiser, and disinfectant wipes to keep themselves and their families safe. It is normal to feel scared from time to time. Feeling worried can prepare us for the threat. However, being in a state of fear can lead to poor decision-making.

There are many uncertainties around coronavirus. With an invisible virus and a lack of testing available, we don't know whether the tickle we feel at the back of our throat is the first symptom; we don't know whether the person next to us is infected; we don't know if we are infected yet asymptomatic. Could we infect our loved ones? If we do catch it, will we end up on a ventilator in an ICU? In the short term, there is much of which to be scared.

We also don't know how long this will last. At the time of writing, we have been locked down in the UK for 6 weeks. The UK government has started to suggest that social distancing may remain in place in some form for the rest of

2020. What will our society look like if the UK remains locked down for this length of time?

Many people are worried about their financial future. "Will I still be employed at the end of the pandemic?" "Will my business still be operational after coronavirus?" Many businesses, particularly in the service industries, will not survive the coronavirus pandemic. What will our towns and cities look like after this is over? Our high streets have been struggling for several years, but can they survive this crisis?

## On a War Footing

Stories from healthcare professionals in China and Italy spoke of a tsunami of COVID-infected patients heading towards the UK (Campbell & Mason, 2020). Warfare metaphors were used to describe the coronavirus pandemic (Brindley, 2020). The similarities are clear, all activities were cancelled unless they supported the fight. The initial skirmishes with coronavirus were in our schools and universities, in our workplaces, on public transport, in our pubs and restaurants, and our entertainment venues; anywhere we could bump up against another human being was now a risky place to be. Describing the pandemic in terms of war may have been a deliberate strategy to convey the level of serious risk people were in if they didn't follow social distancing rules. It may have been used to instill a feeling of British pride: 'We survived the war! We will survive the pandemic! We're in this together!' However, for the key workers who have to leave the safety of their homes every day to go out and keep the country running, putting themselves at risk from this hidden enemy can only be described as terrifying. However, the casualties of these skirmishes were sent to intensive care where the real battles were fought.

## Inside the Intensive Care Unit

The NHS were held up as the army to protect us from the coronavirus and Intensive Care was the field of battle. As the government declared war on coronavirus, the streets fell silent and ICUs across the UK prepared for war. Hospitals turned themselves inside out to create new ICUs to deal with the flood of patients infected with COVID-19; non-emergency surgeries were cancelled; outpatient clinics were suspended; staff were redeployed from their normal clinical duties to become part of the response to coronavirus; the teams who were treating patients in the ICU were brought in from other wards with the briefest of training programmes; The Nightingale Hospital, a 4000 bed specialist coronavirus unit, was set up in nine days*. Hospitals challenged all the accepted norms in order to squeeze as much capacity as humanly possible out of the resources available.

However, it soon became clear that our army was not equipped for the battle. The personal protective equipment (PPE) required to keep the healthcare staff safe from COVID-19 was sparse. Imagine being asked to climb a cliff without a rope; healthcare staff was asked to treat coronavirus patients without adequate PPE. Many continued to treat patients despite the risk to themselves, and sadly there have been a significant number of healthcare professionals that have died from COVID-19. If you don't work in healthcare or on the frontline of the NHS, imagine how you would feel travelling to work every day, knowing you were entering an area where patients had COVID-19, and you weren't being provided with sufficient protective equipment to be safe.

*Whilst setting up the London Nightingale Hospital in nine days was an impressive achievement, it is not without serious criticism. It was opened on 3rd April 2020 and went into hibernation on 4th May 2020. At its peak, it had 35 patients, which is less than 1% of the advertised capacity.

**Adapting to New Ways of Working**

Anticipating the wave of patients with coronavirus forced hospitals to make massive changes to prepare. The ClinComm Podcast (Queen Mary University of London (QMUL), 2020) released an interview with an ICU consultant, Jon Aron, and nurse team leader Chris Ryan. They discussed how the coronavirus forced intensive care units to make sweeping changes to the hospital environment and clinical practice. Established ways of working were abandoned, to be able to prepare for the flood of patients. Hospital wards were converted into surge wards in a matter of days to create maximum capacity for patients who would need ventilators. These major alterations to the clinical environments were motivated by fear and pragmatism. Healthcare staff were scared that they would not be able to cope with the flood of COVID-patients so they created as much capacity for patients with coronavirus that the hospitals could accommodate. These changes had a knock-on effect to the way care was provided.

Due to the increased pressures on ICUs, additional healthcare staff was required to care for patients. Under normal circumstances, all nurses who work in critical care would be required to complete a minimum of twelve months of training and have at least of six weeks of supernumerary experience (NHS England, 2020). However, for the coronavirus pandemic, it was expected that non-critical care staff would be required to deliver nursing care under the supervision of critical care-trained nurses. Ward nurses, non-ICU clinical nurse specialists, non-ICU doctors, medical students, theatre staff, and healthcare assistants were enlisted to support ICU nurses often with *'limited or no knowledge of acute and critical care'* (NHS England 2020, p.1). Instead of the usual one-year minimum training, these healthcare staff were provided with an emergency training, lasting two days. NHS England (2020) acknowledged that the changes to working environments would cause anxiety, including the ICU nurses who were required to supervise them.

The increase in numbers of patients and changes to the skills mix of the team in ICUs inevitably resulted in different working practices. The previously-established nurse-to-patient ratios were revised (Park, 2020). ICU nurses changed from providing one-to-one nursing to overseeing up to five patients at a time. The non-ICU staff supported the ICU nurses to provide the specialist care their patients required. These changes to everyday practice, with minimal training, created anxiety and uncertainty for all involved. ICU nurses not only had to adjust to changing work practices, they also had to adapt to working with different people who had little to no ICU experience.

When things are difficult, we tend to rely on people we know and trust. There is safety in familiarity with the people around you, in knowing people's skill sets, knowing people's strengths, and knowing who you can rely on when things get difficult. The coronavirus pandemic disrupted normal teams and forced people who didn't know each other to work together. The ICU nurses had to adjust to leading people whom they had never met before and had to rely on people to complete clinical tasks without knowing their skill set or their background. Each shift would bring a new team with a different skill mix, and the staff had to adjust and accommodate these changes. Under normal circumstances, this would be anxiety-provoking and draining; during the pandemic it was made even harder by wearing personal protective equipment (PPE).

Due to the highly infectious nature of COVID-19, staff were required to wear PPE to protect themselves, their patients, and their colleagues. Wearing PPE is uncomfortable and difficult to work in for long periods of time. PPE can cause difficulties in recognising colleagues and presents challenges when communicating with patients and colleagues. The Health & Care Professions Council (HCPC) published some guidance about 'Communicating During the COVID-19 Pandemic'. They highlight that PPE significantly reduces the ability for people to see body language, particularly facial expressions, which can reduce the ability to communicate effectively. Healthcare staff should bear this in mind when communicating with each other and adapt their communication style to account for this. They also acknowledged that increased workloads and stress levels of healthcare staff are likely to be particularly difficult. They suggest that healthcare professionals need to support each other and work together to help mitigate the challenges brought by coronavirus.

One of the effects of fear that we mentioned earlier is its effect on decision-making. Being able to make critical decisions whilst under significant pressure is a defining feature of modern medicine. Knowing how to act in a literal life-or-death situation is a key skill of healthcare professionals that look after critically-ill patients. It is therefore important that, as much as is possible, doctors and nurses are not subjected to more stress and anxiety than is already inherent in the present crisis. Theo Usherwood, LBC's Political Editor, was taken to intensive care after being infected with coronavirus, unable to breathe. After he was discharged, he reported that the doctors "*were operating on a completely different level, trying stuff, trying to figure out how they could save my life. And they can't do that if there is chaos and pandemonium*" (Usherwood, 2020). It became a concern for healthcare staff that the fear and anxiety would overwhelm their decision-making and that mistakes would be made. The compounding factors of treating higher numbers of patients, unfamiliar teams, the challenge of working in PPE, and the worry over becoming infected or infecting those around them would make it incredibly difficult to make clear medical decisions.

Several strategies were used to help manage clinical decisions in the presence of overwhelming stress. Clear treatment targets were identified for each patient and printed out to be kept with the patient. This enabled the teams working with the patient to not have to remember five different patients' targets. Team leaders ensured that their staff took breaks to allow some respite. Staff looked out for when their colleagues appeared overly stressed. Dr Jon Aron, ICU consultant, and nurse team leader Chris Ryan discussed some of these strategies on The ClinComm Podcast (QMUL, 2020). Some hospitals converted break areas into relaxation zones or first-class airport lounges for their staff – a place where they could get a break from the relentless pressures of clinical care during coronavirus so they could continue to care for patients (for example, see Brown, 2020).

With the NHS being the centre of hope in the war against the coronavirus, how does the public see the NHS?

**The Perception of the NHS**

During the course of this pandemic, a new appreciation for the NHS has emerged. Healthcare staff have been named '*heroes without capes*', 'the *hidden army*', and the '*virus heroes*'. Every Thursday evening at eight, people come out of their houses or open their windows to applaud the hard work of the NHS. It is fantastic that the public are willing to show their appreciation for the NHS, particularly as satisfaction with the NHS has declined over the past decade.

In 2018, public satisfaction with the NHS fell to its lowest level since 2007 (King's Fund, 2019). Overall satisfaction was 53%, which was a three-point drop from 2017 year and the lowest in over ten years. However, in 2019, public satisfaction with the NHS rose by seven-point compared to the previous year (King's Fund, 2020). Given the public's reaction to the coronavirus pandemic, it is highly likely that the level of public satisfaction with the NHS will have gone up. The NHS will likely come out of the pandemic crisis severely depleted, but more valued by the public. It is hoped that this new public appreciation translates into lasting, positive changes to the funding for the NHS.

**The Aftermath**

The coronavirus has made high demands of the NHS and society. Everything has been thrown at the pandemic to survive the COVID-tsunami. The government stated they will do 'whatever it takes' to beat COVID-19. This approach may well have been necessary, but is it sustainable? Will there be enough resources left to be able to carry on? Ten years of austerity had left the NHS desperately short of resources. There was a shortage of forty thousand nurses prior to the pandemic; how much bigger will that shortage be? Many healthcare staff have come out of retirement to support the NHS, but this is a short-term solution; they cannot be expected to bolster the NHS indefinitely. Once they go back into retirement, what will be left of the regular staff?

The massive personal efforts of individual staff members will take its toll. Long shifts, wearing PPE, being in a state of constant fear, juggling life at home, and being unable to take a break or a holiday will leave staff depleted and drained. LBC presenter James O'Brien (2020) took a call on his radio show from a senior nurse called Nicola on April 7th, who shared, "*We are all broken, we are all exhausted.*" Some staff will be reinvigorated by the pandemic and will feel tremendous pride in the NHS and their contribution to overcoming the crisis (Arnold-Forster, 2020), but others will be left traumatised and broken. How many healthcare staff have pushed themselves to breaking point? What is the effect of prolonged stress, of repeated traumatising experiences, of constantly going above and beyond to their own personal cost? Perhaps we can rely on the next generation of nurses and doctors to keep the system afloat.

Many students of medicine, nursing, and other healthcare professions volunteered to support the NHS during the coronavirus pandemic. Others graduated early to become qualified doctors and nurses to help with the pandemic (Cutter, 2020). Whether students or newly qualified doctors, all will experience things that they would not be prepared for. They will have seen patients struggling to breathe, patients dying of coronavirus, families who have lost a loved one, and clinical staff exhausted and broken. This will be overwhelming and distressing for them. Some of these people that stepped forward to support the effort will be traumatised (Walker & Gerada, 2020). Some will choose not to continue with their training, or may choose to leave the profession that they have invested so much in. Anthea Allen wrote in her weekly diary from ITU (Allen, 2020) that a junior doctor told her, *"when this is done, so am I. No amount of money could make me stay"*. The generation that are currently entering the healthcare professions, Generation Z, have been described as exhibiting higher self-directed preferences when compared with other generations (Howe & Strauss, 2000). This suggests that they may prioritise their own needs over the needs of society. How many others won't want to make that level of personal sacrifice?

### How Can the Effects of Fear be Managed?

The Health & Care Professions Council (HCPC) (2020) have published some guidance about '*Communicating During the COVID-19 Pandemic*'. They highlight that patients, their families, and healthcare professionals will likely have heightened levels of anxiety and stress. Anxiety may impact their ability to communicate, and this is something that healthcare staff should be mindful of when engaging with them. There are some strategies available to help manage anxiety and fear that are specific to the pandemic.

Dalton, Rada & Stein (2020) provided some guidance for communicating during the COVID-19 pandemic that may help to reduce anxiety. While the focus is talking to children, it highlights several key principles that could apply to communicating with patients and colleagues. Communication should be honest and authentic. It is important to provide an accurate account of what is happening for people, so they can process what is going on. That uncertainty should be communicated. Clinicians should be clear about what is known and what is unknown, and should avoid providing unrealistic reassurance. Emotions should be shared in communication. An absence of emotion during conversations can leave people feeling like they can't talk about their feelings. Intense emotions that go unprocessed tend to come out in unexpected ways. In summary, be honest when talking with patients, share uncertainty, and be open to discussing feelings.

The NHS provided some useful guidance for maintaining well-being during the crisis.

---

The NHS guidance for managing anxiety during the coronavirus pandemic:

1. Stay connected with people
2. Talk about your worries
3. Support and help others
4. Feel prepared
5. Look after your body
6. Stick to the facts
7. Stay on top of difficult feelings
8. Do things you enjoy
9. Focus on the present
10. Look after your sleep

https://www.nhs.uk/oneyou/every-mind-matters/coronavirus-COVID-19-anxiety-tips/

---

These ten strategies aim for us to stay well enough so that the coronavirus does not devastate every aspect of our lives. If we can take care of ourselves, stay healthy, stay connected with others, and ensure our loved ones are also cared for, then we can recover from this crisis. These strategies will also help us to feel less anxious, more in control, and less isolated.

**COVID-19: A Cause for Alarm**

During this COVID pandemic, we fear for our own health; we fear our family's health; we fear for those we're looking after. I fear not being able to support my colleagues; I fear not being able to do the best that I can; I fear of losing hope. During this unprecedented time, I fear the effect that long-term fear will have on me and my colleagues; I fear for the state of the NHS after this pandemic has passed; I fear becoming accustomed to my own fear and becoming desensitised to the whole situation.

# The Impact of COVID-19 Across the Lifespan

*David Rawcliffe*

This chapter rapidly examines the impact of COVID-19 on individuals across the lifespan. It considers some of the issues for specific groups, these issues come from COVID-19 itself or in some cases because of Government and individual's responses to the Pandemic. It comes to the conclusion, that many groups are affects by COVID-19 and the fear that it raises.

Please note the areas of people from black and minority ethnic groups and those with mental health problems has not been covered here, as they are addressed at length in the rest of the book.

## (1)　The General Population

The impact of COVID-19 has hit all groups in society, with many famous individuals being diagnosed with and some dying from COVID-19. Some of those that have died from COVID-19 and its complications are: Eddie Large (comedian), Tim Brooke Taylor (Comedian), Dave Greenfield (musician), Fred the Godson (rapper), Andrew Jack (actor), John Prine (singer). Prime Minister Boris Johnson, Prince Charles and Tom Hanks have all experienced the effects of the virus (all cited in Sky News 2020a).

Celebrities are not the only people suffering, of course, with increasing numbers diagnosed and dying from the condition (Table 1). Fear of being ill and becoming a burden on loved ones is a reality for all.

| Table 1: Total World-Wide statistics for COVID-19 | | | |
|---|---|---|---|
| Date | 3rd Week of April, 2020 | 27th May, 2020 | 5th June, 2020 |
| Diagnosed | 3.76 million | 5.556 Million | 6.603 Million |
| Death | 259,474 | 350,212 | 391,732 |
| % deaths compared to diagnosis | 6.9% | 6.3% | 5.93% |
| Reference | World Health Organization (2020) | European Centre for Disease Prevention (2020a) | European Centre for Disease Prevention (2020b) |

## (2)     Pregnancy and COVID-19

Fear regarding the health of both mother and baby is intense, especially if the mother comes into contact with COVID-19. The Public Health Agency of Canada (2020) highlights the effects of fear in pregnancy during the COVID-19 pandemic, noting it can be extremely stressful.

Public Health England (2020a) has placed pregnant women in the 'vulnerable group' as far as COVID-19 is concerned. (It should be noted that women with pre-existing conditions such as congenital heart disease are considered an 'extremely vulnerable group' (Public Health England 2020b).)

There are physiological changes in the immune system during pregnancy, which could be associated with more severe viral symptoms (Mor & Cardenas, 2010) such as those seen with COVID-19; this is especially true during the third trimester, in which women are more susceptible to severe symptoms from viral infections (British Medical Journal, 2020). There is an increased risk to the mother of getting viral infections due to physiological changes in pregnancy (Dashraath, et al., 2020). These changes mainly affect the cardiorespiratory system which is an area that COVID-19 is known to target.

The Royal College of Midwives (RCM) and Royal College of Obstetricians & Gynaecologists (RCOG) (2020) records that the miscarriage rate for pregnant women is the same between those with and without COVID-19. Pregnant women with COVID-19 are admitted to intensive care at the same rate as women without the condition (Intensive Care National Audit & Research Centre, 2020). Both the British Medical Journal (2020) and Breslin, et al. (2020) confirm that the severity of the condition is comparable between pregnant women and non-pregnant women with COVID-19, which is to say: 86% mild symptoms, 9% severe symptoms and 5% critical. Future studies need to look at pregnant women with pre-existing medical conditions and consider this in more depth.

Comparing caesarean (c-section) rates of those with and without COVID-19 is interesting: The World Health Organization (2015) records the normal rate as 10-15%, whereas Knight, et al. (2020) suggest this has raisto 59%.

| Table 2: Risk Factors for Pregnant Women's Admission to Hospitals During the COVID-19 Crisis | |
|---|---|
| 1 | People from Black, Asian or minority ethnic (BAME) groups |
| 2 | Being overweight or obese |
| 3 | Those with pre-existing comorbidities |
| 4 | Maternal age over 35 years |
| Royal College of Midwives (RCM) and Royal College of Obstetricians & Gynaecologists (RCOG) (2020) | |

**Risks from a Mother with Coronavirus to the Baby During and After Pregnancy**

Can the mother pass on COVID-19 to the baby in-vitro? This is called vertical transmission, a process that remains a little unclear. Lamouroux, et al. (2020) suggest that it could be as high as 2% transmission, rising to 2.5% within twelve hours of birth (Knight, et al., 2020); within forty-eight hours, the rate increased to 5.6%.

LaMotte (2020) of CNN reported a small study of sixteen pregnant women who had COVID-19, which suggested that the size of their placenta was reduced because of the virus. Miller, an assistant professor of obstetrics and gynaecology at Northwestern University Feinberg School of Medicine, suggested that despite these smaller placentas (which has implications for the blood flow during pregnancy) all of the babies were born 'healthy, normal, and beautiful'. Nevertheless, he suggests this is an area that should be more closely monitored, and that it is clearly one which may have a huge impact on the anxiety of mothers.

The virus that causes COVID-19 has **not** been found in breast milk. Breastfeeding can provide important food security for the baby (Public Health Agency of Canada, 2020). The World Health Organization (2020b) say that "A woman with COVID-19 should be supported to breastfeed safely, hold her newborn skin-to-skin, and share a room with her baby." It is clear, nonetheless, that this may be an area of real concern to mothers and to professionals.

**(3) Schoolchildren**

The Office of National Statistics (2020a) record that there have been 'no death…in those aged 0-9 years', and only one girl aged 10-14 years old due to COVID-19 since the start of the pandemic in January 2020. While a child may get the condition, it appears as if their symptoms may be less serious. Although in some respects - particularly in terms of children's mental health -

the government assurance that schools can reopen makes sense, there is widespread worry for children, teachers, and parents.

The Department for Education has provided numerous guidance documents for schools (for examples of these see Department for Education, 2020a, b). These include advice about social distancing and personal protective equipment. However, COVID-19 is not the only concern: there is the issue of education and ensuring the viability of this approach.

In many situations, this has enhanced parent-school partnerships as parents help or encourage their child to take part in online lessons. Schools have worked hard to ensure that classrooms are ready, making them social distancing friendly and flexible enough to encourage learning and play.

There is a great deal of fear being expressed by some head teachers and local authorities, as they prepare for the opening of schools to include more pupils. They are worried about the contagion, not to mention the task of maintaining social distancing in the younger students as they see their friends - especially during the early days of the return.

Some students who have returned to their class already are not having their usual teachers, and are not getting the usual breadth of experience as social distancing is expected in the playground.

We know that many children need routines, and that that these routines were radically disrupted when the lockdown was announced. Parents and children established new routines, built in part around online learning. As children return to schools, these new routines will be disrupted again, and new ones will need to be forged.

## (4)    Autism

For me, this section is particularly personal. My son is autistic, and it was difficult for him to suddenly be "locked in." Luckily, he planned ahead and ordered himself a game system so that he could still play and interact with friends. It is also personal because of other family members: my great-niece had to move mid-lockdown because of tensions at home, which are there because she did not have her usual escape space anymore. I also hear of other friends, and the rapid change in routines causing children with autism tension and fear of the consequences.

'Autistic people … are likely to be worried about their own health, and that of their loved ones, while also having routines interrupted, and access to friends or colleagues halted' (Social Care Institute for Excellence, 2020). Jane Harris, Director of External Affairs at the National Autistic Society, says, 'it's harder (for people with autism) to understand what is going on in the first place' (reported by *Clare & Reed (2020)). It is understandable that* Molly (National Autistic Society (NAS), 2020) talks of being 'scared', Ben (NAS, 2020) said the lockdown was 'really hard' and a 'dark time'. Molly's fear is increased because 'I can't control it.' *Ian (NAS, 2020) confirms that he is 'constantly taking his temperature', fearful of getting COVID-19. Claire & Reed (2020) report on a man in a residential care home who is fearful that he will become ill via sick care staff, and that soon the whole residential home will be infected. Amy (NAS, 2020) is fearful that she cannot visit the hospital from where she gets her normal support*

Connor (NAS, 2020) reports *that since the lockdown, his routines have been interrupted and this is causing him to have issues maintaining his 'sense of peace and mental clarity'. Amy (NAS, 2020) says, 'now my routines are all disrupted and I don't know what I am doing – I feel lost'. 'Sudden change has been very overwhelming,' reports Jake (NAS, 2020), noting that aspects of this situation causes him to be 'confused or having a meltdown'; he is fearful that he will lose control.*

*One autistic man who lives in his own flat and needs two visiting caretakers is reported by Claire & Reed (2020) as losing said caretakers as the lockdown was announced. Apparently, the impact on him was not considered in-depth, and simply losing these essential workers will mean his personal routines will change, causing him to face the huge challenge of adapting.*

*Interestingly, some have found the lockdown reassuring. AutisticPb (2020)*
*appreciates the lockdown for the 'peace and quiet, warmth and productivity'.*
*Charis (NAS, 2020) found the lockdown 'great', as she had prepared and*
*surrounded herself with things that entertained her, and that she appreciated*
*being home-schooled and maintaining friendship via online systems.*

We know re-establishing routines takes time, but it is vital. There is less
concern with whether routines will be re-established, and more about when –
and how – these will be re-established. A further fear comes with the worry
that when lockdown routines are relaxed, it could result in a second phase of
COVID-19, necessitating the individual's routines again needing adaptation.

## (5)    Learning Disability

Consideration of the individual with learning disabilities in the COVID-19 crisis
and the fear that it brings is crucial, according to Mencap, who tells us there
are approximately 1.5 million people in the UK with a learning disability. They
continue by saying that the person with a learning disability 'takes longer to
learn new things and may need support to develop new skills, understanding
difficult information, and (may have difficulty) engage with other people'
(Mencap, 2020).

Like most of the population, people with learning disabilities are confused by
the amount of (sometimes conflicting) advice that they are given. Neil (2020):

> 'I have been getting confused about the different information. There
> have been too many different bits of advice and I didn't know what to
> believe. A friend told me I could go outside and that confused me.
> Then my GP told me to stay indoors for 12 weeks and because of all
> the different information I was getting, I had been going out to the
> shops. At times, the police stopped me and told me to go home. This
> was all very confusing.'

There should be consideration put toward the breadth of needs had by those
with learning disabilities. There are individuals who are being cared for at

home by their parents; in their own or independent living situations; or in residential care, hospital, and prison settings. Each person will have their own unique sets of wishes, needs and strengths.

There is a fear associated with the number of people with a learning disability seemingly dying. There is fear over the loss of liberties and human rights as regulations are changed. And there is fear of becoming increasingly socially isolated and not being able to get the help that they need.

**People Dying**

We know that all people are probably at risk of getting COVID-19, and that some of these people will die (National Health Service (2020a)) However, these figures do not seem to be high enough, as the Care Quality Commission (2020a) reported to the BBC that the death count of those with autism and/or learning disabilities between 10th April and 8th May, 2020 is 3,765 people (as compared to 1,370 people over the same period in 2019.) This, it can be seen that there is a significantly higher mortality rate in this period.

| Table 3: COVID-19 deaths of patients with a learning disability notified to LeDeR | | | | | | | | | | | |
|---|---|---|---|---|---|---|---|---|---|---|---|
| | 27/3 | 3/4 | 10/4 | 17/4 | 24/4 | 1/5 | 8/5 | 15/5 | 22/5 | 29/5 | Date not known |
| COVID-19 related deaths | 35 | 80 | 110 | 115 | 75 | 50 | 25 | 20 | 15 | 10 | 15 |
| All deaths | 105 | 155 | 165 | 175 | 120 | 100 | 70 | 50 | 55 | 25 | 35 |
| | | | | | | | | | | | **National Health Service (2020b)** |

One of the contributory factors could be the National Institute of Health and Care Excellence (2020) COVID-19 Rapid Guideline: Critical Care, which established the Clinical Frailty Scale as reported by Walker (2020). This resulted in an "unprecedented" number of do-not-resuscitate orders for learning-disability patients' (Thomas, 2020). Julie Bass, Chief Executive of Turning Point, a learning disability charity that provides residential care, reflected on the number of DNR's for people coming to her organisations being significantly higher since the outbreak: she called this 'illegal' and an 'outrage'. As a result, the Chief Nursing Officer Ruth May and National Medical Director of NHS England and NHS Improvement questioned the way Do Not Attempt Cardio-Pulmonary Resuscitation orders were being written. May & Powis (2020) wrote, 'The Key Principle is that each person is an individual whose needs and preferences must be taken into account individually.' They continue by stating, 'Blanket policies are inappropriate, whether due to medical condition, disability, or age.'

**Loss of Liberties and Human Rights**

Another major move by the government during this period is the changing of the Mental Health Act (1983) via the NHS (2020b) Legal Guidance for Mental Health, Learning Disability, Autism and specialised commissioning services supporting people of all ages during the coronavirus pandemic. This is designed to make it safer to place the person on a section of the Mental Health Act. It increases the time the individual can be detained in some instances. Examples of the changes include detaining someone for treatment, moving from two doctors and an approved mental health professional to one doctor and a mental health professional, or increasing removal to a place of safety by the police from twenty-four hours to thirty-six hours. There are other temporary changes during the COVID-19 crisis, and one of the fears is that these 'temporary' regulations will not be lifted.

Edel Harris (the Chief Executive of Mencap) records that over two thousand people with learning disabilities are currently locked away in inpatient settings against their will. Sir Simon Wessely (Department for Health & Social Care, 2018) made recommendations for reviewing the Mental Health Act, with the idea of reducing the number of people being detained. The Care Quality Commission (2020b) confirmed:

> 'There is a clear case for change: the rate of detention is rising; the patient's voice is lost within processes that are out-of-date and can be uncaring; there is unacceptable overrepresentation of … people with learning disabilities and/or autism are at a particular disadvantage. We are also concerned that we are out-of-step with our human rights obligations.'

## Social Isolation and the Help Needed

In the Scope (2020) survey, 28% of people with learning disabilities say they feel forgotten by the government- which is not surprising. When the planning for COVID-19 started, the Care Quality Commission (2020b) noted that many people with learning disabilities and autism remained in hospitals because there was a lack of community services. Government planners identified that, of those patients that had to be discharged to make way for the influx of COVID-19 patients, 49% would require support in the community or rehab beds. They further anticipated that 1% would need to remain in hospitals (Her Majesties Government / National Health Service, 2020). They point out that the onus seems to be on 'safety' and discharging people quickly, rather than finding the right place for them.

Catalina Devandas Aguilar, UN Rapporteur for the Convention on the Rights of Persons with Disabilities, discussed that social distancing and self-isolation 'may be impossible for those who rely on the support of others to eat, dress, and bathe' (United Nations, 2020).

There are further issues with the way that some people in residential care and independent living situations are supported. Rig (2020) on the Mind website, whose daughter is in residential care, says she is becoming 'very depressed' and he feels the 'care company … (are) not doing anything to help the situation', and that they only allow 'two telephone calls per day'. Others report that they can bring parcels to the door, but do not get to even wave at their child. With the lifting of some of the lockdown restrictions, this may change.

One young man who lives in his own flat recounts that " (SCLD, 2020). He has caretakers who come in, and because he pays them from his personal independence payments, he is seen as an employer of personal assistants. He is fearful that if he were to become ill with COVID-19, his personal assistants will need personal protective equipment, such as aprons, masks and maybe a visor; he is unsure exactly what they will need, and even more unsure how to get these things.

Chief Enablement Officer and a nurse consultant at PBS4, Jonathan Beebee highlights that when caretakers come gowned and masked, the quality of communication will inevitably be reduced (Dean, 2020). Similarly, SCLD (2020) says that 'providing support or care during social distancing/isolation is increasing experiences of loneliness and social isolation'. The Scope (2020) survey noted that 38.5% of their cohorts were concerned about social isolation. Excellent advice from a service user, Neil (2020), was for someone to be appointed to keep in contact with the individual on a regular basis. SCLD (2020) highlights the continued need to provide support and care during social distancing/isolation.

Fear for people, their families, and their caretakers seems to be an inevitable consequence of all these issues.
Dean (2020) says that 'fear of leaving home has increased as time has passed', and Scope (2020) records that 60% of people with learning disabilities and autism are not currently leaving their home.

There are some people who feel the benefit of social isolation, perceiving that there are fewer demands on them (Dean, 2020), and at the same time some people are reacting to the social isolation with expressing themselves in ways that can be seen as causing 'behavioural problems'. This could well be to do with changing routines, insecurities, and the need to adapt.

| Table 4: Selection of Items from the SCOPE (2020) Survey of People with Learning Disabilities During the COVID-19 Crisis. | |
| --- | --- |
| **Social Isolation** | 28% feel forgotten or ignored by the government.<br><br>59% are currently not leaving their home at all.<br><br>38.5% feel extremely concerned about their mental health and well-being if they need to self-isolate for more than three months. |
| **Medical Help** | 63% are concerned they won't get the hospital treatment they need if they become ill with coronavirus.<br><br>40% are extremely concerned about making medical appointments if they have to self-isolate for more than three months. |
| **Help and Support** | 45% say they have had issues getting essential items. |
| **Other** | 26% say they have faced negative attitudes from other shoppers.<br><br>86% reported they are very worried or somewhat worried about the effect the pandemic is having on their lives. |

## (6)    Domestic Abuse

While the government response to domestic violence has been to increase police powers to deal with the situation (Patel, 2020), and supply additional funding toward resources used to support individuals at risk of abuse. While drawing the reports for this section, policies have been developed for children, women, and minorities- though there is little pertinent to men. The World Health Organization (2006) recognises that domestic violence impacts the whole family, and that it can occur between any members.

| Table 5: What is Domestic Abuse (Home Office, 2020) | | |
|---|---|---|
| Domestic abuse is not always physical violence. It can also include, but is not limited to: | | |
| • coercive control and 'gaslighting' | • online abuse | • emotional abuse |
| • economic abuse | • verbal abuse | • sexual abuse |

The Government acknowledges that recent measures announced to tackle coronavirus (COVID-19), such as the lockdown, can cause real fear or even terror for those who are experiencing or feel at risk of domestic abuse. Home Office (2020) includes a long list of organisations that can help. Lavietes (2020) states that domestic violence has risen globally, as many countries imposed tougher restrictions on people leaving their homes. Patel (2020) tells us that the National Domestic Abuse Helpline reported a 120% rise in the number of calls it received in one recent twenty-four hour period.

| Table 6: Weekly Police Arrest in London for Domestic Violence. | | | |
|---|---|---|---|
| Year | Weekly | Context | Reference |
| 2012 | 320 | A major crackdown on domestic violence | British Broadcasting Corporation (2012) |
| 2020 | 100 | The COVID-19 Crisis, Lockdown period | Lavietes, 2020 |

There are a number of contributory factors for domestic violence, but issues of power and control within relationships tend to be the major factor. Increased time together in lockdown and the feeling of not knowing when things will change only makes these issues more acute. An additional consideration is alcohol and drugs, which are known to reduce inhibitions and cognitive abilities (de Paula Gebara, Ferri, Lourenço, de Toledo Vieira, de Castro

Bhona & Noto, 2015). The World Health Organization (2006) suggests alcohol is associated with increases in intimate partner domestic violence. With the increased usage of alcohol and drugs during the lockdown (Griegson, 2020), we can see that increased levels of domestic violence are almost inevitable. Griegson (2020) reports that approximately 50% of drinkers during the lockdown were starting much earlier in the day, drinking for longer periods and more often during the week. Similarly, 40% of those that use cannabis have increased their use during this period.

On the 10th April, Home Secretary Priti Patel (2020) announced increases in funding to help with domestic violence. Her idea was that the perpetrators who caused 'torment and abuse' should 'leave the home' but 'sadly, this is not possible'. Therefore, the money announced was being invested in counselling services for the abused and the abusers, as well as in housing and supporting charities who run shelters, etc. Once people are there, the key is 'to take care of mental as well as physical health and seek support if needed' (Home Office, 2020).

Meanwhile the Ministry for Housing, Communities & Local Government and Public Health England (2020) provides guidance for different types of accommodation. This guidance looks at ways to ensure the accommodation is free of COVID-19 for people living, working, and visiting there. It appears fear for those trapped in potentially violent situations is at least being acknowledged by government. However, the impacts of these measures are hard to quantify.

## (7)    Health and Social Care Workers

The occupations with the highest rate of COVID-19 diagnoses are patient-facing healthcare workers and resident-facing social care workers (Office of National Statistics (ONS) (2020). In June, up to 1.87% of the health and social care workforces are currently recorded as having COVID-19 (ONS, 2020b).

A Sky (2020) news report on the 6th June, 2020 confirmed that a Department of Health and Social Care spokesperson (unnamed) said, 'The safety of our

NHS and social care staff is paramount and employers should follow their legal duty to report the deaths of any staff who die as a result of exposure to coronavirus'.

The Health and Safety Executive (2020) have responsibilities under the Reporting of Injuries, Diseases and Dangerous Occurrences Regulations (RIDDOR) (2013) and are monitoring occupational exposure to COVID-19, which is resulting in dangerous occurrences (release of the virus), a case of disease (where someone gets exposed to the condition and is diagnosed with this), and work related deaths (where an individual's death can be attributed to getting the contagion from work and then dying as a consequence of this).

Employers such as NHS Trusts, social care organisations, and residential care organisations have responsibilities under the Health and Safety at Work, etc, Act (1974) and under additional regulations such as RIDDOR (2013). These include a 'direct duty of care for safety of the employee' and visitors to the organisation, which would be within their capability to achieve (Table 7).

| Table 7: Employer's Direct Duty of Care (Dimmond, 2015) | | |
|---|---|---|
| At common law, the employer has an implied term in the contract of employment to look after the safety of the employee. | | |
| (1) To ensure the plant & equipment are safe. | (2) To provide competent staff. | (3) To establish a safe system of work. |

It was reported on Sky News (2020b) on the 6th June 2020 that the Health and Safety Executives have received 250 fatal disease reports about healthcare workers in the last five months (up to 18th May 2020); this figure can be seen as significant when it is compared to last year, for which there were only 147 cases reported across all industries. Up to ninety-one of Health and Safety Executive reports, including twenty-six from local authorities, are currently subject to further investigation. They are looking at questions such as:

- Was there enough personal protective equipment?

- Was there enough staff?
- Did the staff have the right training?

At the same time, it is reported that there are a number of private legal cases being prepared by families. This is a direct response from people due to their bereavements, and it could be argued that this may lead to organisational fear. With any luck, it will just help the organisations examine their systems and get these right more quickly in future.

## (8)    Older Adults

Prince Charles (Mills, 2020) was interviewed on the television about his experience with COVID-19; you could hear the fear in his voice. While he was candid about the condition, his description of being unable to see his father, Prince Phillip – who is ninety-nine years old – or give his grandchildren a hug was accompanied by tears. He further said that using the internet was not the same. Prince Charles, of course, is not the only older adult who is missing family; there are many who are afraid and unable to receive family visitors because of the lockdown.

Those older adults in care or residential homes are also affected deeply by the non-visiting of relatives; in some instances, this increases already-existing isolation and despair, and they may develop feelings of abandonment. Some of these homes are taking innovative action, such as putting Perspex walls in hallways so that an individual can be visited by relatives, or relying on the internet. With the repealing of some restrictions (and hopefully with good weather), many are arranging visits outside, though with social distancing still in place.

We already knew before the COVID-19 crisis that loneliness affects our mental health (Mind, 2020) (Figure 1). Priti Patel (2020) declared that the lockdown measure was 'leaving people feeling isolated, vulnerable, and exposed, which heightens the impact of loneliness'. Age UK (2020) says, 'Most of us will feel lonely…particularly those in later life… loneliness can define our lives and have a significant impact on our well-being'. Alzheimer's UK, in the person of Jonathan Pryce (2020), has highlighted that things have changed and individuals are 'scared, lonely, and struggling to get vital support'. The Campaign to End Loneliness (2020) was established in 2011 and has recently adapted its website to provide tips for those who are being socially isolated because of COVID-19. Their aim remains to reduce loneliness in the elderly.

**Figure 1: Loneliness and Mental Health (Mind 2020)**

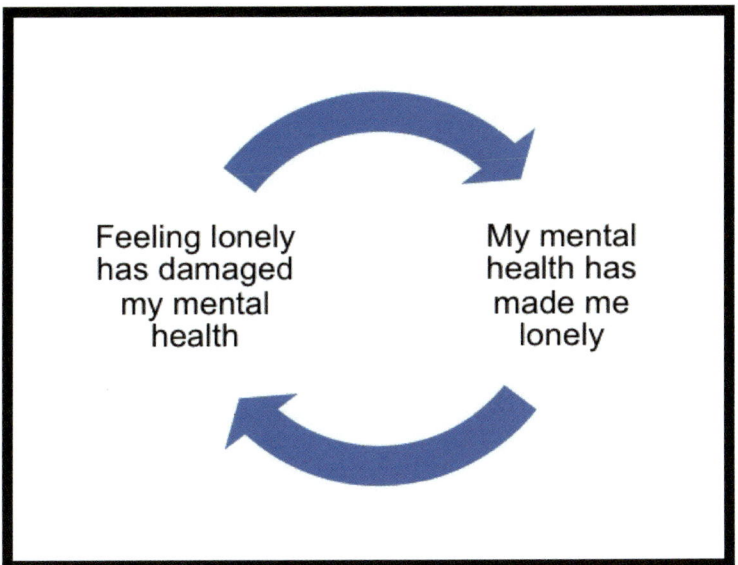

A major aspect of COVID-19 that needs to be considered - in this group especially - is the idea that the advice given to older adults to stay indoors during the lockdown simply increases their levels of fear. It is understandable, and it relates to the individual's responsiveness to the COVID-19 virus. Those who are seventy or older are considered at 'moderate risk (clinically vulnerable)' (NHS, 2020c). However, many of these people will have one or more clinical conditions, such as diabetes, which increases vulnerability. This effectively means age is a contributory factor to possible deaths and is made worse if the individual has one or more pre-existing conditions. The Office of National Statistics (2020b) records that 90.4% of people dying with COVID-19 had at least one pre-existing condition. It highlights both dementia and Alzheimer disease as the most common pre-existing conditions, equating to 20.4% of all deaths involving COVID-19 in the UK. In England alone this figure rises to 37% of all deaths. This percentage is likely to rise further, now that the statistics are including those from care and residential homes, along with the individuals at home.

## (9)    The Issues

From this overview of different vulnerable groups, we can see that the fear caused by the virus has been accentuated by the issues they were struggling with. However, the thing that is most obvious is that people's lives have been changed and will continue to be changed by the impact of COVID-19 related fear. This chapter is not comprehensive. In the future, we must consider other vulnerable groups: those in prison and immigration removal centres, the unemployed, and those in areas of social deprivation and affluence.

# Communication in a Crisis

*Mike Waddington*

**"The truth will set you free, but first it will piss you off..."**

I keep six honest serving-men
(They taught me all I knew);
Their names are What and Why and When,
And How and Where and Who.
**Rudyard Kipling**

This article will explain and discuss the approach my organisation, Central and North West London NHS Trust (CNWL), is taking to communicate with its staff during the COVID-19 Public Health Emergency. Communication is not a front-line activity, but it supports the front line as well as informing and sometimes directing. It also validates the front-line's concerns and experiences, which are the experiences that count.

I will touch on external communications (there is a read across for all communication approaches) but will concentrate on communication with our approximately 7,000 staff (across at least 150 locations in London, Surrey and Milton Keynes); often called 'internal comms' - an outdated term, as the barrier between internal and external is very thin.

There is also an enormous amount of communicating going on; our emergency response reporting structure of Bronze (local level), Silver (service level) and Gold (executive level), was a pump for circulating communication. One rather defining feature has been the rise of 'virtual' and 'distance' working through Zoom, MST and others; training, teams, catch ups (virtual coffee shops) staff networks and weekly catch-ups with service leads and ward managers by the executive.

This digitalisation has enabled a much more flexible working pattern and has psychologically changed the mindset from ICT that felt clunky and old fashioned. The crisis pushed us across the chasm and made an important leap: digital working has been warmly embraced! That said, several people find these meetings more intense, requiring more concentration and thus feeling more tired; this is commonly known as Zoom-fatigue.

We also produced some films for staff – when needed – around wellbeing. For patient use, we have recently used Zoom recordings with slides and a commentary from the top right-hand corner. We have also pioneered a once-a-week 'radio' show; the format allows for poetry, readings, features, 'live from a ward', and a segment where patients can ask questions of guests such as QPR's Les Ferdinand, most recently.

Communication is always about this multi-layered repetition, and whilst these layers are particularly useful, we needed a regular pulse beat directly intervening with staff as our general communication channel.

The main channel we used for staff was a daily bulletin:

- News – topical and current
- Guidance
- Pace
- Orientation
- Realistic expectations
- Recognition of problems and recognition of effort
- Trustwide (authoritative, but with an informality to try to match the personality of the Chief Nurse)
- Plain speaking.

At the time of writing, there have been sixty editions (on fifty-eight days, 12 March to 20 May, with five special second-editions). The five special editions were each devoted to a single topic – PPE (twice), CPR advice (twice), and an appeal about NHS Nightingale.

It was circulated six times a week, not usually on a Sunday (though we produced an issue on each of the four days of the Easter weekend). This is being scaled back to weekdays only (from Saturday 2 May), as the peak of the crisis has passed.

Normal communications services continued, such as the All-Staff Three-Minute Read on Mondays. We also completed ninety design projects (leaflets, webpages, graphics, films, banners, posters, and leaflets). We anticipate this slowing further and focusing more content on 'Recover & Thrive', and the 'new' CNWL will from the crisis. Twice-a-week briefings were sent to our governors and stakeholders. This article answers Kipling's verse, with its appeal for plain writing.

## Introduction

David Goodhart, of Policy Exchange, writing in the Sunday Times (26 April 2020) said:

> 'I watched the BBC News at Ten one night last week, and by the end felt emotionally drained and no better informed about anything than at 9.59pm. On too many nights, the news bulletins…run along these tram lines: here's something about COVID-19; here's someone who died; here's a sobbing relative or frontline hero telling you to stay at home, save lives and protect the NHS. Yes, it's a bleak and emotional period…but I feel an aching lack of authority, explanation and context, and a general infantilisation of the public discourse. Too much communication has become performative rather than informative.'

I agree with this analysis, while accepting a point Goodhart later makes: '… the expressive, emotional public tone reflects real changes in popular temperament in recent decades, and perhaps also a less middle-aged and macho public culture.' (ibid)

No organisation exists in a communication vacuum, and the media fills much of a person's down time. Like many NHS organisations, we even advised staff to limit their consumption of news media (initially only social media) in the interests of their emotional well-being; the incessant emotional rhythm can drive anxiety and worries up.

CNWL began by recognising these traits. In fact, we know that personal stories with emotional impact tend to attract more media interest. During the first month of the crisis, we attracted some media for the experiential stories of redeployed staff – in print and on the radio – and a small piece on the BBC London TV News was well received by staff, who felt it was a good story about how the NHS was adapting successfully.

Thus, our approach was going to be more informing than performing – to use Goodhart's useful phrase. It had to have an emotional content, but one that was calm and even, not shying away from bad news (and prepared to risk some upset).

## Gloria Steinhem

A favourite quote of mine is attributed to Gloria Steinhem: 'The Truth will set you free but first it will piss you off!' (now the title of her latest book.) I frequently use it to describe myself and the approach I take to communicating.

Transparency is vital for a number of reasons. It's about resisting the impulse to be defensive; it's about accountability, but it's also about sincerity. It's a question of trust; you're more trustworthy if the story you're telling is sometimes about errors and the candid apologies that go with it.

CNWL is a very transparent organisation, and at the time of the Grenfell Fire in 2017 (CNWL provides the Grenfell Health and Wellbeing service) we adopted the charter recommended by Bishop James Jones in his report on Hillsborough (November 2017, p 7).

The whole charter is actually a very good guide to communicating.

> I commit to [this public body] becoming an organisation which strives to:

1. In the event of a public tragedy, activate its emergency plan and deploy its resources to rescue victims, to support the bereaved and to protect the vulnerable.

2. Place the public interest above our own reputation.

3. Approach forms of public scrutiny – including public inquiries and inquests – with candour, in an open, honest and transparent way...

4. Avoid seeking to defend the indefensible or to dismiss or disparage those who may have suffered where we have fallen short.

5. Ensure all members of staff treat members of the public and each other with mutual respect and with courtesy. Where we fall short, we should apologise straightforwardly and genuinely.

6. Recognise that we are accountable and open to challenge. We will ensure that processes are in place to allow the public to hold us to account for the work we do and for the way in which we do it. We do not knowingly mislead the public or the media. (Op cit)


**Trust and Trustworthiness**

Baroness Onora O'Neil has written widely about trust, particularly linking trust to trustworthiness:

> "Trust is valuable when placed in trustworthy agents and activities, but damaging or costly when (mis)placed in untrustworthy agents and activities. ... . Information about others' generic attitudes of trust or mistrust that take no account of evidence whether those attitudes are well or ill placed can offer little or no help for those who aim to place or refuse trust well. ... But where we aim not to influence others, but to place and refuse trust intelligently we must link trust to trustworthiness, and must focus on evidence of honesty, competence and reliability. (International Journal of Philosophical Studies April 2018)

The watchword of CNWL was to be trustworthy (honest, competent, and reliable) in the eyes of our staff. That meant a straightforward style, not an officious, bureaucratic, or self-serving, 'corporate' tone, but to advise, listen, and respond. Communication style at CNWL is about showing empathy and reacting sincerely, so that we can be persuasive by being authentic and trustworthy. Communications were raised at the daily Silver calls (service managers and the Cirri's Response Team) and messages were clarified, re-sent, or explained again.

We wanted to say things as they were. Therefore, on 2 April the piece on PPE began frankly: 'Let's be honest – that's not been good, and Claire Murdoch has been pressing (the system) very hard on this..."
PPE (personal protective equipment) and being able to perform CPR (resuscitation) with the right PPE were important. We understood its importance to staff and patients; we had to take into account national stories of shortages, but also crucially wanted to make sure PPE was being used correctly and safely. We had to watch vocabulary; a good example was that some people missed an item about staff testing because it was headed as 'Staff Screening' – many responded but the skim readers missed it. A small but important point.

The British Psychological Society raised a similar point about national messages and how it would be better to refer to 'Physical Distancing' rather than 'Social Distancing'.

**'Keep Yourself Informed, Keep Calm and Carry On**

On 6 March, the Chief Executive wrote to all staff (in her blog, *Talking Trust*):

> Staff are following advice – we recently had a visitor from North Italy coming into a ward, and staff rightly used our on-call system for advice and with 111, did the right and sensible thing.

> So, at the outset thank you from me for all you're doing in your day to day work and for Coronavirus our watchwords are those of the WHO; "facts not fears; science not rumours."

And I want to mention and applaud those staff who've been on the front line in the isolation Unit in Milton Keynes (they used 20,000 face masks over those two weeks) the Camden staff working on community swab testing in UCLH, our Hillingdon Team for the isolation Unit at Heathrow and community swabbing team. Thank you all.

We're in the 'contain' phase right now but moving to 'delay'; so that means if you have been to, or exposed to someone from, the specific areas, you should self-isolate and call 111; if you have been to those countries but outside those specific places, you only need to call 111 if you have symptoms.

My message to you all is to keep yourself informed, keep calm and carry on.

## COVID News

The first edition was on Thursday 12 March and had information from the Chief Executive on the shift from the 'contain' phase of the pandemic to the 'delay' phase. It made proposals about lockdown and its impact on staff – at home and at work. It also mentioned PPE, which was the item that featured in most editions, alongside staff well-being.

## Why Daily?

It's often said that 'people won't read that', and that's as true as it is unilluminating; you cannot expect busy people to read everything that gets put out. The average daily edition of the Daily Mail has 140 pages and clearly very few people would read every page – people dip in, but also always check front pages and major features. We felt our communications should aim to do the same: act like a newspaper with an expectation that people would read most editions, but would mostly pick and choose. The conversation in the organisation would do the rest. We would reach enough people.

A new rhythm was set with Daily Situation Reports (SitReps) and Silver and Gold meetings (seven days a week), so the newsletter was to follow that pattern. Therefore, the newsletters had a metronomic purpose too – it was the drum beat to the day's routine; it was to show that it was led from the top of the organisation as it moved up a gear. That's also why it was produced on a Saturday. We had many staff working from home, as well as hundreds redeployed to other locations, so this was another reason daily bulletins were produced. A new sense of purpose was felt by many staff, several of whom were taken from their usual work into new patient environments they were trained for but not used to.

Many sexual health staff – trained physicians and nurses – moved into Offender Care, some into mental health wards, and many stepped down into Intermediate Care (of vulnerable people discharged from hospital to free up a medical bed). This generated a new sense of belonging, and the cross-fertilisation of experience we have advocated for many years actually came to fruition in the response – broadening horizons and strengthening the family feel of the Trust.

The bulletin was a reinforcer for that spirit, helping bring the organisation together – with policy guidance, but also stories and compliments (see below). It is said that journalism is the first draft of history, and CNWL's emergency response memory is contained in these bulletins.

**Was it Read?**

On 9 April, we had a request to add a contents list so that staff could go back to editions – as they were obviously storing them for later use (despite also being put on the intranet – called Trustnet at CNWL). But it is hard to judge precisely.

On 25 March, we sent out a special edition at 16.48pm asking for volunteers to go to NHS Nightingale. By the following morning, we had 107 people volunteering from CNWL as well as twelve others from outside of the Trust (which also shows there is never anything that is wholly secure – indeed we often write in the expectation it would go wider, though we also included some partners like Commissioners and others in the circulation).

If you consider that this appeal to go to the front trenches needed to be read, considered, and responded to, it showed how quickly news was read and spread. The response gives an indication of the circulation and readership – with its initial spurt and a long tail – i.e. messages having an initial response but continuing to trickle through the organisation.

The responses were as follows:

| | |
|---|---|
| 25-Mar | 52 |
| 26-Mar | 98 |
| 27-Mar | 22 |
| 28-Mar | 7 |
| 29-Mar | 6 |
| 30-Mar | 10 |
| 31-Mar | 6 |
| 01-Apr | 4 |
| 02-Apr | 4 |
| 03-Apr | 1 |
| 04-Apr | 1 |
| 05-Apr | 0 |
| 06-Apr | 0 |
| 07-Apr | 2 |

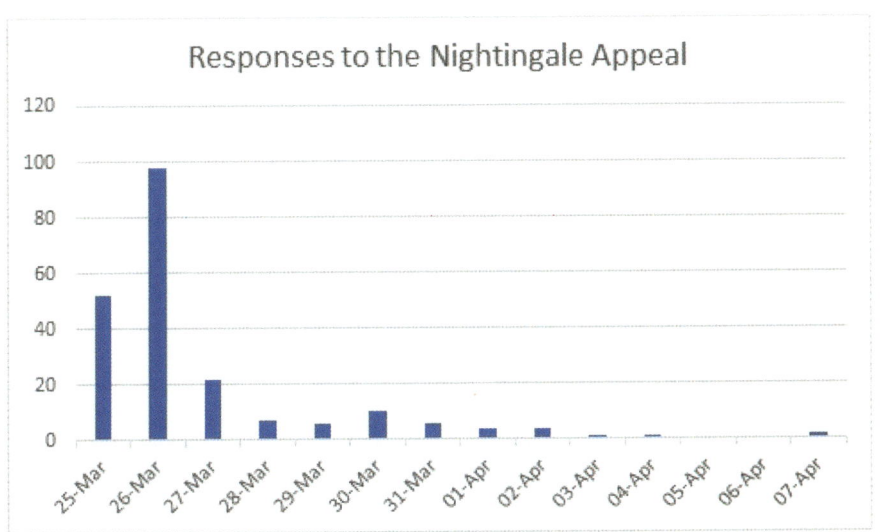

We also had direct feedback, like this one from 1 May (after the critical care surge):

> 'I just wanted to say how much I appreciate these emails - I'm a doctor mainly working in another trust, but I do Special Interest sessions with CNWL so I get the staff emails - and I have found the email updates to be consistently warm, caring, thoughtful and sensible. It makes such a difference and feels like the senior part of the organisation understand how staff are feeling. So, thank you, it is appreciated.'

Or this one from a Doctor in Hillingdon:

> 'Maria, these bulletins are fabulous, well done to all producing them.'

It was also tweeted – as here:

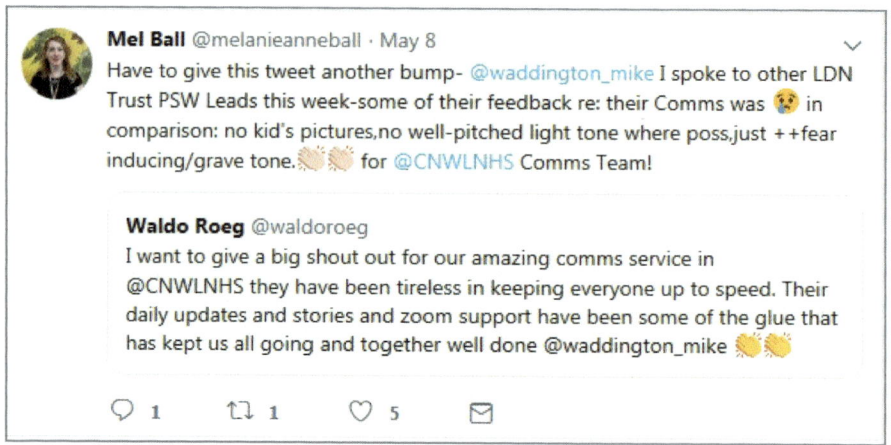

Mistakes also have a good side; it's not uncommon for people to point out typos or errors, which again lets you know where material is being read.

On 1 May, the Newsletter carried a well-being graphic and we received this response (anonymised):

> **From:** XX (CENTRAL AND NORTH WEST LONDON NHS FOUNDATION TRUST)

**Sent:** 01 May 2020 11:57

**To:** CNWL, Communications (CENTRAL AND NORTH WEST LONDON NHS FOUNDATION TRUST)

**Subject:** RE: To all staff - COVID-19 UPDATE – Friday 1 May 2020

PLEASE reference the author of the tree. You cannot take other people's work and pass this off as your own. Dr xx

As it happens, we had permission, but these types of response show it reaches further than you might think. Our conclusion was that it was read, re-read and referred to throughout the organisation; it reached enough people.

## Content

From edition two – Saturday 14 March, when the Response Hub was set up – it was issued in the name of CNWL'S Chief Nursing Officer, Maria O'Brien; to underline it was a Trustwide issue, that it was to be clinically led, and that the nursing staff (around 3,600 of our staff) would be central to our day-to-day response to the crisis.

We adopted the strap line, "we are the NHS" to mobilise around. On Wednesday 18 March, we wrote:

> 'We are all being asked to do extraordinary things, as the NHS is at the centre of caring for those most affected by COVID-19. We do this because we are the NHS.'

The first editions were all about what was happening and the guidance we recommended - PPE featured a lot, partly because national advice changed a number of times; the press began reporting shortages, some staff experienced some difficulties, and some staff were not as familiar with it as they could be (and came to be).

There were also lots of questions about how to socially distance; working from home with good routines, including health and well-being; or hotel accommodation. Some staff reported that a few schools would not recognise staff as keyworkers. The police wanted to see keyworker letters other than NHS IDs. There were offers of free parking, free Santander bike usage, parking, food. A lot of this kind of information was included.

We wanted to show progress, so over time we developed a commentary on the national graphs from the national daily press conferences and produced our own sitreps about patients in our care. We also included figures on the numbers of staff off (at one stage 1,300); over time these numbers fell.

We repeatedly reported about those who were COVID-positive, those who were isolating due to symptoms, and those who were isolating due to somebody in their family exhibiting symptoms- which comprised the largest of the groups. We wished these staff well and directed different messages toward them – testing being an important message to bring the 'self-isolating' group back to work where they were needed.

In fact, we issued a corrective at one stage: So much attention had been focused on the need to get people back to work, that it could have seemed as though we were overlooking those who turned up every day and dedicated themselves to the task. To avoid this, we issued a 'Thank You for Coming to Work Today' poster, reproduced in the newsletter (6 April) and used around the Trust. We reported on service changes and the whole mobilisation effort (redeploying hundreds of staff).

We also started reporting about the Clap for Carers events (nine so far) and Captain Tom (now Colonel) Moore – which was about hope in a dark time, and the appreciation the public was showing. National messaging about social distancing – sometimes interpreted very narrowly and strictly – felt at odds with what we were asking staff to do. Anxiety needed to be managed by talking about the necessity for the work, the importance of PPE (supply and use), IPC - Infection Prevention and Control ('Be bare below the elbow') - social distancing (including asking staff to stop visiting friends at other locations), and always thanking everyone for their efforts.

On Wednesday 25 March, we also asked for positive stories and received an immediate response. We received two messages from different parts of the Trust asking for their child's drawings of encouragement to be published. We hesitated for a day about this – would it appear flippant? Would it run counter to the seriousness of the work we are doing? We had already started to use more graphics in the newsletters, so we decided to try, since it played to the wider objective of 'we are the NHS', linking their work with their families and wider society. From 30 March onward, we acknowledged the growing intensity of the work, the new things staff were having to do, and PPE. We responded to this throughout the surge of cases.

It was very warmly received, and scores of pictures, photographs, messages from abroad, paintings seen in the streets, songs, poems, and hobbies were sent in and we found we were publishing two or three a day. When staff went into uniform (also an IPC measure), a new set of staff photos followed – social distancing or in PPE. These stories rounded off the newsletters on a lighter note, but one to remind them of their 'ordinary' lives and validating their experiences and dedication.

We have some staff who have been in hotels for six weeks, unable to see their families and – in some cases – their children. It is humbling to hear that and should be recorded.

We also carried news of sites visited by executive directors – again to record thanks for the work of the teams, but also to underline that the execs were at the front line too; part of the newsletter was to make all this visible.

**Reaction to the Death of Staff Members**

On 31 March, we reported on the first staff member to die from COVID-19: a 29-year-old care coordinator from our Contact Centre in Hillingdon. Our first thoughts are always with the family, and we based much of what we did on their wishes. Secondly, it was her colleagues who wanted it to be marked, their grief acknowledged, and their tributes made. This was an awful time, but we decided that we had to let the staff know. Word would soon spread anyway, either through social media or through personal links; the person was well known and had other family members working at the Trust. We couldn't be silent.

However, the message could only be general and said:

> 'We are very sad to report that Emily Perugia, who worked for CNWL in Hillingdon, has died.
> Emily worked for the Care Connection Team in Northwood as a Care Co-ordinator and previously had worked at the Northwood Health Centre.
> She was twenty-nine and had been self-isolating because of COVID-19.
> Emily was a very well-liked and popular member of staff and a devoted professional.
> ...
> Emily's mother, Tracey Perugia is the Contact Centre Team Lead. Emily's sister Louise works for the GP Confederation. Emily's brother, Andrew, works for CNWL as a Primary Care Research Co-ordinator at St Pancras.
> Emily was engaged to James Day, who also works in the Contact Centre. They had recently moved into their first home together.
> We send our heartfelt condolences to them all.
>
> The family asks that if anyone would like to donate to a charity in her memory, Age UK, the Animal Welfare Trust or The Guide Association would all be appropriate.'

We were sent this message from a doctor:

> 'About the 29-year-old staff member dying, and was isolating due to COVID-19. It reads as if she died of COVID without underlying conditions.

It's not helpful because it will make staff more anxious. We are struggling to contain staff as it is. Either put more detail in or less detail.

Who puts this stuff together!!!!!'

We also had feedback from some staff who were at home who were worried about the message – some said they were 'frightened'.

We couldn't go into confidential clinical detail, and it was the age that troubled people. On the other hand, the staff who knew this person wanted us to do more.

We discussed it in the 15 April edition:

'We've had feedback about reporting for when staff members involved in the pandemic sadly die. It is very difficult, and we appeal for everyone's understanding.

We want to salute these staff and allow their colleagues to pay their respects and make their tributes. We will continue to report this news to you, as you must hear it from us, not from the media or social media.

On the other hand, some staff find it very difficult indeed and – truly meaning no disrespect – would prefer to move on from the news.

With that in mind, we report immediately below this item, the death of a staff member in Surrey.

These may be very small numbers and very sad occasions but are also examples of dedication and commitment that must be marked, not least for their families.

We are creating a page on Trustnet – our Roll of Honour – where tributes to these staff members can be made by teams, colleagues and friends: details shortly.'

We had feedback that this message landed well:

'In general, staff members have said that the delivery of this news has become so much better and acceptable and they are appreciative and also fully understand the need to inform staff of the sad demises. Personally, I think the (above) is really well delivered and 'satisfies' both needs - reporting and compassion.

I love the idea of the "Roll of Honour". Something that we will all be able to treasure about our colleagues who gave up their lives to keep us safe.

Thank you so much for taking feedback and doing something about it.'

It was a valuable – and unavoidable – lesson in truth; we reported the worst kind of news, and although there was some turbulence, but ultimately it only balanced and strengthened our trust.

## The New Normal

On 17 April, the chief executive wrote to staff thinking about the 'new normal' that would emerge once the peak had passed.

> 'I've been able to visit a number of your teams, but I wanted to write to you all with my thanks to everyone for what you are doing now and though it is far from over, we do need to start to think about preparing for the New Normal.'

She began with a plea about PPE, reminding people to use it correctly. Claire went on to talk about the future:

> 'It is far from over, of course, but things have changed; changed utterly.
>
> We have all been part of the crisis response – every team, every service and every person, from porters, PAs, drivers and admin staff to nurses, medics, therapists, social workers and pharmacists – all

have responded. And we had many people choose to return to the frontline from retirement which was inspirational to see.

But it's also been a great reconnection of physical and mental health, almost a new integrated professionalism has emerged bringing skills together – something we have been reaching for, for years! New working patterns have emerged that helped services and helped at home.

What service changes have we made that have been so beneficial to us and patients that we just would not want to lose? What changes do we need to sustain? Even develop further?

We are setting up a COVID-19 Plan Ahead Team that will work alongside the COVID-19 Crisis Hub, so that we can continue to manage the crisis here and now and at the same time get on the front foot for planning for life after COVID and the New Normal.

Every crisis delivers a legacy; a silver lining to make changes that benefits us all.'

As always, there was a message about well-being:

'The pace we are working at is not going to slow down; it's a marathon not a sprint.

It's important that you look after yourself, each other and your teams. If you are healthy and well, you can offer great care and services to others; visit our Well-being microsite for all the ways to get support to stay well.

I liked from the beginning the 'Going Home Checklist':

- Take a moment to think about today
- Acknowledge what was difficult - and let it go
- Consider three things that went well

- Check on your colleagues – are they OK?
- Are you ok? We're here to support you
- Now switch your attention to home – rest and recharge.

## Interim Conclusions

- The bulletin has been the focal point for communicating and responses from staff.
- It had reach
- The use of pictures and photos showed a good level of engagement from all areas
- It upheld trust values of Compassion, Respect, Empowerment and Partnership
- It was controversial at times
- It offered a transparent position on cases of COVID-19 being cared for and staff members affected.
- It was a trusted source of information on PPE and CPR
- It received positive comments from staff and stakeholders.

## The Team

The whole communication campaign was a team effort and I have a great team. They were dispersed to work from home, which was a great success in increasing productivity. I often say I recruit writers or journalists (including our two designers) and this operation was run like a newspaper, but we also wanted to be an efficient service – responding to requests for updates (from the words to designs to posting on Trustnet and the website, all through many meetings on Zoom). We could not have done it without this wonderful team: Jane Rogers, Amit Bharakda, Jeremey Dunning, Jess Horton, Alisha Nurse, Suze Rodrigues, and Imogen Sweeny.

Thanks to them.

# Holding onto Our Thinking When the World is Gripped by Fear

*Anna Maratos*

'In war the enemy's object is so to terrify you that you cannot think clearly, while your object is to continue to think clearly no matter how adverse or frightening the situation.'

(Bion, 1979 p. 322)

This chapter seeks to understand the United Kingdom (UK) government's response to COVID-19, which was in contrast to that of several neighbours and to the World Health Organisation guidance. In Britain, large gatherings were not banned, and older adults not shielded until quite late in the process. This was partly due to fears of 'lockdown fatigue' and partly a belief that this virus was here to stay and therefore allowing it to pass through the community would help us achieve 'herd immunity' among the fit and healthy.

While this may be a rational strategy, it also felt quite callous; were we meant to brave it out with our grandparents as collateral? While there are multiple complex reasons for the UK government's choice of strategy, one aspect may have been a culturally familiar fantasy of 'independence' and 'omnipotence'. This fantasy is experienced by individuals in adolescence and in healthy individuals is superseded in adulthood by functional interdependence. This paper suggests that perhaps Britain is going through a kind of adolescence of its own; as such, the government was gripped by a 'group delusion' that they could 'beat the virus' and that they themselves would not be at risk of serious illness or death, despite shaking hands and standing in close proximity with hundreds of people.

This delusion of omnipotence can be understood as a psychological defence to protect its proponents from feeling afraid of an uncontrollable, invisible threat which requires a degree of unity, interdependence, and collaboration to be defeated. Cultural forces in the west, and perhaps particularly in Britain, promote independence and invulnerability over openness and leaning on others; stoicism is seen as resilience, while being in touch with one's vulnerability and dependence on others is often associated with weakness. There is something peculiarly British about 'not panicking' which can result in 'not preparing': for example, the 1918 Spanish Flu was not even discussed by the cabinet until it had almost claimed the life of the prime minister, David Lloyd George.

Our own cabinet only took on board our vulnerability as a nation in mid-March, when new modelling came to light predicting that the current trajectory would result in a quarter of a million deaths, at which point the cabinet group suddenly changed course to enforce a lockdown. Although this acknowledgement of our vulnerability had a humanising effect, it felt like a lurch from denial to paralysing terror. This has had potentially short and medium-term health ramifications of its own.

For example:

- People with cancer are not receiving life-extending chemotherapy.
- Others needing operations are deteriorating at home as operating theatres have all been converted into ITUs
- Parents are keeping their children away from Accident and Emergency to avoid burdening the NHS.

The lockdown in and of itself is not a sustainable solution.

What seems hardest to do in the current climate is to acknowledge and stay with the unknowns; the more we feel we already know what the right thing to do is, the less we are able to learn from experience.

## When Anxiety Must Be Suppressed, We Cannot Prepare

When we heard about a new virus which could be deadly and could be spread easily, many of us began to prepare. The death toll in Europe had superseded China's and the UK's death and infection rate started gathering momentum. Many of us became familiar with the concept of 'exponential growth'. This had the hallmarks of 'the big one'. However, there was a sense that a culturally familiar 'keep calm and carry on' approach would prevail in the UK. What actually seems to have happened, at least in London, was that the establishment bodies such as the NHS, schools, and the BBC adopted this approach, whilst many private sector organisations started preparing by splitting teams, moving operations online, and setting up home working. A couple of anecdotal examples from the NHS follow:

On the second of March, at work in a large NHS Trust, I emailed our new COVID-19 hotline to ask for guidance about transferring patient meetings online in the likely event that this became necessary in the next few weeks. I was running a psychotherapy group with vulnerable adults and did not want to have to cancel sessions during a time of national crisis. The response from the email hotline stated what I already knew: 'At the moment there are no restrictions on gathering for events.

However, the advice is changing daily, and should there be any changes this will be communicated out to all staff via Comms'. I had an irrational feeling of being put in my place. I set up home working, consulted with group psychotherapists in the United States (US) who were already familiar with online therapy, and prepared my patients and staff for an imminent move online. On the 16th March, we received the directive that all non-essential face-to-face sessions were to be cancelled with immediate effect – no planning had been undertaken and services were suspended; would planning for this have meant getting in touch with our vulnerability to a looming threat on the horizon?

At about the same time in early March, a colleague at another NHS Trust outside London was drafting up protocols for all surgical patients to be swabbed for COVID-19 and was ensuring the supply of full PPE for all staff operating on any patients where the COVID status was unknown or positive. The initial response from colleagues was that she should stop 'raising staff anxieties', although these protocols ultimately became Trust policy. A number of medical and nursing staff did contract the virus, and some died. We can assume that there would have been more staff deaths had the testing and PPE protocols not been implemented.

These are just two examples among many within and outside the health service where people wanted to prepare but found this went against the prevailing culture. Requests to work from home at the BBC were denied in case this 'sent the wrong message'; teachers began contacting unions about working conditions. It was as if the government narrative – however irrational – had been adopted by many in establishment authority across the country. At the same time, many in the private or third sectors began to 'test' working from home or splitting teams in two more than a week before Britain locked down.

'Keep calm and carry on' prevailed beyond organisational hierarchies too: a group of older adults travelled to Berlin to see an orchestral concert; the prime minister was proud to be shaking hands with people who had the virus; a quarter of a million people went to the races at Cheltenham. Even the Chief Nursing Officer's Conference went ahead so that hundreds of senior nurses were packed into a hotel in Birmingham.

It seems that in all such cases, attempts to prepare for the pandemic pierced the national psychological defence that had been espoused by the government and which had become the national 'social unconscious': that we were not as vulnerable as the rest of the world and we did not need to learn from or lean on them.

During this time of steadily rising deaths, many people including myself were in a state of quiet simmering fearfulness due to the government's seeming inability to acknowledge and/or prepare for a crisis. Older adults, who at that stage we knew were at risk, continued to babysit grandchildren; PPE stocks were not increased; online food deliveries were not bolstered. Even my personal therapy group explored my request for a plan in terms of health anxiety and a mistrust of authority and continued to meet in a small room in central London, most of us still travelling in by tube. Eventually, on the 15th of March, I wrote to the therapist to say I had taken the decision no longer to attend in person and the following day received an email to say the group had been moved online because two people at the practice had symptoms. Despite two months of increasingly clear warnings, the narrative from government and press was that this was an unpredictable shock to the system.

Despite the lockdown, a level of denial still prevailed: an anaesthetist colleague became severely ill after having been coughed on by a patient who had not been swabbed for COVID-19 prior to his operation. Our prime minister chaired the Cabinet Office Briefing Room (COBR) meeting from home after testing positive, but he was the sole member of the group on screen while the rest continued to meet in person. By the beginning of April, four cabinet ministers and their advisors had the virus; Matt Hancock, the minister for health, had recovered but was still holding regular video calls in his office while surrounded by up to twenty colleagues (Thomas, 2020). 229 scientists signed an open letter to the government, warning that its laissez-faire attitude would result in tens of thousands of deaths, but this was not able to be heard by the government.

**Facing Our Fears**

It was only when a paper published by Imperial College London warned of half a million deaths that the government was suddenly able to snap out of its increasingly uncomfortable state of denial. Though this modelling was almost certainly wrong, as it did not take into account the ability of the healthcare system to flex and increase its intensive care capacity at pace, it nonetheless seems to have resulted in a sudden realisation from the government that the threat was real. Almost overnight, the country was put into 'lockdown'. At risk populations were told to stay at home for twelve weeks, while the remainder could leave once-per-day for exercise and work if they could not work from home.

Up until this point, the strategy had been one of prioritising the economy and civil liberties; now it became saving as many lives as possible. Prior to this watershed moment, not even the elderly were shielded; there was a sense that the UK would be less affected in some way and that even if a few people died, we would prevail as a stronger and less-cowardly nation because we stoically 'toughed it out'. After this moment, perhaps there was real fear of the virus itself, or – more cynically – of the career-limiting impact of being held responsible for so many deaths. Whichever it was, the defence was pierced. Fear had a humanizing effect: the laissez-faire stance was jettisoned in favour of a general stoppage.

However, the country seemed to lurch from denial into terror: the modelling, as had occurred in the past with BSE (otherwise known as mad cow disease) and foot-and-mouth diseases, was received as a concrete prediction rather than a hypothetical assumption based on statistics – which could not be based on all the facts as these were changing rapidly. Modelling provides answers when it feels too hard to stay with not knowing what may happen. Six million animals were killed, many probably unnecessarily, when BSE and foot-and-mouth disease entered the food chain.

Despite over two hundred scientists making less concrete and less catastrophic predictions in the run-up, the government chose to listen to the same team from Imperial whose modelling had caused the panic-induced cull of millions of animals a decade prior. Why did they listen to Imperial and not the others? Was it that they offered a confident, assured, and assertive 'truth' rather than a considered, caveated prediction openly acknowledging that this was impossible for any scientist, politician, epidemiologist, or modeller to know? Or was it that the numbers were so appallingly high the government suddenly felt afraid enough to act?

## Why Did We Not Prepare for COVID-19?

It seems likely that we did not prepare for the pandemic, despite two months of notice, because our leaders did not feel afraid; they had entered a state of denial, a highly-effective, primitive psychological defence mechanism. Feeling fear would have meant not only the anxiety of being afraid, but also the ego wound of admitting one's vulnerability and interdependence upon others.

This state of denial also invites a 'knowing' stance: we relied on models by mathematicians as though they were the truth, rather than engaging with the confusing, incomplete emergent science. It seems that the most difficult position for governments dealing with a global threat to be in is to stay with an awareness of not knowing. This unconsciously driven governmental strategy drove an equally-unconscious social denial where 'staying at one's post' was seen by many as the noble and correct thing to do. As a response to this culture, The Health Service Journal was moved to write an open letter entitled 'Please Stay Home Too: an open letter to NHS managers and admin staff' (McLellan, A. 2020). Where did this psychological and social defensiveness come from? I would like to explore this in the light of group analytic theory in the next section.

## Group Analytic Psychotherapy

The UK government response to the pandemic has thrown up issues about how we maintain our thinking and our ability to lean on others, as well as how we take in useful information from the outside world when fearful. As a group therapist, I often work with people who are struggling with a constant background fear which may manifest as 'independence' and not needing others. The group helps individuals practice how to keep their thinking and develop/maintain friendships when battered by emotional storms. It also helps the individual to build 'epistemic trust' (Fonagy & Allison 2014), which is the ability to take in helpful and healthy information from the outside world, rather than being closed off to and mistrustful of these sources of support.

Example

> Alex (not her real name) was a woman in her mid-thirties who had made two serious suicide attempts following a period of severe depression prior to joining my weekly psychotherapy group. She had some friends, but always broke up with any possible partner when he began 'asking too many questions'.

> About eighteen months into the group, Alex opened the session by stating, 'I have something I need to talk about'. The remaining group members – perhaps inappropriately, but warmly – laughed and broke into spontaneous applause: it was the first time she had proactively asked for help since joining.

> Over the following few months, group members helped her explore her feelings around asking for help: when pressed, she said it made her feel 'disgusting' to ask for help. We understood this considering her traumatic backstory of boarding school in a foreign country, the death of a parent in early childhood, and the isolation and forced 'independence' that followed. Closeness triggered intense fears of abandonment and shame of needing others.

> Over the course of two-and-a-half years, Alex emerged as a highly attuned and sensitive group member. Having joined highly sceptical of group therapy, she became committed to the other members and began to be more open. She brought material that 'she would rather have died than share with anyone'. She also began noticing that, outside the group, she was hiding aspects of herself less from her friends.

Alex was subject not only to a traumatic childhood, but also to a culture which values independence over interdependence, thus she felt shame and fear when feeling a normal pull to connect with and gain support from others.

## The Social Unconscious

When it comes to group analytic theory, Foulkes (1948) teaches that our responses and experiences are organised by our social environment past and present, as much as by our families of origin. It seems likely that some of these common defensive processes formed in our leaders when the virus began its journey west and quickly bled into the national psyche, in what Foulkes termed the 'social unconscious'. We were a strong, independent nation – we didn't need European PPE; we had a superb NHS; we were calm. The 'bad' was out there in chaotic Italy and dirty China.

> 'The concept of the social unconscious refers to the existence and constraints of social, cultural and communicational arrangements of which people are unaware' (Hopper, 2003 p. 126).

The UK and US responded more slowly than other countries. Western neoliberal capitalist society promotes independence: wealth, power, and privilege are competed for and are seen to flow from being 'independent'; conversely, pro-social, interdependent behaviours are less valued the higher up the social hierarchy one reaches (Manstead, 2018). An early boarding school education, explicitly promoting independence, is still considered a privilege, despite evidence in some 'survivors' of serious psychological effects akin to having been taken into care (Schavarien, 2004). There is still a cultural tendency to 'push feelings down' and keep going, although this is steadily shifting towards increased openness and sharing of painful feelings. Yet our 'stiff upper lip' coupled with our competitive capitalist society both arguably contributed to our difficulties with acknowledging our vulnerability as a nation, and perhaps also to our difficulties in accepting our need of one another.

This may also have to do with self-image: despite losing our colonies, we were not invaded and occupied in the Second World War, unlike other European nations; there is a sense that 'we stopped Hitler'. For our European neighbours, however, the occupation may have helped them view themselves more realistically as being vulnerable, thereby giving them an ability to keep their thinking and prepare for the current crisis. Central European countries such as Slovenia, for example, who had a recent reminder of their vulnerability through war and revolution in the 1990s, typically locked down early. Greece, after the catastrophic economic crisis of the last ten years, locked down after its first COVID death. All these countries are now opening up again.

A parallel can be found in our individual psychological development: in adolescence, we feel omnipotent and independent; we feel almost immune from harm and take risks. This is a crucial process for us to be able to separate from our parents and evolve our own identities. To renegotiate this, we need to make our own mistakes. If we can mourn our losses, the current pandemic will help us see ourselves in a more realistic light, and therefore enable us to accept help from others in a healthy, interdependent way. Perhaps Brexit also is a necessary moment in our history, giving us the chance to forge a new identity which is more realistic and less idealised: we are not a super-power, with whom everyone will be desperate to make deals; our national treasure, the NHS, though indeed a wonderful resource, could have better prepared for this pandemic – though it was successful at flexing to increase capacity once the pandemic hit.

Perhaps the growing impact of heightening awareness of the dangers of supressing our feelings will begin to shift the 'keep calm and carry on' culture towards an ability to acknowledge our fear: perhaps, 'keep calm and prepare'.

**Interdependence After COVID-19**

With the arrival of COVID-19, we have been forced into a place where we do not know how long this will last or what impact it will have economically and psychologically. We have also been forced to step off the treadmill and look at what is around us; people have connected and collaborated with each other in a new way, despite their differences. Pro-social behaviours of care, empathy, gratitude, and collaboration are returning as the ironic result of social distancing and lockdown. The unknown, the vulnerability, and the fear have fostered a measure of tolerance and appreciation of difference and care in some social circles where this was not previously the case.

The UK did not prepare well for COVID-19 as evidenced by the lack of PPE, the late shielding of care home residents and others known to be vulnerable, and the lack of a coordinated health response. This was likely to have been due to the UK 'establishment' – including the government, Public Health England, and others – having great difficulty in being able to accept and understand our vulnerability to the virus, possibly due to a psychological 'block' formed by our independence-focused culture. The defensiveness of the response was based on a reliance on 'knowing' which, in turn, made it difficult to learn from the rapidly changing and increasingly anxiety-provoking situation. A cultural premium on 'knowing' and independence over interdependence and 'not knowing' likely led to the erroneous over-reliance on modelling, and a difficulty using messier but more useful information in decision-making.

Some benefits to slowing down and facing our fears have been felt in wider society, although this is by no means the whole picture as domestic violence, mental illness, and suicide rates rise as the lockdown extends – triggering early experiences of isolation, abandonment, and (lack of) control. However, where people have been able to embrace uncertainty as even the government is now beginning to do, more of us are able to reach out to each other, take in helpful information, and give as well as gain valuable help with navigating life's inevitable crises.

It is to be hoped that the legacy of COVID-19 may help us swap the bravado and denial for a swift acceptance of reality, and shift our aspirations from an unrealistic fantasy of independence and immunity to a realistic and satisfying interdependence on each other.

# Part 2

## Exploring the Meaning

## of Fear

# Gone Viral

*by Laura Cavill*

I saw a Virus walking tall

Coughing every two metres along China's great Wall.

I watched it hop, skip, jump

(As insidious, sickly as Donald Trump.)

It spread its way across our land

And overnight drowned-out Wuhan.

From there the Virus, named COVID

Attached itself to Italians amid

The oncoming shock and alarm

When Italians arrived home in a terrifying qualm.

People were suddenly passing away

With symptoms as killers attacking their prey.

In Europe days later we dropped like flies.

'Twas then with sudden bewildered cries,

"Corona? China? Bats? 5G?

All of us shouting but without harmony.

We locked our children behind four walls

We shut down our Malls

We began to fathom the scale of our fate-

Urgently buying toilet rolls before Twas too late.

Most of us were fed details

Of continuing deaths.

Sadness, anger, fear, millions bereft.

Most followed ruling for two metre 'dance'

Some ignored it, taking their chance.

Conspiracists bred confusion by way of news

In which they believed it was all a ruse.

We clapped, cheered for NHS staff

And slowly the country allowed us to laugh

A little, connect with strangers

And volunteer for ranges

Of help we could choose.

Still, so many, globally solemnly refuse

To let the Corona, the Virus of doom,

Slither its way into our room

And infect, destroy, kill without conscience.

Those aggrieved speak with love not vengeance.

We are trying to keep as safe as best we can.

To be selfless and kind to our fellow man.

We may never know the truth at Wuhan.

Be bitter not, but share lovingly

your grief.

As far as you can and spare a thought no matter how brief,

For all of us who did our best,

All of our loved ones laid to rest

Take pride in your efforts no matter how small.

But don't look back over China's Great Wall.


LEC. 8/5/2020

# The Rhetoric of Fear and the Narrative of Hope in the Wake of COVID-19

*Dr Ryan Kemp*

I am writing in my home during the United Kingdom's COVID-19 lockdown. Outside, the sun is shining; it is a beautiful spring morning. It is also Easter, and my thoughts are not just about the philosophical and psychological aspects of this situation, but its spiritual dimensions as well. For Christians, this weekend laments the killing of Jesus, but also celebrates His miraculous resurrection. It is dark at first, then out of this darkness comes the light of a new life. My thoughts are on the darkness of this lockdown, along with the separation and loneliness that follows this process. I cannot shake the hands of my colleagues, hug my friends and family, worship with my Quaker friends, and cannot partake in any community events. Yet there may be a light that will shine on humanity in due course. Perhaps it will be a miracle, or perhaps not, but right now things are dark. People are terrified, or at least anxious. A nation – a world – in a state of fear and anxiety. What will be born of this fear in the near and long-term future?

From a psychological perspective, fear initiates the innate action potentials of survival. If the object causing the fear is apparent and observable, then it is perceived as a threat and designated very primitively as an 'enemy'. Retaliation is the most obvious response unless the threat is perceived as extreme. In other words, unless the enemy is extremely powerful, we humans take up a position of antagonism against others who threaten us. Thus, during this health emergency, we hear world leaders using the rhetoric of war. Evoking the usual martial metaphors, Emmanuel Macron has described the COVID-19 response as 'fighting a war against an invisible enemy' (Guardian,

2020). And yet this enemy is invisible and not trying to attack us in the usual sense. So where will this tendency for retaliation go if we cannot direct it against this virus? Will it turn against others who can shoulder the blame? A good example is President Trump blaming the Chinese and the World Health Organization. From history, we recall Hitler blaming the Jews for the troubles of post-war Germany. A political scapegoat is extremely useful, and the public tends to fall for it.

However, fear is not universal; many feel only mildly anxious. If you were to see a psychologist about your anxiety, they would likely explain to you the fight-flight-freeze response mechanism. It is hypothesised that if you were faced with an immediate threat – a bear or lion, for example – your nervous system triggers one of three reactions: You would either move away (flight), attack the threat in order to survive (fight), or unconsciously feign death (freeze). Each response has an evolutionary, unconscious biological pattern of response. You are given this explanation to allow you to understand what you are experiencing, that you are not able to prevent these responses and therefore should not judge yourself. It is the secondary, self-critical processes which are often more pernicious than the initial feeling of anxiety. You can't control the spark of fear or anxiety, but you can control what you do with those emotions.

The difference between fear and anxiety, at least as psychologists see it, is that with fear the object of threat is directly apparent. In the case of anxiety, this threat is absent. When psychologists work with patients diagnosed with anxiety disorders, they spend time teaching them about threat responses, but in most cases, anxiety is often fuelled by 'nothing'. Patients will readily imagine a threat, such as the possibility of attack, picking up an infection, or simply predict that 'bad things will happen'. Anxiety-based rituals, common in Obsessive Compulsive Disorder, often serve to protect others from harm – usually family and loved ones. All of these threats are absent by definition, which is why the most common response to anxiety is avoidance. In anxiety treatment, the patient is advised to stop avoiding the threat, while noting the absence of the expected negative outcome. In these circumstances, the patient has to expose themselves more and more directly to the perceived threat. By going through this process, the patient discovers that their appraisal of the threat was inaccurate and, most importantly, that their body reacts differently to that exposure. So, the situation would be: there is no threat; and even if there is some threat it poses no harm; please expose yourself to it to discover this truth. However, the COVID-19 situation is unique in that the threat is not imaginary and the advice is to avoid it.

To some extent, the behavioural change needed by policy-makers is exactly the opposite of what is usually required to treat anxiety disorders. There is a threat; it is invisible, but exists; it is very dangerous; please use avoidance as your main tactic to help counter this threat. The message to health and other key workers is not the same because it is vital that they keep working to ensure health and other key services are maintained. Thus, they are seen as heroes, the soldiers of this 'war', out in the trenches being exposed not just to the virus but also to exhaustion, death, and infinite grief. They are on 'the front line, fighting this unseen enemy'.

What we have had so far in this crisis is a rhetoric of fear and avoidance. To be clear, I am not being critical of this discourse; it was necessary and responsible. Yet discourses of fear are limited, and they divide people. We are being forced to be literally divided and this rhetoric of fear is dividing us further. What is now crucial to consider is what a narrative of recovery will look like and how it will be constructed.

What I wish to explore is how societies and communities respond to collective traumas, and how we might respond to the trauma of COVID-19. I am particularly interested in the emergence of meaning, and whether this can serve as some sort of inoculation against the effects of this virus. Not a literal, physical protection, but the protection that establishing meaning can give to those that have suffered a trauma. Thus, I am concerned with a societal trauma and how an inclusive narrative, which constructs an emergent collective meaning, can in some way deliver us from this tragedy.

We should consider that we will likely see some enormous economic impacts, post-lockdown. Government debt levels will soar; there will be mass unemployment and a significant economic depression. Taxation is likely to rise substantially while services to the poor are curtailed. It is potentially possible that the economic impacts of the lockdown will kill more people than the virus itself. What will the rhetoric of the virus be then? Who will be the enemy and what will the retaliation be? I won't be speculating about that, but will discuss what factors may build our communities and our social body in a way that does not necessitate any kind of scapegoating of groups or nations. I am thus interested in community cohesion and how it can be fostered.

**What Happens After Collective Trauma?**

It is possible to consider the present COVID-19 emergency as a collective trauma. Whole nations, communities, and families are suffering. As we are currently still going through it, we can only speculate about what will unfold during the event and what will follow. Yet we may be able to predict this, based on collective traumas of the past. Perhaps the most obvious parallel to the current situation is the suffering of the population during a protracted war, such as the second world war.

The impact of WWII is still visibly apparent in the United Kingdom (UK). It is celebrated annually during November, now being almost mandatory to wear a red poppy badge. The national psyche is incredibly sensitive to the memory of this war, and I would go so far as to say the UK national identity was forged during those war years and what followed. Despite this, seventy-five years have passed since the war ended. Indeed, during the celebrations mid-lockdown, there were reports of social distancing restrictions being breached. During the COVID-19 emergency, we hear call for a 'blitz spirit' to emerge as a way to struggle through to victory. NHS workers are lauded as if they were soldiers because they work 'on the front line'. In the USA, WWII is remembered as the 'good war', which was clear in its moral positioning, fought by the 'best of generations' (Gallicchio, 2013). It is not altogether clear why the collective suffering of millions has led to such an idealisation of this war. No doubt victory is part of the process and the subsequent discovery of the Nazi atrocities made the moral position clear. Yet I want to highlight the community-building that the war necessitated. 'Back at home', the war was fought through collective effort which joined communities together, moved the genders towards more equalisation, and was supported by a national narrative that very few disputed.

The 9/11/2001 terrorist attack on New York is another case in point. This was a direct violent act, which promised more attacks. Thousands died and many more were injured and gripped with fear. And yet the expected flood of traumatised individuals did not emerge, or certainly not in the numbers predicted (Updegraff, Silver & Holman, 2008). Somehow, a collective narrative was forged which allowed a growth in solidarity and a relative agreement on the steps that followed. A meaning emerged that the vast majority of the populace could find purchase onto and which buttressed their recovery. This raises the question about how meaning emerges and is constructed.

**Constructing Meaning**

French phenomenologist Merleau-Ponty argued that the human subject is 'condemned to meaning' (1982. p.xix), which was his way of articulating that it is impossible for humanity to live outside significance. In this discussion, we are concerned with meaning **in** life as opposed to the meaning **of** life. There is now a vast field of psychological research (see Czekierda, et. al., 2017 for a review), and it is clear that meaning is vital for community life, human well-being, and the cultural soul of the nation (King, et. al., 2006). In simple terms, meaning is the symbolic and emotional salience that particular beliefs and behaviours hold for us. In many cases, this is derived from the local and macro-culture in which we are embedded. This macro level of meaning has been religious for thousands of years, although western subjects are now far less religious than individuals and communities in developing countries.

Neimeyer (2004, p.53-54) contends that humans must maintain a self-narrative which he defines as 'an overarching cognitive-affective-behavioural

117

structure that organizes the "micro-narratives" of everyday life into a "macro-narrative" that consolidates our self-understanding, establishes our characteristic range of emotions and goals, and guides our performance on the stage of the social world'. Fundamentally, humans need to seek meaning through shared narratives and collective behaviours (Becker, 1971). Survival in the face of adversity requires humans to constantly encounter fear, anxiety, and the possibility of death. From these challenges, individuals develop personal meaning which congeals over time into a collective narrative, which defends that society against dread and the existential givens of life.

Social symbolic significance is thus created out of a combination of historical facts combined with shared myths, beliefs, and rituals. These embodied practices are more or less taken up by individuals. It could be argued that social and political revolutions happen when individuals no longer embody the collective narratives of that culture. This can be seen in the revolutions, which happened in so many Eastern Bloc countries in the early 1990s. This is equally true regarding the failure of banks, when customers no longer believe that the bank is solvent. This results in a 'run on the bank' and the failure of the bank, no matter what the real situation was before the collective fear emerged.

Within families and small communities, micro-narratives are maintained by actual people and their behaviours. The death of these individuals challenges the coherence and validity of these meaning structures. Large-scale death is thus far more devastating than singular deaths, not just because of the pain of loss but because of the damage that is done to the very symbolic fabric of life. Death tears the fabric of meaning that sustains communal life. Recovery is then a re-weaving of these meaning threads into a coherent whole again. The heart of this restitution is a new or reconstructed narrative (Neimeyer, Burke, Schmidt & Rosner, 2010).

## Collective Trauma

It has yet to be definitively determined whether the COVID-19 emergency constitutes a trauma, and if it does, how wide that trauma will be spread. Like other mass events such as wars, some individuals are more affected than others. However, I am going to proceed as if this unique global event constitutes a widespread assault on our lives. 'Collective trauma refers to the psychological reaction to a traumatic event that affects an entire society' (Hirschberger, 2018 p.1). This reaction then seeps insidiously into the awareness of victims, and over time a realization occurs that their community either no longer exists or has been irrevocably changed (Erikson, 1976). This potentially creates a disabled collective body, unable to perform as the host of its members (Somasundaram, 2014). We can see this manifest in individuals and in communities, but perhaps it is equally in the ecology which harbours us, in the very world itself.

The ecological position would see 'traumatic events as ecological threats, not only to the adaptive capacities of individuals but also to the ability of human communities to foster health and resiliency among affected community members' (Harvey, 1996, p.5). Issues like racism, sexism, poverty, and isolation can thus be seen as environmental pollutants while community cohesion, collective values, beliefs, rituals, and traditions act as communal gifts that support resilience.

Recovery can then be enhanced by reducing isolation, fostering social competence, enhancing individual coping, and promoting belongingness (Harvey, 1996). Conversely, failure to recover can be seen as a deficit in the community environment and the collective assets therein. Leaders can mobilise assets in different ways to different effects. They can set and direct the discourse which flows through the community after traumas are suffered. For example, Abramowitz (2005, p.2117). studied two communities in Guinea which responded to the aftermath of war in different ways.

'One community created a rhetoric of resistance and revitalisation while the other adopted a position of defeat with a narrative of shame and anger.

For the latter a period of moral chaos and disorientation followed. Abramowitz notes that "opening a discursive space for talk, memory, and mourning, be it through local or western therapies", is uniquely important in facilitating the emotional recovery of a community' (p.2117).

Thus, recovery is a combination of actual help (medical, practical, social) coupled with a narrative which fosters community strength and cohesion.

This narrative thus sets up a coherent account that allows the other aspects of recovery to make sense. This 'making sense' is nothing other than the creation of meaning in the face of tragedy. Hirschberger (2018) argues that, after a collective trauma, meaning is established by:

a. Passing down culturally-derived teachings and traditions to the community or nation.
b. These teachings and traditions amplify existential concerns and embed the trauma into a symbolic system of meaning.
c. This symbolic system fosters a sense of a collective self that lasts through time promoting a sense of meaning that mitigates collective existential threat.
d. Any sense of historic collective self increases group cohesion, and group identification also enhances meaning creation.
e. A profound sense of meaning perpetuates the memory of the trauma, preventing it from being forgotten or trivialised.
f. The collective trauma becomes the epicentre of group identity and the lens through which members view their environment and society in perpetuity.

What is unclear from this process is how the meaning is generated and how much leaders, artists and thinkers can influence its creation. However, what can be observed, both at the individual and collective levels, is that trauma initiates a search for meaning. If those of us who have a voice, even if it is through writing essays like this, do not claim that opportunity, the process will happen nonetheless and a more chaotic form of narrative of failure might emerge. So, we turn to the issue of that creation.

## Constructing Meaning Against Trauma

In the aftermath of trauma, victims respond with two primary understandings of meaning that help them with crises and coping post-trauma: Meaning as comprehensibility and meaning as significance (Janoff-Bulman & McPherson, 1997). As such, any meaning constructed and communicated after this emergency must be understood by the population and likely communicated in multiple ways over an extended period. In addition, it must be important to them and to how they are imagining their future. It is important to foster a sense of hope and possibility for individuals, families, and their communities. For a trauma to be transformed into a meaningful narrative that transforms death and suffering into something coherent and life-affirming, many elements are needed. The first of these elements is that the story needs to be acceptable. Might it be possible that what protects against community-level collective trauma is the construction of meaning that the whole community accepts?

In addition, this meaning needs to penetrate to a level of self-confirming significance. As Hirschberger (2018 p.2) argues, the 'creation and maintenance of meaning comprises a sense of self-continuity, a connection between the self, others, and the environment, and the feeling that one's existence matters'. It is easy to understand how some survivors will see their existence as mattering little. Those in marginalised groups will be especially sensitive if their group has been significantly affected. I am thinking of the elderly and those in ethnic minority groups.

Further, the meaning needs to be able to work at an individual, community, and national level. In 'recovery, the survivor assigns new meaning to the trauma, to the self as trauma survivor, and to the world in which traumatic events occur and recur' (Harvey, 1996 p.13). This way, the world itself is healed, not just the survivors. It strikes me that the world is in some dire need of healing right now.

Also, this emerging narrative must address the suffering and loss that the population has endured. It must be honest and open about the mistakes made and the protections needed in the future. More than anything, it should not downplay what has happened, whether this is outright denial or the more subtle playing-down of the impact's extent. It perhaps does not require a Truth & Reconciliation Commission, so successful in post-apartheid South Africa, but there should be some form of open forum in which the pain and loss can be aired. Experts should also be given the space to articulate the extent of the impact, both on individuals and on communities. The truth deserves to be spoken.

Yet not all suffering is exclusively negative. Strength itself is built through suffering (Janoff-Bulman, 2004), and there is now considerable research documenting the 'growth' that often follows traumas (Schubert, Schmidt & Rosner, 2016). Survivors often discuss a renewed spiritual faith that comes in the wake of adversity. Indeed, spirituality and religiosity were found, in different ways, to be protective factors amongst survivors of 9/11 (McIntosh, Poulin, Silver & Holman, 2011). The assumption that struggling with major difficulties in life can lead to positive changes and sometimes radical transformations is part of ancient myth, literature, and religion. Influential clinicians and scholars of the twentieth century also pointed this out. Victor Frankl (1959) developed an entire system of psychotherapy based on meaning creation, which originated in his experiences of Nazi concentration camps.

This terrible event has prepared us for future pandemics and the suffering can be viewed as having been worth it, if it protects the public in the future. This message could reimagine the losses sustained as a form of sacrifice, which can be taken up in a transcendent manner. I would suggest this element, which might place the losses in the realm of the mythic, is also connected to the issue of collective values. Each nation, community, and family explicitly live out its values via its decisions, behaviours, and discourse. If the meaning generated by the recovery from trauma could harmonise with these values, the more likely that this would allow a wholesale adoption of this narrative. I should point out that this sort of moment is not one for inventing values that are not inherent in the lived ecology of the place being considered. These must be existing and deeply held values.

A final element needs to be the establishment of a new sense of community cohesion built out of a new identity. People have died to give a future to those who remain. That gifts us, whether we desire it or not, a new sense of self. If the trauma has ripped at the fabric of our lives, then meaning can serve as the weave of essential connection, recreated at a special sacrificial moment. The essence of meaning is that it connects us to ourselves, to our community, and to our world.

In summary the following elements are needed to weave the new fabric of our society:

- A narrative that make sense, has significance, and is acceptable.
- It should connect to the future, giving hope as its message.
- This message should be coherent with the values of the population.
- It should foster self-continuity and the place of this self in the world.
- The details should be transparent and honest about the losses and sufferings caused.
- It should allow for this tragedy to be connected to learning and fortitude.
- Leaders should convey a message which leads to group cohesion and builds connection.
- What is developed should tie together or weave on top an existing collective sense of identity.
- A practical response, in terms of aid given, should embody and be true to this narrative.
- Blaming and scapegoating should be avoided.

The final point may be the most difficult. Most collective traumas involve an aggressor or perpetrator, but in this emergency, that 'enemy' is an unseen virus. That has not stopped individuals and governments from filling that void with conspiracy theories and outright lies. This hearkens back to something I described earlier: that it is a natural response to fear, anxiety, and suffering to attribute this to an aggressor. This evolutionary mechanism serves the advantage of protecting the individual and the community against future attack and losses. How to account for scores of dead people? It cannot just be the result of nature or government failures. There must be a secret process at play – be it the 5G rollout or a plot by the Chinese government. It is the responsibility of leaders and anyone with a public voice to counter these divisive claims and attempt to instead foster a spirit of togetherness and solidarity.

The final issue that needs consideration is the question of who creates and spreads such a meaning. My first answer is that it is the role of leaders. However, this is a complex argument because, in most modern societies, leadership is diverse and dispersed. In times gone by, the national leader and the state religion would be able to communicate and dominate the message. Newspapers would relay such a narrative and it would be powerful. Today, however, there is a crisis of legitimacy around both political and religious leaders, especially in the UK. Therefore, I would argue that these individuals must play their part, but so too must business leaders, media owners, those who have large followers on Twitter and Instagram (and other social media platforms), and also intellectual leaders.

Just like the creation of meaning is a weave of many colours, the speaking out in the face of tragedy is more likely to be a choir of many voices. The extent to which those many voices harmonize will determine how this deeply resonant voice is heard and how it is incorporated into the psychic life of the nation, neighbourhood, family, and individual. We have started this crisis with a message of fear, now we need a story of hope and resilience. On the other hand, in a world of social media, we are all given a voice to share our opinions and views. To hand this task solely to leaders is perhaps too easy and too limited. We can all play our part and should help this reconstruction out of tragedy. We all have a role and responsibility in creating this new narrative.

# The Experience of Fear in Society and How it is Interpreted

*Brian Sheppard & Nolene Sheppard*

"The ultimate core of any community does not lie in the right pure and beautiful notes, but rather in its left and dark centre"
(Bataille, 2001)

You wake up one morning to a world that is a different place in which to live: It is a new world completely distorted from the one you remember. Where are the beautiful notes? The changes occurred in front of your eyes. We all question ourselves: 'Is this the reality of the worst nightmare in our century?' 'What do I do?' 'Who can I turn to?' 'Will I lose everything – my mind, my body, my heart, and my soul?' You realise you are not alone in this paradox. Fear is rapidly taking over, and you question the reality of your life and living. Subjectivity and objectivity blur in a world that once seemed beautifully normal, but is now a dark and chaotic place.

In the present pandemic, lessons about fear need to be heeded from the psycho-social aspects of previous pandemics and from both the perspectives of psychology and sociology. We will consider the psychology of fear, whilst sociologically we reflect upon the impact of globalisation, and the influence of social media will be evaluated as possible contributors of fear in the 21st Century.

The knowledge that unresolved fear can impact ones' ability to cope often stops people functioning fully. We need to learn lessons in how to adapt and how to cope. We can learn lessons from a group that has achieved this well, those approaching the end of life or near-death experiences. We can further relate this to the management of the fears raised by the present pandemic of COVID–19.

## Psycho-Social Lessons from Previous Pandemics

The Ebola Pandemic (Coltart, Lindsay, Ghinal, Johnson & Heyman, 2017) had successive waves that increased the levels of fear. 'Fearonomic is the direct or indirect effect on the economy due to misinformation' (Shultz et al., 2016, Bali, Stewart & Pate, 2016). In Sierra Leonne, the fearonomic effect had a substantial impact on the economy and the utilisation of healthcare provisions. This can also be seen in the present pandemic, as people are in lockdown, many shops being closed, and government paying 80% of people wages. Furthermore, healthcare provision throughout the country has been reorganised and expanded so that there are more intensive care beds, including the emergency Nightingale Hospitals.

During the Ebola outbreak, the impact of fearonomics caused people to self-medicate by consuming large amounts of salt water and defying quarantine to obtain holy water from Lagos (Bali, Stewart & Pate, 2016). It can be argued that the government closing places of worship addresses some of these issues. The question is, what will happen when some of the lockdown regulations are lifted and these places are opened? Will we be tempted to breach even the social distancing regulations of keeping two meters apart? And if this happens too quickly, what will the impact be on getting a second or subsequent wave of coronavirus? Will we be the same as when the Ebola Virus came in waves? And how will this then impact future levels of fear?

O'Leary, Jalloh and Neria (2018) confirmed that Ebola sufferers had two main areas of fear: that of contracting the disease and the fear of being stigmatised for having or having had it. They confirmed that 95% of Ebola victims had felt discriminated against by someone else. The idea of stigmatising groups was highlighted by research by McCaulty, Ministry, and Viswanath (2013) into the H1N1 panic in Mexico, April 2009. They discovered that post-pandemic out-groups were identified in Mexican Indians and those from a Latino background. They defined these out-groups as marginalised factions forming part of the minority. Such stigmatisation tends to increase the level of social marginality already experienced by this group and their sense of belonging to the society is reduced. Furthermore, being stigmatised and discriminated against significantly impacts the individual's level of self-confidence (Karafilakis, et al., 2015; O'Leary, Jalloh & Neria, 2018) and this, in turn, impacts the individual's responses as effective members of society.

## The Psychology of Fear

Blanchard and Blanchard (2008) assert that the psychology of fear is concern with our thoughts and behaviours. It is our automatic response to a perception or feeling based on exposure to visual or oral stimuli.

Perceived and actual threats to life or an aspect of life can result in fear (Struyf, Zaman, Harmans & Vervliet, 2017). These threats start from a sensory input – such as seeing, hearing, smelling, tasting, or feeling things – that then triggers memory. These past experiences are stored in the centre of our brain, which prepares us for future threats. Elliot and Richardson (2018) maintain that early life experiences shape the way we respond to any kind of external threat. Walters, Carew, and Kandle (1981) argue further that fear results in emotional and behavioural responses which are designed to protect us or prepare us for danger. Thus, fear will result in us preparing to 'fight' and conquer the danger or to 'flight' and avoid the danger.

The behavioural response to fear has to do with the actual expression of emotion. The majority of our response to stimuli or human reaction is due to sociocultural norms. For example, a smile signifies happiness and a frown signifies sadness. Most of these socio-cultural responses are universal. So, in the face of fear, it's normal for us to freeze, run away, or to avoid it altogether.

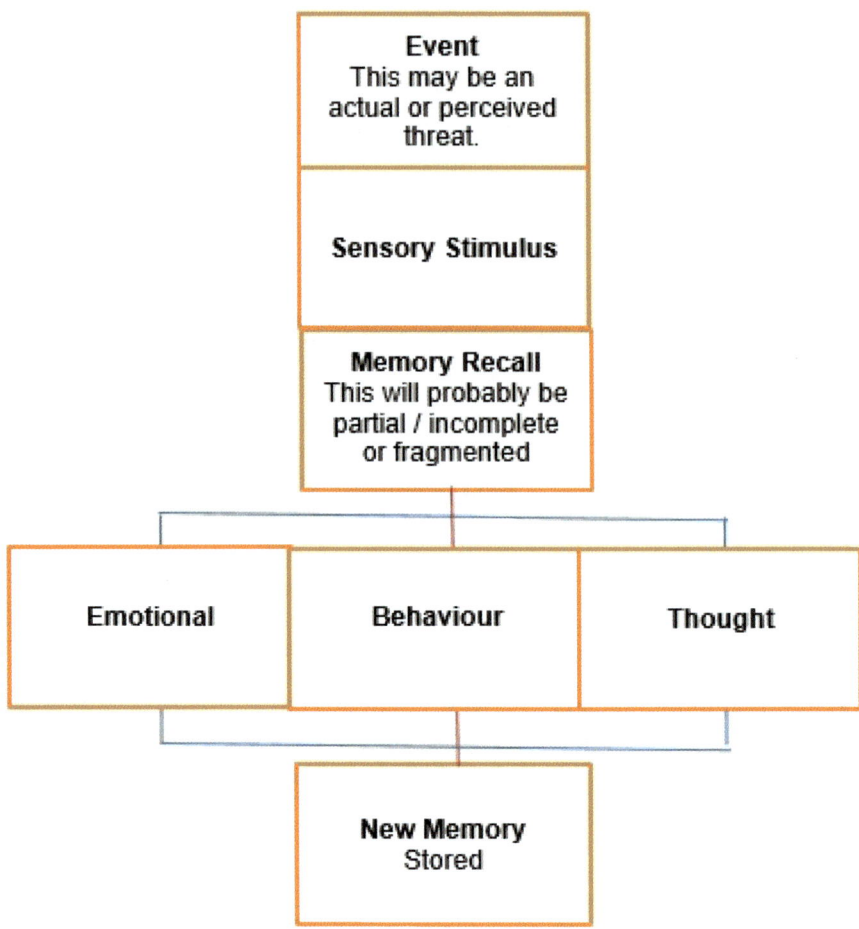

**Figure 1.0**

Our brain stores interconnected networks which consist of some long-term memories (Asok, Kandal & Rayman, 2019). In Figure 1.0, this is where memory recall happens. These networks are then connected with certain responses that are encoded with certain events. Every time these networks are stimulated by the media, the codes associated with certain negative responses are enforced and reactivated, thereby strengthening the plurality of these responses and leading to a reinforcement of negative memories. The distorted reality created this way by the media and politics is one with strong intentions, causing conflict among societal groups and individuals alike (Asok,

Kandal & Rayman, 2019). The media tends to enhance fear and excitement in people by distorting the truth (Klaidman & Beauchamp, 1987).

Our internal psychological states will influence our reaction to fear (Elliot & Richardson, 2018). Examples can be seen in the table, including: reactions to childhood environment and early life stressor factors, our present emotional state, memory of similar experiences, gender differences, level of resilience, social support, and our own belief systems. Thus, fear in the psychological life of the individual has many factors, which makes it complicated to understand.

On a micro level, the perception of fear and stigma associated with having an illness, especially a contagious illness like coronavirus, perpetuates fear in society and causes people to respond in a certain way. The question remains, 'how does the perception of fear effect our response to fear, and does this perception distort the reality?'

Perception refers to how we interpret the world. Research done in the past investigated whether people's perception of fear or the over-generalisation of fear increase the fear response and intensifies the amount of fear attributed to the initial response.

In some groups – such as those who suffer from anxiety, phobia, and those with post-traumatic stress disorder – the perception of new danger on top of their normal sense of danger can heighten their overall levels of fear.

For example, it was demonstrated that individuals suffering post-traumatic stress disorder tend to experience an inflation in fear response when exposed to any stimulus that have overlapping traits to one's experience (Kinchin, 2005).

For example, Shawn is an ex-soldier, diagnosed with post-traumatic stress disorder. Since then, whenever Shawn leaves home, he experiences panic attacks, shortness of breath, stomach aches, and palpitations whenever he is exposed to intense noises. This has an adverse effect on his mental and physical health. Shawn suffers depression and tends to isolate himself. This brings about additional problems which affect his ability to get a job and be more independent. Shawn now relies solely on the benefit system, as well as health and social care.

## The Sociology of Fear

Globalisation is 'an intensification of worldwide social relations, which link distant localities in such way that local happenings are shaped by events happening many miles away and vice versa' (Giddens, 1990). Here, the pandemic can be seen as a globalised concept, with researchers across the world spending time and energy finding a reliable test for the condition, as well as a vaccine. In fact, the virus is so impactful that normal standards for research are being compressed to try and find this vaccine faster, and once it is discovered there will be the issue of producing enough of this to reach the world.

Sumiala & Tikka (2011) investigated the impact that circulation has on specific social and cultural environments. They were interested in finding out how social media and circulation transform the landscape of peoples' mindset and behaviour within this global village. In this context, circulation is the rapid rate at which information is shared on social media (Lee and LiPuma, 2002). The circulation of four school shootings were tracked, including: Columbine in 1999, Jokela in 2007, Virginia Tech in 2007 and Kanhajoki in 2008 (Chyi and McCombs, 2004; Newman, Cybelle, David, Mehta and Roth, 2004; Muschert and Carr, 2006; Muschert, 2007a, 2007b; Kellner 2008; Raittila, Koljonen and V'aliverronen, 2010; Sumiala and Tikka, 2011).

The intertwining and overlapping of the content that was being shown made it exceedingly difficult to decipher the truth. For example, the killers first shared content on YouTube, before being further circulated by amateurs who might have used the same material before adding their own take on the events. After the shooting took place, professional videos were aired by broadcasters, which in some ways perpetuated what had been previously shown (Lee and LiPuma, 2002). The constant copying, sharing, repeating, and circulation on social media platforms has an impact on our social reality by increasing and impacting perceptions of fear (Bataille, 2001). Klaidman and Beauchamp

(1987) maintain that the media is responsible for creating and contributing to fear and panic within society. All of this can be seen in the spread of COVID-19 information and misinformation via the media, including social media.

From a political perspective, the anticipation of fear tends to have an impact on one's political beliefs and the support one has for specific government policies. It can be noted that the fear of being infected has been increasing in the global pandemic that mankind faces in 2020. This is increased by over-conceptualised ideas based on little knowledge or fake news, thus causing a lack of trust alongside increased greed, selfishness, and – most of all – fear.

## Social Media and Fear

The sharp increase in the use of smartphones, laptops, tablets, and other handheld devices have made social media more accessible, which inadvertently has an impact on how we interpret the rest of the world. Some of us are suffering from the 'Fear of Missing Out' (FOMO) (Przybylski, Murayama, De Haan & Gladwer, 2013). Some scholars account for this as the 'pervasive apprehension that others might be having a rewarding experience for which one is absent, and is characterised by the desire to stay continually connected with what others are doing'. JWT Intelligence (2012) say FOMO is characterised by a persistent fear or anxiety of missing out. This concept can be broken down to what other people are doing that you are involved in or what other people know that you do not know.

Conick (2017) suggests that most people are becoming addicted to the use of smartphones and devices through social media. A survey conducted in America by Perrin (2017) revealed that 96% of 18 to 29-year-olds live in households with at least one smartphone, whilst 51% contain three or more smart phones. With Facebook being the most visited site, regular users of social media can easily become addicted to the internet. This is often because users tend to log on to manage loneliness and isolation. On a positive note, people in the lockdown are visiting one another and participating on a broad range of online Zoom parties. In this context, the use of social media is a positive thing.

Carleton (2016) posits that the 'fear of the unknown' is most impactful, which is possibly the ultimate fundamental fear. He demonstrated that those with a perceived absence of information at any level of consciousness had higher levels of fear. Again, it can be argued that the government's daily briefings on COVID-19 and coronavirus are trying to address some of these issues, although many complain about too much information that is presented in a confusing way.

For example: John is an apprentice carpenter who is temporarily out of work. John does not have a lot of knowledge about the existing virus and tends to rely on social media. He has a habit of believing everything he hears or sees on social media. These constant visual and oral stimuli tend to leave John with a feeling of restlessness, irritability, and anxiety. The amount of fear John might experience is now elevated further, putting John at risk of developing anxiety of some kind.

**Learning to Manage Fear**

There is clearly a need for the individual to learn how to manage their levels of fear. Penman & Ellis (2015) explored strategies for encouraging people to cope with fear when experiencing life-limiting conditions. Hammen (2016) examined emotional responses related to early childhood experience, chronic stresses, and how to turn these into maladaptive and adaptive coping strategies.

Maladaptive coping skills refers to participating in negative practices to reduce stress, such as getting drunk or using drugs (Hammen, 2016). It is known that during the lockdown there have been increases in domestic violence, which have been associated with the abuse of alcohol; both are maladaptive coping skills, the latter also increasing fear in their victims.

Moss (1993) defines adaptive coping skills as various strategies that one can utilise in the face of adversity. In other words, various strategies one might use to reduce stress. Penman & Ellis (2015) identified four main factors that people use to manage their fears:

1) Drawing on resilience
2) Maintaining relationships
3) Gaining the ability to keep one step ahead
4) Engaging in spirituality

During our lifetime, it is almost inevitable that everyone will face a traumatic event (Joseph, 2012), so the individual needs to learn about resilience. Macedo (2014) states that 'resilience is an individual's ability to maintain or regain his/her mental health in the face of significant adversity or risk of death'. Drawing on resilience and inner resources has to do with focussing on one's past coping accomplishments and focussing on one's strength (Penman & Ellis, 2015). They gave an example of a palliative care patient who struggled with cancer in the past. The patient was able to draw on his past experiences and reflect on past positive outcomes with cancer. In COVID-19, the individual can draw on the knowledge that most people who become ill are recovering. They can further draw on feelings and thoughts where they have survived a stressful situation in the past and they can heed public health advice, such as maintaining social distancing or wearing personal protective equipment.

Penman & Ellis (2015) stipulated that a lot of patients experience comfort by having friends and family around. One patient reported that he always had a better night's sleep after church members visited and prayed for him. Having friends and family around also increased hope and acted as a temporary distraction from reality. It also helped lift the mood and promote mental health and well-being. Managing health relationships or positive relationships is seen as being one of the main factors in building well-being (Seligman, 2011), as these relationships allow us to share our fears and concerns in order to recognise and resolve said fears. In the lockdown, individuals are spending less time with their work colleagues, family, and friends, except those that they live with. However, the use of technology means that we can still meet with friends and family, we can write emails and, of course, the traditional old-fashioned letter. In all of this, it is possible to maintain those positive relationships which help us grow.

Gaining the ability to stay one step ahead, Penman & Ellis (2015) continued by stressing how important it is for clients to be given ample information in a timely fashion. This allows clients to have a substantial amount of time to make an informed decision. This also empowers the client to take control of the situation, gaining the ability to 'keep one step ahead'. The New Economics Foundation (2006), in their *Five Ways to Wellbeing*, highlighted 'keep learning' as a way forward towards mental health. In this crisis, it could be argued that the government is giving people instructions of what they need to do in order to stay informed. However, some examples from officials could be interpreted as breaching the best advice, thus resigning their role. Broadly following the main advice from the government seems to be working, as the number of deaths appear to be steadily dropping. The major concern is if there will be a second wave after lockdown is lifted. Previous pandemics warn that this is likely to happen.

Engaging in spirituality and religious activities, Eckersley (2007) believes that there must be a greater spiritual dimension in life today, for mankind to rise above the fearful times we live in. Seligman (2011) believes that this spirituality should be learning to work towards the greater good of society. So, when people are volunteering to shop for the elderly neighbourhoods in this COVID–19 crisis they are working towards this greater good.

**What Have We Learnt?**

During the COVID-19 crisis, we can learn lessons from previous pandemics and crises. The psychology and sociology of fear also has a lot to offer. The psychology of fear includes emotional, thinking, and behavioural responses. We further draw on our memories, which can increase or reduce the impact of the present crisis. In the sociology of fear, we considered the impact of globalisation, circulation, social media, and politics – aware that they each have the possibility of raising fear, but knowing that these very factors can help resolve some of the issues.

Finally, we drew on lessons learnt from people facing life-limiting crises, some of whom learnt maladaptive ways of coping and others who developed adaptive coping skills. The maladaptive methods were noted as being destructive, whilst the adaptive ways helped the person to grow; individuals can learn these lessons to help them deal with the impact of fear during the crisis. These lessons included learning about resilience and using the past experiences to face future trials. Ensuring that they have relevant information to make informed choices should reduce their levels of fear. Maintaining and developing positive relationships during lockdown will need effort and the use of technology to try and promote communication. The development of spirituality is also seen as useful, which is working towards the greater good.

# Humanity in Crisis-Fear Perspective Amongst BAME Groups

*Ntsoaki Mary Mosoeunyane*

"A solitary dream can transform a million realities -The desire to reach for the stars is ambitious, but the desire to reach hearts is wise"
(Maya Angelo cited Dillon, 2014)

Fear and anxiety are shared human emotions triggered by various unpleasant experiences. The Cambridge English Dictionary describes fear as an emotion induced by perceived threat or danger while anxiety is described as an emotion characterised by feelings of uncertainty and tension. Some liken the fear and anxiety to a 'tsunami' (Campbell & Mason, 2020). The biopsychological impact on individuals includes a change in blood pressure, sweating, dizziness, and an array of physiological imbalances with negative consequences to well-being. These emotions are common denominator with no regard to status, ethnicity, race, or culture. In crisis and heightened anxiety, people typically pull together and hold the humanity bonds that provide courage and resilience to navigate coping. As COVID-19 news develops and people seek understanding, anxieties can provoke either negative or positive stances to cope.

Unfortunately, while we were still in the moment of sharing human crisis with humility and kindness, the pandemic provoked some distressingly disproportionate statistics in mortality rates within Black and Ethnic Minority (BAME) communities (Public Health England, 2020). Media coverage and other resources also reported that BAME Health Care Professionals (HCP) have high death rates compared to their white counterparts. Incidents of racism and xenophobia towards BAME communities have also circulated through media, particularly increasing blame culture towards people of Chinese origin. This implies that fear during the crisis has many layers, and experiences portray certain behaviours. Siddique (2020) reported in the Guardian, highlighting actions taken by the major of London, Sadiq Khan, who has joined hundreds of signatories in a letter to the prime minister (PM) calling for comprehensive investigations into race and health inequalities. Omar Khan (2020), also reporting at the Guardian, further stated how the pandemic is bringing the harsh realities of racism and health disparities into a sharp focus, putting race at the top in a list of social determinants of health. Many may jump to conclusions due past experiences, putting race in the forefront.

> 'The patterns we're seeing – a disproportionately high number of BAME deaths from coronavirus – are not random, but instead track existing social determinants of health. … In other words, their employment and housing circumstances mean they are more likely to be in contact with more people and so are more at risk of getting COVID-19' (Omar Khan, 2020).

However, there needs to be a careful, well thought-out investigation before any credible conclusions are drawn. Existing empirical evidence relating to some of the factors contributing to high risk in BAME groups will be significantly considered. It is equally important not to underplay how individual, systemic, and structural racism has shaped people's lives through history.

This chapter seeks to explore the narrative of fear and anxiety from a BAME Health Care Professional (HCP) and Health Educators, from an educational standpoint as well as hands-on in the front line of COVID, to establish how their role was played out and what educators need to do to reshape the narrative. It will put into perspective how the news about COVID unfolded, address known empirical findings on risk factors amongst BAME people and their disposition to COVID, and further borrow existing data and anecdotal conversations to address ways in which racism is seen as a "determinant of health" and reflection of social inequality. The author will build from her own writings described in her book, My Life in England (Mosoeunyane, 2015), and build on the research she conducted into the impact of racism on the well-being of BAME professionals. It is important that we prepare for the aftermath of COVID, as people could be faced with post-traumatic stress disorder (PTSD), flashbacks, nightmares, increasing anxiety, etc. What could the harsh realities of COVID-19 mean for the well-being of minorities now and in the future?

**The Current Narrative: COVID-19 News**

Before we jump to conclusions, it is imperative to understand what research highlights about the underlying factors that put BAME HCP at a higher risk of COVID-19 when compared to their white counterparts. Factors such as the social and economic inequalities (finances, employment, neighbourhoods, housing, education, precocity) will be put into perspective, while further exploring how to think differently about other possible explanations.

When the news broke, reports from the World Health Organization (WHO) (2020) concerned a new strain of coronavirus (COVID-19) that began in Wuhan, China in November of 2019. People were dying due to respiratory failure from pneumonia-like symptoms, only more severe due to the impact on the lungs. The report stated that lungs get plugged by excess mucus due to inflammation occluding air entry and gas exchange, with consequent organ failure and death. The world was awakening to yet another human crisis that would cost lives. Reports point to the downplaying of the disease to reduce panic among the public. Unfortunately, this led to some delays in response for preventative measures and treatments.

The first positive cases in the UK were announced on 31st January, which was business as usual at that point. By the 2nd March, the first known deaths were reported by NHS England (2020) and Public Health England (2020). At this time fear and anxieties coupled with uncertainties, creating horror over what could possibly be the worst nightmare in our lifetimes. Yet speculations about the nature of the virus being an epidemic or pandemic continued well over two months. When the disease began to spread globally, it was finally declared a pandemic on 11th March 2020 (WHO, 2020).

While everyone will experience some fear and form of anxiety during a pandemic crisis, past empirical evidence points to heightened anxieties for those who are unable to tolerate uncertainty, as a study involving the Influenza H1N1 pandemic in 2009 revealed (Wheaton et. al., 2011). Depending on the causes of triggers for these emotions, navigating the challenges will differ from person to person, and varies according to multicultural perspectives.

Several factors can influence how people respond to the threat: age, mental health challenges, comorbidities, and many more. When the news about COVID-19 transpired, the whole world understood that this virus was one that did not discriminate according to social class, ethnicity, race, or geographic factors (except for the identified physiological variables above). There was also some relief that humanity has no colour, class, status, etc. Unfortunately, our response to the virus told a different story. Survival was the only thing that mattered as we all watched in fear. In fact, as we watched, people in high celebrities, prime ministers (John Major), and even those within the Royal Family (Prince Charles) came down with the virus.

There was a lot of misinformation as 'panic psychology' transpired through social media across the globe, with consequent increased anxieties. Hoaxes travel faster than the speed of light, and people buy into these conspiracy theories with further psychological injury. A lot of myths developed around the novel coronavirus, with speculations that poor economies like India and Africa seem to be relatively spared. Myths regarding the demographics were spreading, with some claiming Black people had immunocompetency to the virus. To date, in accordance with available statistics across the globe (Table.1), most of the poor economies have the lowest number of cases and deaths, with a few reporting zero cases by the third week of April 2020. Death rates for those confirmed with COVID-19 in Africa are still low, and some countries in Africa and the Caribbean report no deaths and high recovery rates. For instance, Rwanda reported 273 cases; 163 recovered and zero died, while Lesotho had zero cases by 8th May, 2020 (WHO, 2020). Sadly, these figures are increasing (see Table 1).

| Table 1: Worldwide Data | | | | | |
|---|---|---|---|---|---|
| **Region** | **3rd Week of April** | **31/12/2019 - 27/5/2020** | | **Population number (% of world population)** | **Density per Square km** |
| | **Number of cases** | **Number of cases** | **Deaths** | | |
| **Europe** | 1,654,345 | 1,862,304 | 169 385 | 741.4m (9.6%) | 128 |
| **Americas** | 1,586,129 | 2,571,974 | 149,023 | 1.002b (13.1%) | North 20 South 32 |
| ***Eastern Mediterranean** | 237,323 | | | 502.8 m (Approx. 6.1%) | - |
| **Western Pacific** | 157,447 | Asia 992,377 | Asia 28 077 | 1.7 b (Approx. 21.8%) | Up to 150 |
| **South-East Asia** | 86,294 | Oceania 8,611 (1,000,988) | Oceania 130 (28,207) | 655m (8.5%) | Although Oceana 5 |
| **Africa** | 37,717 | 119,775 | 3,590 | 1.216b (17.2%) | 45 |
| **Globally** | 3,759,967 (Deaths 259,474) | 5,555,737 | 350,212 | | |
| ***Eastern Mediterranean** is part Europe, part Asia and part Africa. | World Health Organisation (2020) | European Centre for Disease Prevention (2020) | | | World Bank (2020) |

There was growing talk via social media that Africa was spared from the calamity, despite having no credible or valid sources to support such claims at the time. There was a relief that, if Africa and other poor economies are spared, it prevents more serious consequences of the viral impact, as the health systems would not sustain the people. Religious beliefs, spiritualism, and many other beliefs became the basis for such speculations. As the humanity of the story unfolded, everyone was able to share anxieties. A lot of people from Africa and the diaspora began to believe that, for whatever reason, God had spared Africa, and that in Europe there had not been any known reports of people from the BAME who had died from the virus. I recall some of my white friends asking me to confirm whether or not black people were immune. Of course, at this time these were speculations born of observations, and not with scientific evidence or statistical reports. From the WHO (2020) statistics above, Africa still shows low cases, with latest death reports rating exceptionally low and easily outnumbered by recoveries.

It was not too long before alarm bells were raised and scientists, politicians, and critics began to look closer at the demographics of COVID-19. The world watched as the pandemic cases in the US escalated far beyond Spain and Italy. Black communities were hit harder despite making the least of the total population, which created a lot of scrutiny to the President and his office. It became clear that deaths according to race and ethnicity showed disproportionate figures, as the mortality rates became higher within those of Black and Ethnic Minority (BAME) groups (Kendi, 2020). The same picture within the United Kingdom was being mirrored. BAME people in the UK make up 3% of the population, and yet 6% have died from COVID-19 (Public Health England, 2020). 'Recent statistics suggesting that a third of critically ill with coronavirus were from ethnic minorities have highlighted the greater risk' (Omar Khan, 2020). The Royal College of Psychiatrists (2020) also highlights high mortality within BAME health care workers, settling around two-thirds despite only making 20% of the overall workforce. Various speculations and theories emerged, seeking to explain these disparities.

While BAME people were dying at an alarming rate in the western world, cases in Africa, India, and other poor economies remained extremely low. Some reported no deaths four months into the pandemic, e.g. Lesotho. Several factors could have contributed to the low cases, such as resources, under reporting, etc. It is apparent that they kept up to the rest of the world in lockdown measures. It is surprising that the media has not paid much attention to the positive aspects of low cases, nor show any interest in investigating why regions like Africa and India are not seeing an escalation of infections and deaths. Is there anything different for people of Black and Asian origin living in the west? It will be interesting to explore what we can learn from such statistics. Could racism be a major factor in how COVID-19 has impacted lives?

Historic empirical evidence on how race plays at health inequalities is well documented. The current situation is one that is rapidly evolving, and it is too early to provide full picture due to a lack of complete data. A lot of work is being done, which is providing some guidance through BAME forums (Royal College of Psychiatrists, 2020).

Increasing anxiety and mixed emotions have led to criticism of the government for underplaying the pandemic. Stories of risk factors for BAME began to populate every news outlet, increasing pressure on the government. That led to a government initiative to explore the variables underpinning mortality rates from COVID-19 amongst BAME groups as an urgent matter. The pandemic has brought out the greatest darkness, but it is out of darkness that hope is born (Snyder, 2002). Many people came together in various forums for conversations, education, and research; an indication that people felt the need to influence change, which itself provides a chance for positive growth and fosters hope for collective voices to build a better NHS. Crisis can be devastating and turned our world upside down, but some good can come out of it. We can already draw attention to the outpouring of kindness to HCP, help offered to neighbours, or supermarkets giving NHS workers priority shopping. Society has been seen clapping hands every Thursday at 20:00 to show gratitude to the HCP heroes who spend their day saving lives.

Looking closer, society bore witness to how the NHS heroes were portrayed by various media and social outlets as 'white' through the imagery presented. Yvonne Coghill (Stephenson, 2020), the Director of the Workforce Race Equality Standard (WRES) and the president of Royal College of Nursing, highlighted how there has been no recognition for BAME HCP, despite putting their lives at risk to save others (Stephenson, 2020). She further reiterated that racial discrimination is manifesting at a time of global crisis and how the NHS heroes are 'whitewashed'. A number of conclusions or speculations can be linked to chance; perhaps reporters took pictures of available staff at the time, or there was blind bias on choosing staff. Nonetheless, the BAME HCP have felt left out of the positive presentation of being heroes.

When a need was felt to deal with the growing COVID-19 crisis, a new hospital was suggested, named after Florence Nightingale. This created questions on the value placed on BAME Nurses such as Mary Seacole, who equally contributed to NHS in her pioneer work, and how this would be a high time to acknowledge such work.

## What We Know About BAME Risk Factors

Persistent with existing empirical evidence, various health challenges such as diabetes, high blood pressure, and kidney failure are prevalent in BAME groups, with South Asians rating highest (National Institute for Health and Care Excellence, 2019). These comorbidities may explain some of the statistics available on COVID-19 mortality rates. While it is too early to make conclusions, this links physiological challenges to COVID-19 risks. The evidence indicates that disparities in health and social care mostly relate to social constructs embedded in systems of complex ,discriminatory practices, and that these disparities land this group in the risk brackets. BAME HCP comprise a huge number of the NHS workforce, most of whom work on the front line, and are underrepresented within the executive level of the NHS structure (Kline, 2015). This further highlights that these groups often hold positions that disable challenging and unacceptable practices. Various arguments about culture, lifestyle, health behaviour, and religion playing a role in quick transmissions of COVID-19 have yet to be validated through research. For instance, Asian families tend to live together as family groups, something that is a strength in survival but may impact negatively in infectious pandemics. A few GPs have also reported how some BAME patients do not visit the medical centres due to fear of being treated unfairly, mentioning factors such as language barriers, cultural practices, and more.

Historically, racism has manifested in many situations and challenged BAME people with inequalities in health, education, housing, and employment, to name a few.

Professor Andrews (2016) highlighted how, fifty years after the UK Race Relations Act (1965), Blackness in Britain is framed through the lens of racialized deficits, constructed as both marginal and pathological. This fits into the typical negative stereotype of a black person. Liang, Nathwani, Ahmad, & Prince (2007) report that in many studies, a feeling of representation enhances collaborative relationships, eliminates feelings of isolation, and creates positive outcomes. This should afford health educators, health scientists, health care professionals, and policy-makers to come together to challenge and reshape the NHS as an inclusive leadership organisation.

Moss (2019) highlights inclusive leadership as something assuring all team members feel they are given a sense of belonging, value, respect, and fair treatment. Feelings of inclusion not only enhance well-being but also increases loyalty and productivity (Salvatore and Shelton, 2007). It is worth mentioning that the COVID-19 crisis has caused a surge of collaborative work within BAME groups, with many forums for discussions being set across many NHS and partner universities like never before. A promising collective with a shared sense of influencing social change. There is a sense of urgency to seek solutions to support BAME groups in organisations and communities. Out of darkness, a new light can be the source of hope. Positive Psychology (PP) research has demonstrated that there is a possibility of potential growth, even in challenges (Ivtzan, Lomas, Hefferon & Worth, 2015).

## Lessons from the Past

The NHS has faced scrutiny over discrimination for many years. In West, Dawson & Kaur (2015), The King's Fund was commissioned by the NHS to assess the scale of this problem. While the organisation has seen initiatives combating or reducing discriminatory practices, it is sad that a lot of the initiatives have faced obstacles in implementation due to several factors. Among these many factors, it is apparent that unless we bring our unconscious to the conscious, changes in law/policies become a 'tick-box'.

The Equality Act (2010) is often referred to in disputes where an organisation accused of discrimination claims it abides by the regulation. Denial at the existence of racism by most of the white people, including NHS staff, and resigned acceptance from BAME staff only perpetuate racial bias (Liang, et al., 2010). Many studies point out that a collective consciousness of society is key in creating racism awareness, as many people minimise its existence, especially white people that turn a blind eye to its existence (Mancini *et al.*, 2015). Some evidence also points out that you do not have to be white to perpetuate systemic racism, as such practices are wired into our psyche.

**Figure 1: Percentage of NHS Staff Experiencing Discrimination at Work, by Ethnicity and Area. Location: England. Time period: 2018 (NHS England, 2019)**

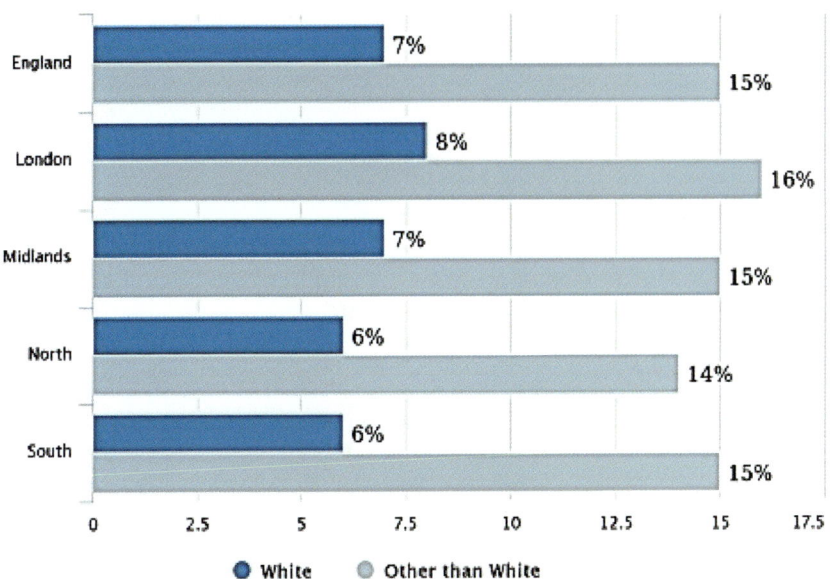

This report on racial discrimination was produced a couple of years after The Kings Fund "Making the Difference-Diversity and Inclusion" report in 2014 by West, Dawson and Kaur (2015), and recommendations were put in place. While this summary reported on discrimination in different variables, racial/ethnic discrimination was the highest on BAME groups. The discriminatory practices were from patients, relatives, the public, and staff members. Amongst others, the recommendations included to enhance individual teams as well as the organisation were:

- Collectively confronting discriminatory behaviour more effectively than members of targeted groups alone;

- Training programmes in which participants agree to several specific goals for their behaviour and attitudes (and review their progress) are more successful than interventions that focus on simply educating participants or encouraging discussion;

- A particularly successful intervention asks people to take the perspective of those in target groups – e.g., 'If I spent a day in this organisation as a black person, I would probably experience…;

- Educate people and leaders about the subtler aspects of discrimination, including negative humour, harassment, and ridicule without overt discriminatory content;

- Include and value different perspectives;

- Regular feedback on performance in relation to the objectives;

- Clear roles and a mutual understanding of these roles;

- Shared team leadership where the hierarchical leader does not dominate, but supports and facilitates;

- A culture of valuing diversity (not just talks);

- Cultivating positive, honest racial dialogues and patterns of listening to and valuing all voices;

- Team leaders who reinforce the value of a diversity of voices, views, skills, experiences, and backgrounds.

While it is crucial to provide equal opportunities to reflect the diversity of an organisation, there should be no illusion that giving people of BAME positions solves the problems of systemic racial bias. If one is unable to challenge unfair practices due to fear, the bias will prevail within. This illusion of 'ticked boxes' further minimises the reality of discrimination and, more importantly, why we should pull together as a collective human voice. Could the challenges learned from the crisis help reshape our collective thinking, and create an inclusive NHS? Are existing structures to support 'ethnic health' working? Could this be an opportunity to explore multicultural perspectives in well-being?

COVID-19 has exposed the ongoing failures of the NHS in effectively using its policies to eliminate unfair practices. This story was captured by the Guardian, as the head of BMA called government attention regarding the vulnerability of these groups to COVID-19. While correct PPE is required for all staff working with COVID-19 patients, some reports have surfaced that some minority groups are not being provided with proper gear, or are forced to go to areas of higher risk. The director of the Royal College of Nursing made similar comments and reiterated a need for PPE for protection of all its front-line health care professionals.

While racial discrimination exists within all UK structures – like education, private organisations in the cooperate industry, and many more – no one anticipated such disproportionate mortality rates amongst HCP, with the higher rates claiming BAME doctors, nurses, and other auxiliary HCAs. This is alarming for an NHS system that depends on foreigners to sustain the health of its nation. We must acknowledge that such practices hurt everyone, which may result in sense of internalised oppression and a negative impact on well-being (low self-esteem, self-worthlessness and disengagement) (James et al., 2008).

The NHS could be ripped of essential HCP if the oppressed feel unsafe, or errors may happen when people feel such pressures. To be willing to risk one's life for the sake of others takes a high moral value. When coupled with an unsafe practice such as lack of PPE, this can trigger different levels of fear (Bar-Dayan et, al., 2010). In a study regarding the Flu H1N1 pandemic, it was found that the willingness of HCP to risk their lives was mediated by trust of their colleagues, workplace preparedness, PPE, and other safety measures.

## Historic Realities of BAME Disparities

Initial understanding of the virus was that it does not discriminate between individuals, other than regarding the underlying risk factors mentioned earlier. In the shared humanity of pandemic fear, it became apparent that society is divided, even when confronted with a common enemy. It is legitimate, given the multidimensional complexity of racism, that fear and coping demand a different approach for BAME HCP. Processing pandemic fear and navigating micro-aggressions calls for a repertoire of outlets – or what is called adaptive coping mechanisms – to ameliorate racism (Mallott and Schaefle, 2015). Navigating the fear of getting infected and constantly appraising biased attitudes causes damage to mental well-being (Brondolo et. al., 2009).

The impacts to family and friends can be diminished as we continue to be resilient in navigating COVID-19 challenges. Highlighting issues of race in this crisis is not meant to exclude others. If anything, it seeks and hopes to challenge our collective consciousness – our humanity – to find solutions. Like soldiers, the HCP are on the front line of battle, risking their lives to protect us. Open dialogues about race are very difficult, thus the story of BAME communities' place in society is often left out. Even though there is vast empirical evidence, these are often left to academics or researchers in specific fields such as the biopsychosocial scientists, and hardly as part of normal conversations.

The COVID-19 crisis has demonstrated that such conversations can no longer be avoided or diminished. Several studies posit that society – especially white people – chose silence in race dialogues due guilt, unconscious assumptions, or simply seeing it as a problem of the 'other' (Brondolo, Verhalem, Pencille, Beaty & Contrada, 2009). Some also posit that white people aren't sure what to say, afraid they will be accused of racism. Unless we understand that racism hurts all of us, it is difficult to bring different groups together.

Regardless of the pre-existing mythical speculations, the pandemic is clearly revealing systemic racial inequalities in health access and wellness (Hagelskamp and Hughes, 2014). For generations, research has highlighted how the structural factors of race and racism has disadvantaged BAME groups in all areas of their lives (Mallott and Schaefle, 2015). Once again, the NHS faces challenges in many aspects of the procedures and policies that guide practices within the care sector. Research has pointed out the alarming realities of discriminatory practices and how they affect a person's treatment within the medical system (Kline, 2015).

The outbreak of a highly communicable disease has a substantial impact on front line HCP. Not only are they faced with increasing workloads and uncertainty regarding pathogenicity but are also immersed in the crippling fear of getting infected. Lack of preparedness, demand to develop new skills, and being moved to areas of unfamiliarity will further exacerbate that fear. Adding insult to injury, there was a growing concern about the lack of personal protective equipment, despite government initiatives in providing for the safety of the staff.

Past studies on pandemic-related fear have not looked at BAME as an exclusive characteristic. The disturbing and worrying death rates called for the attention of the public, HCP professional bodies, the British Medical Association (BMA), The Royal College of Nursing, and others in urging the government to investigate why BAME HCP are more vulnerable to COVID-19.

People harbour racial stereotypes in deep ways, as they are embedded in the subconscious mind and practiced without thought to actions that inflict harm in deep ways (Lowe Okubo & Reilly, 2012). Ms Cooper – the head of equality, diversity and human rights – called for a centre for ethnic health, after claims of NHS being 'white-washed', which she stated during an interview with the Nursing Times (Ford, 2020). She further reiterated how BAME nurses felt they were being put in high risk areas. This comment reinforced the report that was produced by Kline (2015) in the article *The White Snowy Peaks of the NHS*, which alludes to how discrimination is played within the NHS. This is what overrepresentation of positive images and underrepresentation looks like, which shapes how people are viewed daily. In various reports, Kline (2015) has highlighted the underrepresentation of BAME within NHS, with its executives not reflecting their clientele and its discriminatory practices. It also posits that leadership bodies which are significantly unrepresentative of their local communities, such as NHS Trust Boards, will have more difficulty ensuring that care is genuinely patient-centred. Underrepresentation of 'positive' Black people is a big challenge, as it places this group of people in a negative light.

What are ways we may perpetuate racism within practice? Perhaps by not speaking out against injustices such as unfair treatment of a colleague, being pushed to high-risk areas without appropriate PPE, being refused sick leave, and being threatened in one way or the other. Evidence points to higher incidents of unfounded reports for BAME doctors and nurses within the General Medical Council and the Nursing and Midwifery Council in comparison with white colleagues (Uduak and Aliya, 2010). Challenges that BAME HCP face are complex because they are less likely to raise concerns over unacceptable discriminatory behaviours, discrimination around FIT testing for PPE, and many more (Royal College of Psychiatrists (RCPsychi), 2020). The RCPsychi (2020) points to how the existing paradigm for understanding the impact of inequalities on BAME staff set by WRES (2019) may heighten COVID-19 related risks. This contributes to increased anxiety, stress, isolation, and low confidence due reduced exposure to learning. In emergency healthcare delivery, white HCP professionals come to the aid of a white patient over the patient of BAME. (Hagelskamp & Hughes, 2014).

**How Does Racism Hurt Everyone? It is a Business for All**

It is important for society to have an understanding and appreciation of the damage our racialized reactions and practices cause. It is also important to remind ourselves that racism is not over with, and that BAME people are not obsessed with playing the 'race card', but actually call for a mindfulness of stories. It is time to move away from emotional rhetoric or hopeful thinking and start to look at the societal value in affording a fair chance for all; to understand that racism and any type of discrimination holds us back. We pride ourselves as a diverse society with policies that challenges any discriminatory acts or behaviours. Unless this translates into our human connectedness, the laws, policies, and rules will remain aloof to our existence.

Some examples of harm to all can be drawn from various resources. Research within medical health studies, psychosocial sciences, and education highlight how HCP from the BAME groups fail to report medical errors due to fear of victimisation, unfair disciplines, and being laid off from their job (Penner, Dovido, West, Getner, Albrecht, Dailey & Markoval, 2010). Further research posits that their diminished existence within a 'white' NHS perpetuates mistrust, lack of faith, and broken human spirits (Kline, 2015). In the height of global fear, these anxieties are all-consuming and challenges the moral responsibility of duty, as well as fear of being laid off for not turning up.

An opportunity of teaching within higher education in health studies afforded me a chance for involvement in various conversations within HCP BAME forums and students. The forums are channelling their attention into what needs to be done to support HCP, enabling BAME staff to express their concerns freely. In all the forums I had the opportunity to join, many expressed fear and anxieties relating to unfair treatments. It became clear that the expression of fear and anxiety are both anticipatory and real, coupled with huge uncertainties. Anecdotal stories have emerged, with some BAME HCP reporting that they felt the pressure of being removed from their normal area of practice to be put specifically in suspected or confirmed COVID-19 wards. Other concerns included inappropriate PPE, feeling compelled to work, being afraid to take time off for feeling sick (as they are threatened with a visit to HR), feeling their work is at risk if they take sick leave, and many more stories. While it is possible to dismiss such statements as perception, empirical knowledge has long pointed to the difficulty of naming and shaming daily microaggressions because it is often hard to provide evidence (Brondolo et. al., 2009).

Our journeys throughout our lifespan are shaped by the stories we tell and by understanding our existence in line with qualitative research. It is often stories that impact and shape positive social change. While 'others' may not understand, those whose lives are shaped by discriminatory practices cannot diminish such experiences to just perception (Barnes and Lightsey Jr, 2005).

The BAME forums are currently providing the space for constructive, honest, and authentic discussions that some consider not only a strategy forward but also a part of coping. 'Being able to talk about one's experience in a space of freedom and attention provides some buffer of coping', claimed many voices. The energy felt in the BAME forums was positive, hopeful, and seen as a way to provide resilience (Snyder, 2002). Many expressed feeling happy that they could express their experiences without fear.

## Beyond COVID-19

While it is imperative to positively acknowledge the steps the government has already taken to support BAME HCP, it is equally important to maintain consistent and long-lasting strategies far beyond the crisis. This is a 'moment' in time. Breaking news in confidence, building and cultivating a trusting relationship with employees of the NHS, safety for all – this is the business of all organisations. Navigating challenges of COVID-19 are those that will stay with us into the long future. Some more resilient people will live beyond it and return to normal lives, despite the socioeconomic impact. Coping should be thought of for the present and the future, as many will suffer from post-traumatic stress disorder (PTSD). Society at large will have long lasting consequences from the COVID-19 pandemic, whether they be economic, political, work life, psychological, or a completely new way of looking at our world. It is important to think carefully about what has been learned to provide long-term support for the HCP at large, and in enhancing a new way of collaborative work amongst HCP from all groups. There is a hope for human connectivity, in creating 'a safe for all' NHS.

It is important to remember that coping with the pandemic has multidimensional layers for BAME which are often overlooked. Organisations such as The Royal College of Nursing (RCN) and the British Medical Association (BMA) have since called out the government to explore the causes of high mortality rates within BAME HCP (RCPsychi, 2020). Some anecdotal references point to the failure of BAME staff to attend well-being initiatives set by psychologists, health therapists, and more. Some say their failure of attendance is due services not being tailored to their cultural and personal needs. Most psychological measurement devices in use within psychology and counselling do not reflect the minority, as they were developed and standardised primarily by white people, thus they may be inappropriate and pathologising (Jasinkaja-Lahti, Liebkind, and Perhoniemi, 2006). In the fight against COVID-19, everyone fears for their lives and their loved ones. To ameliorate the underlying multifactorial issues challenging BAME HCP, research efforts should be geared toward understanding and investigating individual and collective factors that may buffer/mitigate the effects of discrimination and eliminate marginalisation (Brondolo et al., 2009).

**Conclusion**

There is no doubt that the fear and anxiety relating to the COVID-19 crisis has impacted all of us and have changed our way of thinking forever. It is more so for the Health Care Professionals on the front line, especially with the reality of BAME mortality rates claiming colleagues, parents, friends, and other loved ones. It is a hopeful vision that the lessons learned will help shape society, especially the NHS. All initiatives to combat and investigate underlying factors for those at-risk groups will see new light in building individuals and teams. A stronger, united, compassionate, and well-prepared nation, should we face another health crisis. The challenge, as well as the new energy the crisis created, is one that will shape all conversations regarding multidisciplinary working and will regard BAME as the backbone of the NHS.

# The Fears of Providing Nursing Care in a Pandemic: Nursing Students' Perspectives

*Dr Prasundcoomar Ramluggun*

Fear can be either a conditioned or an evolutionary adaptive, behavioural response to a real or perceived threat. In nursing education, students may experience a fear of their academic studies and practice. This fear is gradually lessened as they learn to cope with their anxieties following incremental exposure to practice settings and their academic work as they progress through their programme.

There are a myriad of factors for how fear manifests itself in nursing students, which varies across nursing fields of practice. These can include exposure to death and dying, breaking bad news, managing challenging behaviours, exposure to complex procedures, and raising concerns. These factors can result in a socialised risk awareness which requires that the fear of caring be carefully managed, and at times masked by adopting a brave front. In their nursing practice, student nurses would have been involved in infection prevention as well as control, containment, and isolation of those who were seriously unwell.

However, the fear of nursing amidst the unprecedented challenges of a pandemic – which etymologically (the Greek word *pan*-all and *demos*-people) means it affects the entire population – such as COVID-19 is something these students would not have experienced or been fully prepared for. This chapter will explore how the students have developed their own clinical scheme of reference to conquer their fear and care for their patients during this life-threatening pandemic. Their personal battle and determination will be illustrated by their stories and quotes (mainly from final-year students), which they have kindly given me permission to share in compiling this chapter. The chapter will conclude with implications for preregistration nursing educational imperatives.

## Responding to the National Call of Duty and Fear

The initial call from the Health Education England for final-year nursing students to either take paid employment to bolster the healthcare workforce or defer their studies has had mixed responses. Some students felt a sense of resolution and trepidation as they responded to the call of prematurely starting their careers on the front line during a pandemic. They were nervous, but also excited to test their knowledge and skills while looking forward to learning new ones. Some welcomed the paid employment opportunities, having missed out on the previous nursing students' bursaries. However, other students' apprehension for this new paid employment arrangement was understandable. Under the new arrangement, although students will not be supernumerary, they will be supervised and enabled to complete their practice-learning requirements. However, such assurances did not completely alleviate their fear.

> *'Even under normal conditions, when we are on placement, we see how stretched the wards are and how difficult it can sometimes be to be supervised when you are classed as supernumerary – and staffing level can be a big issue anyway. So then to go into a situation which is going to be worst and you are no longer supernumerary, which means you are going to be accountable for what you are doing. You start to think when they already struggle to supervise you under normal condition how are they going to manage when the ward is much worst with the virus.*

> *I know we are being supervised but the expectations are that we are going to be able to do the tasks we are allocated to. As a final-year student, of course, there are things you should be able to do independently, but because you are counted in numbers, there may*

*be an assumption that you can get on with whatever you are allocated to.*

*Most staff members where I am on placement have tested positive. My supervisor has tested positive, and he is someone I have been in constant contact with. Now I am fearful of what would happen to me if I have also caught the virus. Who is going to supervise me and how I am going to finish my placement on time?'*

When faced with adversity in an uncharted territory, it is easy to become overwhelmed with feelings of helplessness. Some felt that this disregard to their needs and their inability to assert their personal choice in the call of duty was unfair. Paradoxically, some students felt empowered by this call and demonstrated a readiness for their practice in a time of altruistic need.

Fear has been described as an emotional state in reaction to uncertainty and the threat of harmful effect (Smith and Ellsworth, 1985). The fear of COVID-19 in the students could be interpreted as the primitive behavioural responses of either withdrawing (flight) or defending themselves (fight) on the front line of care. Fighting the external threat was preferred to the flight mode by most of the students, but as posited by functional theorists, this option is influenced by personal circumstances (Blanchard and Blanchard 2008).

In some parts of England, the fear of not completing their studies on time left these students with opting into this scheme as the only option. Feelings of desperation, anxiety, worry, and discontent were prevalent, depending on their personal circumstances. Some students' personal circumstances as matured students with caring responsibilities for their family meant that their only choice was to opt out. They felt they were the forgotten few, with not much consideration given to their personal situation. They argued that their decision to opt out was not received with the same acceptance and compassion as their peers who rallied to meet the challenge of the virus. They felt pressured to opt in and described a range of emotions in deciding to make the right decision for themselves and their family, while at the same time dealing with the uncertainty of finishing their nursing education.

*'It was a very difficult and emotional decision to make... it was scary...
lots of stress and tears, lots of discussion with the family. I had to take
into account my family, as a part-time student, working full-time by
opting in, I did not have anyone to look after my children.*

*It felt like we were being pushed into opting in, and opting out was
the wrong decision to make, because as student nurses we should be
able to go in and help out and that is what I should be doing even if
it's extremely scary.*

*There was lots of uncertainty as how your role was going to be in that
kind of placement... this makes the decision to opt out harder.'*

Additionally, there were a few students who voiced their discontent and felt
angered to be used in this way. Does this mean these students lacked
courage, determination, were seditious, and should not also be supported for
the stance they have taken? Or should their honesty be encouraged for
demonstrating the courage to stand up to what they felt they were unprepared
for? It raises questions about the legitimacy of the call on students to tackle
the coronavirus, the resulting fear of uncertainty that was inadvertently
created by the changes, and the disruption to the nursing education
programme.

For international students, managing the responses to the virus was even
more challenging. Their perception and reactions to the evolving state of
knowledge about the virus seemed to have been significantly influenced by
the overexposure to news broadcast in the media. In examining the role of
television in society, cultivation theorists such as Gerbner (1998) suggested
that repeated exposure to the media can subtly influence the audience
perception of reality and accentuate the risks and consequences for their
safety concerns. As exemplified by an international nursing student, the
elevated fear of the virus was accentuated by being infected or became a fatal
casualty of the virus.

*'For me, continuous broadcasting on the social media and news channels about the virus outbreak, strongly suggesting staying at home to be safe. My family not being around to support me if I suffer from the virus and constantly thinking 'what if I die without my family around to perform last rites and ritual.' Overall, to me it was not the fear of virus or dying; instead it was the fear of dying alone away from loved ones.'*

Thus, the students' deliberation to respond to the national call were influenced by a myriad of factors and reflects Dewey's (1991) position on how we think:

*...The very inevitableness of the jump, the leap, to something unknown only emphasizes the necessity of attention to the conditions under which it occurs"* (Dewey, 1991, p. 26)

This raises another question at a time when the phrase *'we're all in this together'* has gained so much prominence, when we are all shouldering the burden of this pandemic crisis: Is it right to be critical and judgmental of others' inactions and questioning their moral stance for opting out? The students have come to rely on the comfort blanket of a nursing student and having this suddenly ripped away in a non- supernumerary role, although being supervised, can be daunting for some of them. Stress and anxiety have been widely reported in nursing students (Turner and McCarthy 2017) and some are more vulnerable than others due to pre-existing mental health conditions (Ramluggun, et al., 2018). Hence, it is important to recognise that individual students react differently when faced with the additional challenges of COVID-19. The students should be encouraged to be self-compassionate and be reassured that it is fine to be scared and to use a safe space to acknowledge their emotions without any feelings of guilt or shame.

## Death Anxiety and Fear

The fear of becoming infected and infecting their families – especially those who are at high risk of the pandemic – was a constant worry and a few students chose to opt out. The greater susceptibility of Black, Asian, and

Minority Ethnic (BAME) students to die from COVID-19 was an understandable concern for these students. Remarkably, this concern did not seem to have amplified their fear. They appeared more intrigued by why this disease was affecting their ethnicity in western countries such as the UK and the USA. Nevertheless, they had an understandably heightened awareness of their own safety and that of others when they have lost loved ones to COVID-19, as described by a BAME nursing student working on an elderly care ward.

> 'Most of the staff of BAME background have tested positive, and most people I know who have tested positive and been hospitalised have not come back alive. I was so apprehensive and really, really scared of this disease and the fear aggravated because of my family. I have two relatives who have died of COVID and this is always on mind. I woke up every morning, thankful that I am still alive. People younger than me or older than me are dying. I am on a placement with the most vulnerable people providing personal care. One minute they don't have the virus and the next they have tested as positive. Being on the front line at this particular time is the greatest challenge of my life.'

The prospect of caring for patients that are dying from an infectious disease during a pandemic is a frightening thought for even the more experienced staff, but more so for less-experienced staff and nursing students. Positive risk-taking is inherent to nursing care, but such risk is mostly minimal and manageable. Depending on the students' field of nursing practice, exposure to managing a deteriorating patient would not usually be a new experience. However, nothing prepared an adult nursing student in her second year of practice to what she experienced on a COVID ward.

> 'I was working on a COVID ward on a bank night shift with twelve COVID-positive elderly patients. I went on my break around 4.30 am within an hour after coming back from my break, five of the patients died. The doctors in and out of the ward confirming the patients' deaths. I have not been able to come of my flat for a week after this, I

*was so scared by what I saw how people were dying so quickly one after another. I have cared for dying patients before, but for almost half of the patients to just go overnight was shocking. Nothing prepared me for that, it was very scary especially when you are constantly left on your own by their bed observing them, checking their breathing.'*

Death anxiety is a phenomenon that has been reported in healthcare workers and its expression is influenced by sociocultural factors such as age, gender including religiosity (Lehto and Stein, 2009). While student nurses, their supervisors, and other health care professionals endeavour to provide the highest quality care for dying patients, their death-related fears – as illustrated by this personal account may negatively influence their disposition to providing care to those at end of life (Matsui and Braun 2010).

**Personal Safety and Fear**

The feeling of vulnerability was exacerbated whenever the personal protection against the virus was being compromised by either not having the necessary equipment for the virus, not having confidence in the efficacy of PPE, and not being able to adhere to the guidelines for its use. Most of the students were concerned about the level and degree of protection against the virus.

*'My main concern was what was being offered for our safety and protection. The fear for me was how I was going to be protected when I am in placement. Because of my children, I was worried about bringing in the disease home, that was my biggest fear. If I bring this disease to my children, I will never forgive myself.*

*We are the mercy of this virus, the PPE does not give 100% protection against this virus, we can't even breath properly, when we are communicating with staff, we draw our mask down, we take them off in the restroom. So, the guidelines are not really practical, we can't breathe properly in these masks.'*

The workforce concerns over inadequate provision of PPE can result in healthcare workers' moral and ethical tension on whether to take care of patients when they feel they are not being adequately protected (Heron, et al., 2020). The principles of adequately responding to the psychological needs emphasise the consistent access to physical safety needs (British Psychological Society, 2020).

Furthermore, maintaining personal safety was also a challenge, especially in mental health settings. Communication is important in any healthcare setting, but a positive and meaningful encounter between the patient and the nurse is at the centre of mental health nursing care. Displaying warmth, compassion, and sensitivity in effectively communicating with the patients while keeping social distancing can be very trying. It goes against the fundamentals of therapeutically engaging with patients who are emotionally distressed. It can be practically impossible when managing severely disturbed behaviour, as observed by a final-year mental health nursing student on an acute adult mental health ward.

> *'Maintaining the two metres apart was a challenge in one-on-one observation and interaction with patients. There was one time when this patient became disturbed and very agitated, verbally aggressive, and physically threatening. The patient had to be put on hold, there was no way we could maintain this safe distance with the patient.'*

The students have not been educated and prepared for this new dimension of their therapeutic encounter with their patients. Working in different ways while caring for vulnerable and distressed patients requires courage, compassion, creativity, and the resilience to withstand the challenging interaction dynamics to maintain the nurse-patient relationship. It requires imaginative discovery and development of novel ways to reshape the principles of therapeutic engagement in care.

## Compassion, Courage, and Resilience

'The 6 Cs' of nursing (care, compassion, competence, communication, courage, and commitment) was a call to embrace these values (DH 2012). Here, the focus is on caring for patients with compassion and the courage to initiate changes to improve their care and embrace new ways of working. Resilience has been described as the ability to stay in control and balanced when dealing with stressors such as conflict (Pines, et al., 2014). Courage was perceived as doing the right thing and speaking up where there are concerns about poor care (DH, 2012). In a pandemic, the personal strength and resilience to advocate for staff and patients' safety raised a fundamental ethical question about healthcare workers own personal safety in caring for others. Nonetheless, some felt they had the psychological safety (Edmondson 2003) to openly raise their concerns without fear. As stated by Nelson Mandela:

> 'I learned that courage was not the absence of fear, but the triumph over it. The brave man is not he who does not feel afraid, but he who conquers that fear.'

This pandemic will undoubtedly have a lasting and enduring effect on healthcare workers and its psychological impact could be as virulent as its physical effects. Some nursing students are already beginning to reflect on their own strengths and limitations.

> 'What I have learned about myself is that I am not very courageous in dealing with stuff like that. Hopefully I would have gathered enough courage to get back to placement. Getting in contact with other people and seeing how they are managing this will give me confidence. What would have prepared me is to be told what to expect before my shift. I heard people are dying from the virus, but I did not realise how fast, it was terrifying. It's like going to treat a patient's wound, if they tell you beforehand its very bad, it prepares you for it because you know the situation.'

Some have found a safe space in their network to share their concerns, finding ways to help others problem-solve and soldier through by building and maximising their resolve and control over this pandemic.

> *'What has helped me is talking to other students who have children. This has helped me to relax a little bit, and speaking to family members because I had to move my kids out of the home and take them to relatives. Our WhatsApp groups have been very helpful, when I talk to students and receive their encouragement to carry on with our placement and hear how they were coping in their own placements with COVID patients. If we had a landline number that we could call this would have been useful.*
>
> *The next time something like this happens just face it and do what I can and don't run away from it, more practice of such situations will help me. There are carriers of this virus everywhere, you need to acknowledge this, remain positive and confront it rather than running away from it.'*

What is shown by the nursing students' accounts is how understandably frightened they are by this virus as they continue to carry out acts of considerable courage on the front line of care. Although they reported a range of fear, most of them were persevering in their placements. However, fear manifested itself in different ways and with varied subjective reactivity, and therefore some of them initially struggled to confront and overcome their fear. Emotional processing (Rachman 1980) has been used in exposure therapy to explain how fear is activated by a combination of factors, including the meaning of the fear, information, and avoidance of the feared stimulus (Foa and McNally, 1996). The significance of emotional abilities in positively influencing judgement has been widely reported (Benson et al 2010). How we effectively understand ourselves and others, our ability to express ourselves when relating to others, and how we adapt and cope with the demands of new situations has all been attributed to emotional intelligence (Raghubir, 2018). Emotional intelligence and resilience have been associated with the better handling of death and suffering in healthcare settings (Holston and Taylor, 2016). Hence, it would be useful to empirically explore the students' existential coping mechanism and their emotional intelligence in processing their prolonged exposure to this pandemic.

## Educational Imperatives

The dilemma for nursing education is how to encourage nursing students to provide the safest care, while remaining safe themselves, at a time when they have lost the routing of their usual support mechanism, social connections, and educational opportunities. This challenging situation also calls for the preparedness of students and their resilience for a physically and emotionally-taxing disease. How students receive and perceive information and thereby make decisions is also important to understand. The nursing education providers (mostly universities) have had to manage the intractable options offered to the students, including the drip-feeding of information as it is provided by the relevant bodies. Together, universities and their practice partners have had to manage the sheer complexity of the disruption to students' programme.

The Nursing and Midwifery Council (NMC) (2020) view that nursing students will not be disadvantaged by the options they were given is misleading, as it did not fully consider the varied placement patterns across universities (Ramluggun and Anjoyeb, 2017). As described by the students, there was limited consideration of the different stages of final-year students' programme, some of whom may be part-time students, including a lack of clarity on how they will complete their education and compounded by the dichotomy of the available options, which they found unhelpful.

> *'There was so much uncertainty in how the course will continue and when we will be able to graduate.*
>
> *The information at the start was not clear enough. I don't think this was the University's fault, but they just jumped in with two feet and didn't think of all the situations ahead. As an opt out perspective,*

169

*there has been much support and information only that if you have*
*opted out, you will have to defer. The plan put in place is*
*predominantly for students who opted in, and we've been sitting in*
*limbo. Now we don't know how we are moving forward. The Health*
*Education England took the choice to complete our unpaid placement*
*away from us.'*

Studies that examine students' fear and anxieties about their clinical
environment suggest an awareness of predominant fears and concerns, and
how learning activities are structured prior to clinical practice and realistic
ideas about clinical placements (Cowen, et al., 2018). The benefits of
resilience on nursing students' well-being (Li and Hasson, 2020) and its
development in preregistration nursing education has been advocated
(Amsrud, et al., 2019).

*'I have found the workshop on self-care and resilience and the topic*
*on stress in nurses, for which I am reviewing the literature for my*
*dissertation, very useful to manage the challenges I have faced so far*
*in this pandemic crisis.'*

Studies that examine students fear and anxieties about their clinical
environment suggest an awareness of predominant fears and concerns, and
how learning activities are structured prior to clinical practice and realistic
ideas about clinical placements (Cowen, et al., 2018). The benefits of
resilience on nursing students' well-being (Li and Hasson, 2020) and its
development in preregistration nursing education has been advocated
(Amsrud et al., 2019).

For some, this period of their practice may be an enriching experience which
would strengthen their resolve to deal with adversity in their career, whereas
others may emerge with emotional scars which would need time to heal. For
future employers and higher-education providers, this has implications of
recognising early trauma-related symptoms that may surface. Although

nothing would have prepared the students for this unprecedented experience, this pandemic has further underscored the importance of ensuring that nursing students are adequately equipped to meet the emotional demands of their programme. It is the collective responsibility for higher-education nursing providers to enable students to develop their resilience so the inability to cope is not perceived as a failure on the part of the individual student (Traynor 2017).

Therefore, a conceptual framework on resilience – such as the existential model, which captures the authenticity of how students thrive in adopting the identity of a nursing student during times of hardship – would be useful to examine appropriate strategies for preparing nursing students to manage challenging situations. It would be also useful to explore the concept of emotional intelligence in the students' ability to persevere while regulating their emotion and positively influencing others' emotions (Cherniss et al, 2006).

**Conclusion**

This chapter has provided a snapshot of the new fear engendered by COVID-19 for nursing students and the fullness of their experience. Their sobering accounts depict by no means a linear sum of choices and decisions, but the outcomes of unending vacillation and wavering decision-making in opting for the extended clinical placement. Although this virus has created a rift between those who opted in and out, there is a palpable sense of unity among the students. It seems that there is a shared understanding among those who have found the resilience and mental fortitude to opt in, or have understandably faltered due to personal vulnerabilities, including those who have questioned the opt in option with a pronounced degree of cynicism.

For those who opted in, risking their own health while coping with their own fear, they have had to adapt to changes in their studies and find the right balance to contend with this new challenge. In conquering their fear and battling this disease, they have managed to keep a whole load of emotions at arm's length, along with experience from the unimaginable sufferings they have witnessed and the resolve for other challenges they have faced. They have been proactive and creative in finding new ways of forestalling worry and manage their emotional distress by forming a close-knit network with their peers. They have also surmounted the initial apparent vagueness and confusion about their education that has been created.

However, the anticipated aftermath of their emotional experience will not be known until further down the line. Hence, there is an obligation on the education and healthcare providers to support these students and newly registered nurses to manage any emotional aftereffects of this pandemic. Studies of the pandemic's impact on the students' learning and the support received would be useful to these organisations, so they may better prepare and support nursing students for a sustainable healthcare workforce in any future pandemic crisis.

# A Personal Reflection on Fear

*Maggie Pratt*

The quote from Harry Potter, *"…much of what you fear is fear itself…."* (Rowling, 2007) is an inescapable reality. The recent outbreak of COVID-19 has sent the world in to a spin. Consequently, there are a lot of people working on the front line who are fearful of what is happening and what is yet to come. Their everyday lives have been interrupted and shattered by a formidable unseen enemy, bent on destroying the human race! So, why then are we fearful of what we cannot see? Surely, we have all faced fear before? Without a doubt I have, and I'm no different from anyone else – no superhuman armour or blind faith in my infallibility. Why then should you read beyond this point? Well, if you do, there's a chance that one or two of the things I've faced (and been scared by) in the past might just resonate with you. Moreover, some of the ways I've tried to quantify and deal with my fear may just work for you too.

To start with, we really need to know what we're talking about when we use the word 'fear'. Fear can be defined as one of several universal human emotions affecting both the brain and the body and eliciting in us a natural reaction to either confront it or run away. Everyone has heard of the 'fight or flight' response, and you might think we're born with an intrinsic fear of things like fire or spiders. Human babies are only naturally scared by loud noises or falling, so it's actually fair to say that everything else we learn to fear is shaped by our upbringing and environment. It's easy to see why some things that are intrinsically dangerous will tend to be scary – being in a burning building or standing on a cliff edge, but why spiders or snakes? Is it because they can bite? Perhaps, but most do not, nor are most in any way dangerous to humans.

Fear can therefore be irrational and extend to a whole host of things or situations – a scary movie, the thought of starting a new job, meeting new people, public speaking, etc. None of these things will hurt us physically (so long as the new job isn't being a cage fighter, or you don't fall off the stage whilst giving a speech)! However, the list of things we fear is almost endless and will vary in intensity from person to person. An individual's perception of fear resonates deep within their psyche and running away just isn't an option most of the time. Guess we'd better get on and deal with it then!

My relationship with fear (and I call it a relationship because of the way we have danced with each other as I faced new situations) began during the late 1980s. At that time, I was a young teenager embarking on a new career as a police officer. I was full of fear – fear of not fitting in either at work or on the streets (I was the first black female officer stationed in a rural area), fear of not being able to do the job (I felt I had no experience and had led a very sheltered life), and fear of facing aggressive and complex situations (I'm five feet, two inches tall and don't cut a very imposing figure). Moreover, I feared rejection from my family and friends. All the training I received could not prepare me for the way I felt, because I didn't – no, *couldn't* – accept that it would help. Police officers are trained in self-defence and techniques to keep themselves (and members of the public) safe in the most dangerous of situations. However, this type of training only led to me being even more fearful – thinking that around every corner was a mugger, or behind every door was someone intent on causing me harm. To my way of thinking, everyone was either a victim or a perpetrator and I developed a not so healthy suspicion that members of the public were suspects first, innocent bystanders second.

As a young probationer, I clearly remember a constable, who was acting as my mentor, excitedly telling me we were going to the scene of a suicide. Oh, the dread and fear that filled my mind! I'd never seen a dead body; what would it be like? Would it smell? Would I have to touch it? I didn't even want to see it, and I felt sick to the stomach at the thought. To make matters worse, the dead body was hanging from a tree! My heart was pounding and all I could think about was 'why?' You might think that's good – a young police officer thinking 'why did this person commit suicide', but no, I was simply thinking 'why me?'

The drive to the location was a blur. I could hear my partner talking, but I wasn't listening. I barely remember cutting the body down from the tree or examining the torso for any signs of foul play. I do remember my mentor telling me the whole experience was 'character building' and that I should 'just get stuck in, like any of the lads'. Humph!

Without a doubt, the fear that day took a hold of me. Even though I knew I couldn't feel like this every time I dealt with a suicide victim – or anything else that scared me – being so young, I had no idea how to deal with it. I didn't have any coping mechanisms; I didn't even know such things existed. It would take a lot more brushes with danger and scary experiences for me to reach out for help and come to terms with myself and my fear. Age and experience help, for sure, but there are shortcuts and techniques that can be applied to 'speed up the process'.

Writing now about my experiences of some thirty-or-so years ago is quite ironic, because reflecting on what happened to me then is actually part and parcel of just such a coping mechanism. Reflection is an important aspect of how humans come to terms with fear. Looking back on how we have handled situations is a useful way of adapting how we respond to similar situations in the future. A popular model of reflection often used in the field of nursing is the Driscoll (2007) model of reflection, in which we're asked three fundamental questions: 'What?' (the event), 'So What?' (why was that event significant), and 'Now What?' (how will you use what you have learned in the future). You may not think it, but you typically reflect on events most days, and it helps to cope with the normal stresses and strains of everyday life. However, when it's a significant event (like COVID-19) and one that has caused you particular anxiety, it pays to take time out to really think hard about the issue – why it caused you real or tangible fear and what you might learn from how you managed it.

A little aphorism I learned later has helped me to reflect on a great many situations – and not just those involving fear. The questions to ask yourself are 'What Went Well? Even Better If?' (abbreviated as WWWEBI). I like this a lot because it dwells on the positives of a situation rather than the negatives. Reflecting on how you coped with a particular situation can be soul-destroying if all you do is focus on what you did wrong, what a mess you made of it, and how bad you now feel. Doing that doesn't help, and you'll quickly bring your reflection to a premature end without getting any benefit from the exercise. Worse still, you'll risk depressing yourself in the future by reflecting on the next scary situation.

Looking back to my 'reflection' on that first suicide case, I realise now that it was a destructive experience because all I thought about were the negative aspects. Moreover, I thought about it for weeks on end, instead of allowing myself sufficient – but not too much – time to dwell on it. The poor man's face appeared in my dreams. He was my first (and, sadly, not my last) and I did not know how to cope with my fear and feelings.

After a while, I found that talking to my peers and sharing my experiences lessened these emotions. It's often said that people who repeatedly deal with trauma, crisis, or other scary situations develop a 'thick skin'; it's true, to some extent. In reality, it's a way of the body and mind protecting oneself, and in my case, as the years went by, I became desensitised and detached to incidents involving the loss of life, no matter how tragic the circumstances. Coping with imminent fear and danger became a distant challenge. 'Black humour' – or 'gallows humour', as it is often termed when relating specifically to death – also played a big part in me coping with extraordinary events; the jumper in front of the train, which left me picking up bits of body along the train track, was a source of grim humour when I sat down with fellow officers to eat a kebab (body parts in a bag, still in the back of a squad car).

176

Those on the front line sometimes rely heavily on what may otherwise appear to be inappropriate humour, as a way of coping with mental stress and anxiety. Today, we're facing the unprecedented crisis that is COVID-19, but you only have to search social media to find clips of nurses dancing and singing on their wards. It's nothing new, either. During the first world war, soldiers made light of the terrible sights they beheld and acts of barbarism they experienced through their jokes, puns, or satirical songs. This became known as 'trench humour' and was a way of dealing with the stress that could only be appreciated by fellow soldiers who had experienced the same fears.

In Harry Potter and the Prisoner of Azkaban, Professor Lupin tells his students that a Boggart (or shapeshifter) will assume the identity of whatever they fear the most. The only way to deal with a Boggart is to imagine something ridiculous, and thus reduce it to something humorous. Okay, I know that's only a film (and my second reference to Harry Potter, so you can see what sort of films I like), but the principle is the same: Laughing in the face of death maybe sounds a bit clichéd, but finding some reason to see humour – however dark –might just help you get through some tough situations.

Sometime after I left the police service, I decided upon a complete career change and entered the world of nursing. Death and mutilation held no more fears for me, but new fears were soon to replace them! As a trainee nurse, I was terrified of making a mistake where the consequences could be catastrophic. The thought that if I wasn't careful, I might actually kill someone with a dose of the wrong medication, an overdose of the right medication, or some wholly inappropriate medical intervention was scary stuff. Going through nursing school was a real challenge – not only because I was one of the oldest (and pretty set in my ways) but also because I'm dyslexic (in fact, never one to do things by half, I also suffer from dyspraxia and dyscalculia – the 'full set', so to speak). Most of all, I feared academic writing – and with good reason. How on Earth could I possibly write an assignment of academic quality when I'd left school over thirty years earlier, with little in the way of qualifications and a lasting belief that I was 'intellectually slow'?

However, I was to find that help was at hand and that times had certainly changed from when I was a police officer. Instead of the 'grin and bear it' mentality that characterised so much of my police career, the support that was on hand at University was outstanding. I was given IT tools with which to dictate (rather than type) my essays and additional learning provisions were made available to me. My mentors and tutors took time to explore how I was coping, and not just to judge the outputs of my learning. All the counselling and support mechanisms the University had to offer were laid at my feet, and suddenly the fear of not being able to cope academically faded into the distance. I no longer harboured a fear that 'I was too stupid' to write a dissertation, and after three years, I somehow managed to leave University with a First-Class Honours; a very proud achievement, but not just for me. You see, my success was really a reflection of the all the support I was given by all those who helped me cope with my fears and anxieties.

The sad truth is that despite huge advances in understanding and appreciating the importance of mental health and well-being, there are still far too many social stigmas around reaching out for help when you need it, even when it's readily available. The 'stiff upper lip' or 'character-building' attitudes I experienced in the police still pervades society today, where needing help can sometimes still be seen as a sign of weakness.

So, my message is simple: don't wait until it's too late to talk to someone and get help – professional or otherwise. Just talking to a good listener can help, but there are plenty of professionals with a wealth of practical advice, so get as much of it as you can and as often as you need it. Nothing you're facing and nothing you're feeling hasn't been felt by someone else before. I'd like to say that my experiences have helped me conquer fear, but the truth is that it never really goes away.

As a qualified nurse I encountered new and traumatic situations, but I was struck by some advice I got from one of the most unlikely of sources. A few years ago, I was listening to the radio when something just clicked into place. The discussion was about stoic philosophy and its origins in ancient Greece.

Yes, I know it all sounds a bit heavy – and ordinarily that would be the point when I'd switch over to Virgin, Heart, or Magic – but on this occasion, something kept me tuned in.

You see, the basic idea is that once you accept that external events are beyond your control, you can focus on what you can control. Everyone has heard of the Serenity Prayer by St Francis of Assisi, which was translated by American theologian Reinhold Niebuhr (circa 1932-33): 'God grant me the serenity to accept the things I cannot change; courage to change the things I can; and wisdom to know the difference'. Well, it's the same principle. If we can't control the fact that we're in a COVID-19 crisis, then there is no value in concerning ourselves about the how's and why's. However, what we can control is how we respond to the crisis, and how we use or control our fear.

Now, there's a whole lot more underpinning to this philosophy, but it's interesting to note that there's been a huge resurgence in the sales of stoic philosophy books since the outbreak of COVID-19. In fact, the Roman Emperor Marcus Aurelius (from The Gladiator – another favourite film of mine) was an exponent of stoic philosophy and wrote a book called *The Meditations* during one of the worst plagues Europe has ever faced. The Antonine Plague was likely caused by a Smallpox strain that lasted around fourteen years and killed over five million people – eventually, even Marcus himself. However, his book has never been out of print since, and while I'm not suggesting anyone rushes out to buy a copy (or rather orders one online), it is worth taking a moment to consider this: If we can't control some of the major events that shape our lives – be it the Antonine Plague nearly two thousand years ago or COVID-19 today – then should we focus instead on how we cope with fear, illness, anxiety and loss? *The Meditations* becomes a kind of 'manual' in our toolkit for practicing mental resilience and brings me back to my opening quote: '*…much of what you fear is fear itself…*'. I always knew watching those Harry Potter films would come in useful one day! A stoic would say that it's not the virus itself that causes our fear, but the way we interpret or judge it to be scary. In other words, fear does more harm than the thing we're scared of.

By the same token wisdom, patience and self-discipline are virtues that can help us quantify and contain that fear. Learning from how others respond is a key skill and even fictional characters can be role models (roll on, Harry Potter). The idea that fear can be irrational was as well known in the ancient world as it is today, and it's fascinating to think that for all the scientific advances humans have made over the centuries, we can still be afraid of a spider that we categorically know cannot harm us. Most of us will survive COVID-19 – the statistics are in our favour, but we still tend to focus on the worst-case scenario, which can have a hugely negative effect on our emotional or physical well-being and quality of life. Trying to come to terms with the reality of the situation and not entertaining our worst fears is no easy task, but it's crucial to maintaining or re-establishing a sense of perspective.

So, now I teach student nurses as an adult nurse lecturer. I'm not on the front line and I'm not living with the constant fear of contracting COVID-19 from the patients I'm treating. I can't pretend to have ever been in that situation – very few of us ever have been. The fears I face now are for my students. I cannot see the virus and I cannot keep my students safe from harm. They're the ones working tirelessly to support the NHS while also trying to complete their studies. They're the ones putting themselves and their families at risk, and I admire every single one of them for it. The fears they face are real and can become overpowering if left unchecked. So, what else can you try, yourself? Well, one thing to do is perhaps try and compartmentalise your fear. Think about it as a tangible thing that you can put in a box and let out when you've got the headspace to deal with it. Using fear to keep you alert may help, but don't try and comprehend the full horrors of what might happen; instead try breaking it down into small, bite-sized chunks. Think about how you're going to manage a particular problem, get through an hour, or even a day. Don't dwell on the full magnitude of all that could go wrong.

Fear will always walk with you, hand in hand as your silent companion, but you can learn to not succumb to it. Indeed, on occasion it can drive us to great things and be a source of moral fortitude and encouragement.

Who hasn't been moved by the fundraising efforts of Captain Tom Moore and the generosity of the public in donating millions of pounds to NHS Charities? Adversity generates tragedy, but also lifts the human spirit through acts of kindness or courage – be it on the part of health care professionals, bus drivers, postal workers, refuse collectors, or police officers. If you can focus on what's going well, even if it doesn't feel very big or important, it can help you stay positive. This pandemic will end – how you respond to it is down to you and, ultimately, that's got to be a good thing.

# Part 3

## Conquering Fear

# Fear

Fear
It lurks in the shadows
Fear
Fear is a thing that whispers in your ear
Fear it tells you that you are alone
Fear
It's worry about the unknown

Fear it is an enemy,
Fear it only exists if you let it in
Fear it's a game you can't win
Fear it can't survive in your light
Fear it creeps up in the night
Fear it offers sadness and tears
Fear it's a creature of the darkness
It grows in your mind

Fear
You can leave it behind
It's needs you to be weak
Fear doesn't want you to speak
Out, but you are not alone
Fear is a parasite
Get it out, pull it out
Leave it behind you
It's there behind you
Face it, grab it
Crush it, it's in your hands
Drop it on the ground
And trample it down.

Thought today was the day you would succumb
But nope,
You're still here
Live on, fight another day
Fear is nothing compared to Hope.

*Sue-Ann Anderson*
*27 years old woman who's no longer held captive by fear.*

# A Narrative Account of an Arts Psychotherapies Service Response to the COVID-19 crisis: Challenges and Recommendations

*Claire Grant & Dominik Havsteen-Franklin*

This chapter describes perspectives from the academic and practice arts psychotherapies leads within a large NHS Trust in the UK. This was written from the perspective two leads with experience in senior management, research, and clinical practice. The first author is an art therapist and consultant, and the second author is a music therapist and Head of Profession. As part of the core psychological provision, the arts psychotherapies service employs arts psychotherapists, arts psychotherapies trainees, and honorary professionals to deliver specialist care and treatment for patients across mental health services.

The chapter is written during the time of crisis, when the peak has been reached, but the end of the crisis and lockdown remains unclear. The authors take stock of the changes that have taken place to a community arts psychotherapies service during the COVID-19 crisis, referring to the changes in staff provision and practice. During this time, clear lessons have already been learnt, observations made, and inquiries have resulted in broad recommendations which are relevant to health services where there may be similar events taking place. These recommendations relate to how, at an operational level, the clinical work, staff capability, and capacity to adapt are kept in mind and responded to during and after a pandemic.

## Arts Therapies

Arts therapists provide psychological treatment for some of the most vulnerable mental health patients. This chapter will describe how and why major changes to practice took place, such as introducing tele-arts psychotherapies and moving group work to one-to-one. Anxiety, uncertainty, unpreparedness and feeling unsafe were some of the initial experiences of the staff group in relation to the impact of COVID-19. Once changes began to be made, significant questions arose about the conceptual difference between seeing the arts made through a screen and made in person; boundary issues to do with the spaces which the therapist and patient occupied during the sessions; sudden changes to group work being transferred to working with individuals; how nonverbal expression could be understood and what the threat of COVID-19 meant for patients and staff. This chapter offers a narrative account of the change process in community arts psychotherapies provision and the challenges that were faced that we believe are relevant for all therapists where COVID -19 has had a significant impact.

Arts therapies are a group of professions that span various fields of healthcare, are regulated by the HCPC and are trained at MA level. With a broad training, driven by an in-depth understanding of relational change through arts, arts psychotherapists are trained to work within a range of contexts where practice can be adapted according to specific relational issues and physical conditions (Havsteen-Franklin, 2019; Odell-Miller, Hughes, West & Cott, 2006). A culture in arts psychotherapies within UK health settings has developed that draws on innovation and extended thinking to resolve complex issues to do with patient engagement (Edwards & Elwyn, 2009), evidence informed treatment (Alegria et al., 2010; Byrne et al., 2018; Crawford & Patterson, 2007; Van Lith et al., 2013), and working in a multi-disciplinary context (Robinson & Cottrell, 2005). There are areas in mental and physical health where patient choice of treatment is required to inform decisions about effective outcomes (Edwards & Elwyn, 2009; England, 2014). However, the patient choice, in some circumstances, is determined by how they make an informed decision; for example, where people struggle to engage, verbalise, communicate, and identify their needs. For this population, arts psychotherapists provide a viable treatment for people who are more able to connect, be explorative and develop relationships through using nonverbal mediums (Evans, 2008). In arts psychotherapies, the nonverbal expression through making images or music or using drama or bodily movement facilitates a capacity to form emotional bonds with others through a personalised aesthetic expression (Cumbie & Rutherfoord, 1994; Korakidou & Charitos, 2012; Sajnani, 2012; Salas, 1990).

## Why COVID-19 Challenges Therapeutic Assumptions

Despite the adaptive nature of arts psychotherapies professionals, COVID-19 presented unexpected challenges. Seeing the unfamiliar in the familiar is a hallmark of the creative mind (Overall, 2015), but not as easy to achieve. In this context, the unfamiliarity of the conditions required to manage COVID-19, such as social distancing and the use of new technology, presented significant challenges. Arts therapists work with sensed mediums within a social proximity. COVID-19 is an unsensed virus transmitted via small droplets from the nose or mouth usually discharged when coughing, sneezing, or speaking. COVID-19 can be fatal for physically vulnerable people, however, at the time of writing, the mechanisms are not entirely known, including the number of virus strains; mutations; or why some people are affected more than others, such as Black, Asian, and Minority Ethnic groups. The total mortalities in the UK was reported to be 31,241 as of the 9th May, which is known to be a significant underestimation given that COVID-19 related deaths are underreported in care homes and the community.

How is this relevant? The focus of the media has generally been about containing the physical impact of the virus, reducing the death rate and the 'R' number. However, it is reported that in some areas, the psychological impact of social distancing and the exposure to the threat may have as big an impact as the virus itself, especially for healthcare workers, for whom there has been a high prevalence of compassion fatigue and burnout (Greenberg, Docherty, Gnanapragasam & Wesley, 2020; Guile, 2020.; Ho, Che & Ho, 2020). If we consider some of the most important factors that improve mental health through the use of arts psychotherapies, these are primarily introduced through the musicality of relational proximity (Pavlicevic, 1997), engaging with creative and nuanced ways of reflecting on and changing the aesthetics of relating (D. Havsteen-Franklin, 2016), and by enabling an embodied interoceptive approach to developing a personal language through the arts (Fotopoulou & Tsakiris, 2017). This involves being with the emotionality of relational closeness and what this means, in order to be able to establish trusting and collaborative relationships (Taylor Buck & Havsteen-Franklin, 2013).

COVID-19 impacted on several important factors regarding physical social proximity that intuitively worked against core principles of therapeutic practice. These were primarily social distancing, disruption to regularity and structure of appointments, and an uncontained threat to people's lives that requires a physical intervention. Under normal circumstances, these factors would be considered outside of the scope of arts psychotherapies' core practice. In the scenario of COVID-19, the assumptions regarding reliability, keeping patients safe from significant threats, and providing interventions focused on face-to-face relational work through creative mediums were profoundly challenged.

### How Did Arts Therapist's Working in CNWL Initially Respond to the COVID-19 Crisis?

When COVID-19 was announced, there was an exceptional reaction from arts psychotherapists that demonstrated the impact of rallying together to reflect on what will be helpful for the patient, staff, and organisation. As trained innovators, the response was varied and wide and required careful facilitation to look at what would be efficient, effective, and manageable within a complex environment. Arts therapies leaders and supervisors drew upon feedback from clinicians about what was happening and planned the next steps. On March 13th, 2020, before the lockdown was announced, in one face-to-face supervision group that we were offering, when asked what was happening for supervisees, the members expressed feelings of shock, numbness and anxiety. Within days of the announcement of a COVID-19 pandemic, arts psychotherapists considered urgent issues about how clinical work would be guided under entirely new circumstances. The question of 'what next' for some less-experienced clinicians was unimaginable and for others, pragmatic questions about practice were arising, such as: 'How do we protect ourselves and patients from COVID-19? Can we safely move to tele-arts psychotherapies? Will practice be the same? What mental health issues will emerge or be exacerbated by the crisis? How will any COVID-like symptoms be understood and managed within the therapeutic frame? What would the practitioner do if they became unwell?' The feelings of urgency were palpable, an underlying fear of the pronounced instability that threatened the core principles of therapeutic practice, recovery, and organisational cohesion. The group represented profound and important perspectives on how we move forward and became increasingly pragmatic about tacking the problems of an 'invisible enemy' (Fardin, 2020). Suddenly, we were all affected in a way that we were not prepared for.

During this early stage of the pandemic, a supervisor observed a first area of impact; the supervision group pace was faster, the physical demands of being prepared for the unexpected, and the sympathetic nervous system being triggered in the face of danger. The second invisible impact was the cognitive stress of quickly making complex decisions where there was no ideal answer, but constant compromises that felt incomplete. The third invisible impact was on the weight of the emotions. The threat of COVID-19 was either defended against through an experience of 'feeling numb' or being 'in shock', where the reality was not faced, or arts psychotherapists expressed compassionate concern for colleagues and patients. The immediacy of this response in supervision indicated to professional leads that there was a high degree of instability emerging in the system that required attention. These conversations at an organisational micro-level developed into formal operational conversations within care quality meetings, which initiated protocols and a higher-level, systematic collation of people's experiences of clinical work using tele-arts psychotherapies as a solution. The conversation that began,

'What is happening?' resulted in the mobilisation of a range of systems and procedures to enable practice to continue.

**Responding to Change**

How do we generate a sense of safety in times of crisis? Anxiety and distance had become predominant factors within the change process where COVID-19 had heightened the sense of risk and vulnerability in the staff. How do we accept this as part of a process of mobilisation? Some arts psychotherapists felt redundant, as their primary therapeutic skills relied so heavily on attunement to the nonverbal communication that could barely be achieved through tele-arts psychotherapies. The development of playful interactional subjective spaces within the therapy to explore resources and relationality was considered impossible outside of the arts psychotherapy's clinical spaces.

Our professions focus on the importance of the full range of expressive cues – tone of voice, expressive movement and micro-movement, facial expressions, and nonverbal interactions. Video conferencing can help meet the human need for this kind of social connection (see Berge, 2017; HTA, 2016; Krout et al., 2010; Middleton, 2019). However, the limitations of online arts psychotherapies are also acutely felt. We cannot fully access the multiple expressive cues that we usually 'tune in' to as we navigate our place in relation to others: video conferencing reduces the group to a selection of individuals carefully enclosed within boxes, we don't see the whole person, people 'disappear' due to unstable network connections, we don't pick up relational dynamics that we resonate with or jar against when we are physically next to someone, silences can lose their communicative function and the accompanying facial and bodily expressions are poorly construed on a small screen. How have therapists managed these issues in their clinical work and their experience of working life?

On March the 25th, we completed guidelines for the safe transfer of clinical work to tele-arts psychotherapies. The draft was circulated to all arts psychotherapists and comments were assimilated. On the basis that there was such uncertainty about whether treatment outcomes could be achieved, the protocol described tele-arts psychotherapies as 'supportive' for the most vulnerable patients. A survey was rapidly put in place to be completed by the 10th May (Figure 1). Alongside this, we developed a 'red amber green' rating scale based on a measure piloted in early intervention services (Ashir & Marlowe, 2008) to assist clinicians in considering which patients they should prioritise for tele-arts psychotherapies.

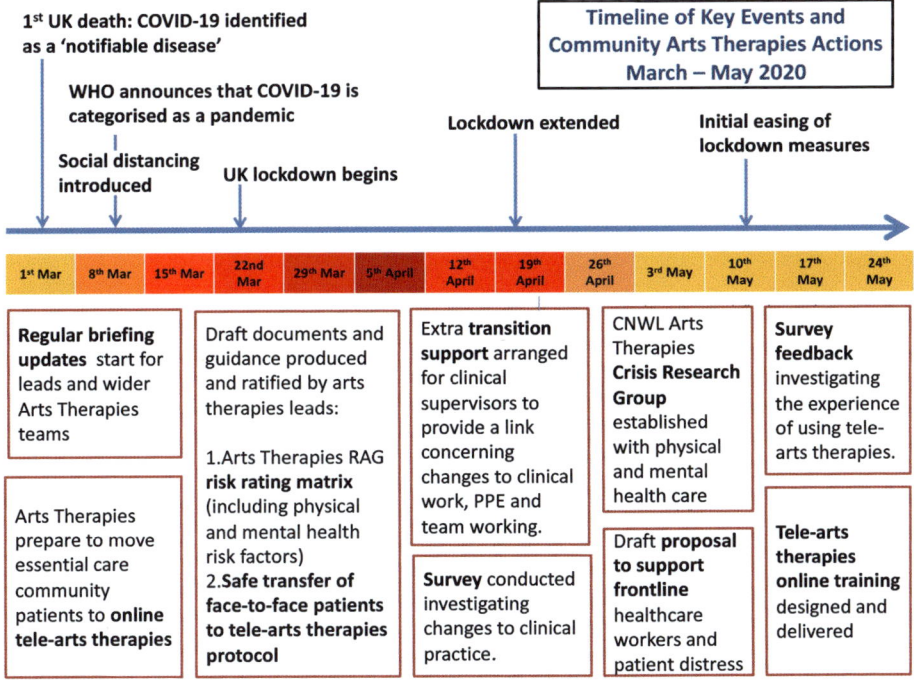

**Figure 1: Timeline of COVID-19 events and responses of arts psychotherapies services in 2020**

## Tele-Arts Therapies

COVID-19 has had an unprecedented impact on mental health services (WHO, 2020). The patients referred to arts psychotherapies in CNWL NHS Foundation Trust have severe mental health issues, which are either impacted on by their struggles to communicate their experience or the illness itself has had such an impact on their functioning that their verbal communication does not immediately offer a clear picture of their experience and needs. These patients are often at high risk of self-harm, suicide, or violence towards others, often due to social disconnection, stigma, and trauma. These are the people who often do not easily access verbal therapies or who commonly disengage from mental health services. During the COVID-19 crisis, these patients are at considerable risk due to their condition being exacerbated by social conditions, media, and isolation.

Arts therapists rarely employ tele-arts psychotherapies except under some circumstances where distance has proved to be the main issue, for example, with war veterans in the USA or rural physicians (Levy et al., 2018a; Middleton, 2019). Within a profoundly different social context, arts psychotherapists working in London UK mental health services were being asked to rethink their practice delivery. We gathered evidence of the effective use of tele-arts psychotherapies, but engagement from the arts psychotherapists was gradual and generally considered by those who did engage as a method of using talking to prevent deterioration rather than as treatment. The assumption was that talking would be less effective than using arts-based methods for a population that had not engaged well with talking about their experience. However, what emerged, and didn't appear to be correlated with experience or position of authority, was a range of innovative approaches from a number of arts psychotherapists who made evidence informed adaptations to their practice to deliver arts psychotherapies online. In art therapy, therapists began to support image making online, or receiving images emailed by the patient for use during an online session. Visual journals reflecting daily experiences and were brought into online sessions and creative exercises were introduced, including online arts resources.

Music therapists collaborated on song writing and singing, played music with patients online or during phone calls, and drew upon shared experiences of musical appreciation. Dance and dramatherapists used narrative and bodily movement to articulate emotional expression and experience.

A new repertoire of arts-based online interventions began to be developed in line with evidence-informed methods (See Chipps et al., 2012; HTA, 2016; Reviews, 2018) that continued to draw on evidence and pragmatic ways of responding to the crisis (Levy et al., 2018; Miscall Brown & Sorter, 2008). Most patients reported that this was extremely valuable during a time when there were increased stressors and vulnerabilities.

**Arts and Health Packs**

At the same time, the CNWL arts in health team supported the development of 'arts and health packs' comprising a range of art materials and paper. Included in the clinical pack were depression and anxiety self-reported outcome measures, a mindfulness exercise, and a letter explaining why the arts and health pack was being offered at this time. Feedback from patients was extremely positive.

One patient, a young woman with a diagnosis of borderline personality disorder, described using the pack as a 'daily journal'. She described feeling safer making the work at home. During an online session, she showed the therapist an image of something like a bird's nest drawn in coloured pencils and chalks. She said that inside it felt 'chaotic and anxious', but outside she could see light. She felt that during the image-making, she worked from the inside out, noticing the changes in her feeling states. After drawing, she said that she felt better, and although she was very worried that the therapist would think it 'wasn't good enough', she was relieved when the therapist appeared to tune in with the experience of being in such an enclosed space, disconnected from others, whilst feeling hopeful that someone will be able to make contact. Her mother had been very depressed when she was a child and her father had left without warning when she was seven years old. The disturbance caused by experiencing others as being unreachable exacerbated her concern that she would always be isolated and lonely. Using the arts helped her to facilitate an experience of her emotions and helped her make sense of how the social distancing had impacted her capacity to compassionately self-soothe (see Gilbert & Irons, 2004), meaning that she was able to better accept her feelings, build connections with people and make sense of her felt experience.

## Arts Therapies in a Time of Crisis

Sinclair and Haines (1993) state that during crises involving deaths of people, there is a potential for miscommunication and fragmentation of the work group as an organisational defence to avoid feelings of shame, guilt, and fear. Due to self-isolation, social distancing, and higher levels of stress, the workforce is vulnerable to fragmentation and to preserve stability is likely not to be working to full capacity. During a time when the organisation and the work group is potentially destabilised, there is also a requirement to meet existing clinical demands as well as a new stream of work responding to a major threat to people's lives. The Centers for Disease Control and Prevention (U.S.) (2005) mapped social disaster responses to help communities anticipate and prepare for the impact of social trauma. The first stage is described as an often-heroic rallying response to the problem that draws people together in action, followed by an optimistic 'honeymoon period', quickly followed by disillusionment and loss. During this stage, the organisation and community is at its most vulnerable, and this time can last months, if not years. The Centers for Disease Control and Prevention (2005) reported that a healthy outcome is for the community to work through change and loss, a process of grieving. During this time, there are numerous triggers that can bring traumas back to the present and potential fragmentation and splits as the community relive a shared impact of the disaster (Figure 2).

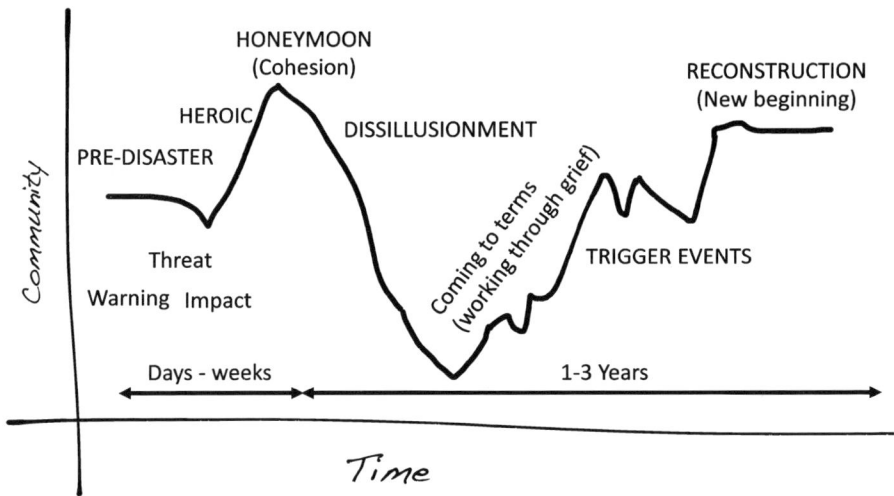

**Figure 2: Community Trauma Response (adapted from Centers for Disease Control and Prevention (U.S. , 2005)**

During the increased period of disillusionment, a common dialogue for the arts psychotherapies concerned what to prioritise; practice as usual, prevention, or responding to the impact of COVID-19? Similarly, what are management to prioritise in terms of receiving feedback? Our baseline understanding of good clinical practice has had to change, given the extraordinary circumstances. For some arts psychotherapists used to focusing on the relational change in the clinical room or using arts as methods of highly skilled nuanced communication and expression, the change from face-to-face practice to tele-arts psychotherapies is as radical as suggesting a surgeon conduct their work in the neighbour's kitchen.

As far as possible, we kept services functioning as usual in unusual conditions. The feedback about the use of tele-arts psychotherapies, management and clinical support was extremely mixed. This was to do with a number of factors, but mainly the therapist's personal relationship to the crisis, family commitments and responsibilities, shielding those vulnerable to COVID-19, support available, and how connected they felt with the service provided. Under these conditions, many of the anxieties and uncertainties about professional role, identity, and service were exacerbated through the physical distancing. However, there was also an increased use of video platforms and telephone to maintain contact within the arts psychotherapy's teams. The demand for contact was more than would have usually been the case. This is not to say that uncertainties about professional roles are necessarily a problem: the NHS is constantly changing, and professionals are required to adapt and change to the context, as well as consider transferability of skills and changes of language, philosophy, and ethos. Therefore, being anxious at times enables an engagement with complex professional issues related to role and responsibilities. Despite fears associated with loss of professional identity, as well as feeling deskilled or disorientated, all arts psychotherapists continued to see their most vulnerable patients or play a role in facilitating change and were supported by colleagues to do so. Their roles now extended to working even more closely with community mental health services, taking crisis calls, and conducting follow-up appointments for at-risk patients.

Given that the unusual characteristics of this professional group also contain radical innovators and adapters to change, the response to the tele-arts psychotherapies transition was extremely mixed. When the survey was collated, most arts psychotherapists had been working with patients using these adapted approaches for 4-6 weeks. 67% of arts psychotherapists responded to the survey. The key themes emerging from the survey were that it was too early to know what the benefits were and how to use tele-arts psychotherapies most effectively, given that there had been no formal training and the transition was conducted through protocol and supervision and had largely been driven by a range of leads working in parallel.

However, given the levels of uncertainty, there was a successful transition with 73.1% of clinicians stating that the transition was 'manageable or quite easy'. Clinicians were in various stages of transition, with 32.1% of respondents having only provided between 1-10 sessions online, and the same number having provided more than thirty-one sessions.

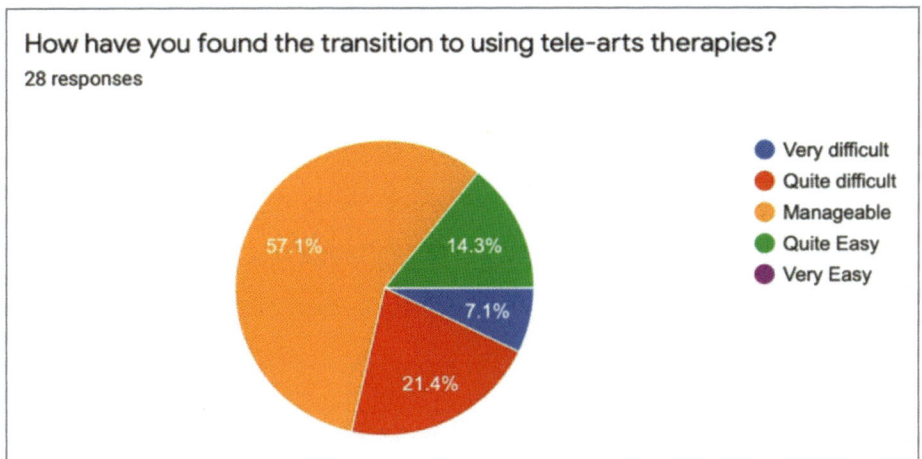

**Figure 3: Arts Therapists' experience of the transition from face-to-face work to tele-arts psychotherapies**

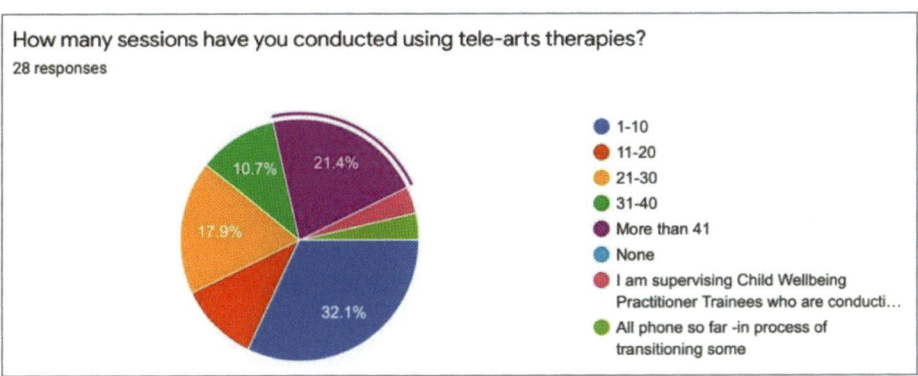

**Figure 4: Arts Therapists number of sessions conducted**

This was surprising, given that the change was rapid and that group work had been the main format of delivery. Now 96% of respondents had transferred the treatment to individual sessions. 81.5% of respondents said that they felt that tele-arts psychotherapies were having a sustainable impact on preventing crisis and deterioration, 63% said that tele-arts psychotherapies impacted on the patient's capacity to mentalize and 56% believed that tele-arts psychotherapies impacted on affect regulation. Within such a short period these findings are important in considering the confidence in the work, even if there is grave uncertainty. However, 76% of respondents felt that crisis prevention and deterioration could be achieved within a significantly shorter period if the work had been conducted face-face. Given that the period of tele-arts psychotherapies being evaluated was a 4-6 week window following the onset of the crisis, the fact that the preventative work was believed to be observed during this early stage of a national pandemic is a remarkable achievement. 72% of respondents said that they would need further training, especially in how arts could be used (83.3%).

**Learning from the Crisis**

The NHS is usually slow to make changes due to the importance placed on a project or social-based clinical and economic impact through consulting stakeholders, considering options available, and ensuring that there is sufficient buy-in from implementers (Bate et al., 2004). In the social conditions resulting from the COVID-19 crisis, changes were forced out of necessity that would have otherwise taken months, if not years to introduce on the scale required. Yet, what have we learnt so far? One of the main learning points for the arts psychotherapies services is that engagement and innovation is supported by people that you may not expect to be so interested or involved. Some clinicians stepped up and articulated responses that were visionary. Some clinicians presented nuanced innovations and embodied change. Resistance was part of the culture, that had to be included within the dialogue to understand what was being lost and to identify key risks to services and patients. However, clinicians engaged with change, despite their deepest fears. This crisis not only highlighted the importance of listening to the vulnerabilities and insecurities of the workforce to help us be sensitive to the risks, but also brought into focus a progressive, creative, and collective drive towards healing for the group, organisation, and society.

A crisis like COVID-19 shakes the ground upon which people have built their professional identity and practice. Attending to these vulnerabilities, whilst also carrying change, is not something that should only happen in a crisis. As the pandemic progressed, compassion, mindfulness, and hearing the voices of emergent innovators amidst collective anxiety were highlighted as potential approaches to enabling helpful changes to dynamic systems that had been in crisis before, albeit not on the same scale.

**Recommendations for Arts Therapies Practice During and Immediately After a Critical Incident**

The preparedness of arts psychotherapies services to respond to organisational change requires agile and engaged leadership. Below are our recommendations, based on our learning, for people in leading positions or for people who can support leadership and can impact the delivery of therapies during an acute crisis.

| **Initial Phase** The initial phase is defined by a stage of uncertainty when an impact is known, but the details regarding the scale, extent and longevity of the impact are unknown. | 1. Keep up to date with information about the incident, the organisation, safety and wider issues happening locally and nationally |
| --- | --- |
| | 2. Arrange frequent communication channels to ensure that information is accurately and speedily disseminated |
| | 3. Ensure rapid decision-making processes are in place that are linked to professional and managerial leads. |
| | 4. Instate extra support as a conduit to inform management about the experience of the changes |
| | 5. Adapt practice ensuring that risk and safety are prioritised, e.g. that there is a mental health and physical deterioration monitoring and prevention strategy for patients at high risk |
| | 6. Write clinical guidance and protocols as 'live documents' and disseminate ensuring that all managers and leads are conscious of changes that need to be made and how this can be safely implemented. |

**Table 1: Initial phase recommendations**

**Mid Phase**

The mid phase is defined by an increased understanding and knowledge about the nature of the threat enabling modelling for the service in relation to longevity and impact.

| |
|---|
| 1. Draw on existing evidence and knowledge for working effectively during critical incidents and integrate into the working models |
| 2. Use novel methods of employing the arts (e.g. working with forms of technology) underpinned by evidence infomed theory and practice |
| 3. Evaluate impact of the change through efficient methods such as surveys or staff consultation. This will also give an indication of how people are and how they are engaging with change. |
| 4. Adapt the team business continuity plan/critical response plan, drawing from the learning gained during then crisis |
| 5. Begin to develop a post-acute phase medium- and long-term strategy, including what will be part of a 'new normal'. It is important to recognise that services will not resume as usual after the crisis due to socio-economic changes and the learning gained from the crisis. |

**Table 2: Mid - Phase Recommendations**

The dynamic changes during and after a significant crisis are relevant to a range of professionals facing similar challenges. Changes to communication, leadership, and adaptations to clinical practice are inevitable during and after a critical incident, crisis, or disaster that affects the provision of healthcare on a wide scale. There is limited evidence for best practice during this time, and much of the learning needs to be acquired through practice. The aim of this chapter has been to provide a narrative from two leads in the organisation – a narrative that maps key issues relating to working with a critical incident, which posed so many challenges to conducting practice as usual, and the basic assumptions underpinning practice as usual.

# Courage in the Face of Fear

*Margaret Rioga*

When I first embarked on my journey of being a mental health nurse, the other students looked at me with the raised eyebrows and shocked looks that said women should not be working in mental health. My family has a strong nursing history, which began with my grandfather, and for me this was what I wanted to do and had seen during my childhood and young adult years. So, I pushed forward with the training, and on graduation, I chose to work in forensic services. In other words, I chose to work with adults who had committed criminal offences, but were also diagnosed with a mental health condition.

I was a five-foot, two-inch female nurse working on a male admissions ward with individuals who seemed like they were seven feet tall! My first day on the ward was terrifying, with all the first-day fears of wondering if I would remember everything that I had learned at university, if I would be able to work with my colleagues, and how to feel about the clients on the ward. It was all a maze of worrying thoughts and questions, but as soon as I walked onto that ward, I knew that I had conquered the hardest part and now it was time for me to immerse myself in the work that I had been training to do for three years.

In the work of Aristotle (ca350 BCE/1999), courage is explored as the midpoint between cowardice and rashness. There is a belief that people are either cowardly or rash, and when faced with a particular situation, there is a great drive to act, which aligns with physical courage (Lester, Vogelgesang, Hannah, & Kimmey, 2010). Physical courage can be understood as the act of overcoming a fear or physical harm in defence of self, family, or country

(Putman, 2010). It is often seen in situations when people risk their lives for the benefits of others, such as caring for the sick in circumstances as trying as a pandemic. In the current climate of COVID-19, we have identified key workers as 'courageous' because they are going out to support those in need of care and treatment and in delivering our key services. This chapter will explore different kinds of courage, how the emotion of fear can trigger acts of courage, and through this, support not only ourselves but also the whole community.

Courage in healthcare has been explored by philosophers as early as the 1950s, with Socrates being recognised as one of the founding thinkers (Kilburg, 2012). Following this, there have been several studies which have developed through the 1980s and then more recently into the 2000s. Over the years, courage has had many definitions, most of which were initially influenced by soldiers going into battle and facing their fear, hence this underlying theme that courage is a result of conflicting forces and standing firm against one's fears (Rate, 2010). Therefore, when we think of courage, we automatically associate this with soldiers, fire fighters, and police – and now, because of COVID-19, we increasingly align courage with nurses and healthcare staff. Children have been painting rainbows, putting posters on their windows and bus stops, and we have all be clapping for our nurses and healthcare staff.

In reviewing the literature, the definition which I identified with was from Woodard (2004, p.4 – 5), who defines courage as:

> *'the ability to act for a meaningful (noble, good, or practical) cause, despite experiencing the fear associated with perceived threat exceeding the available resources'*

This definition recognises that courage *supersedes* fear, in that it is the voice of inner calm that drives you to move forward, even when you know that you are going out to work as a porter, bus driver, train driver, or delivery driver and may encounter someone who has COVID-19. Courage is the coat of armour that we put on when we face situations that could potentially be a threat to us, our loved ones, and – as we have seen more recently – our wider community.

In the work by Seligman and Peterson, (2004) courage is viewed using a 'Character Strengths and Virtues' classification: bravery, perseverance, integrity, and vitality. 'Bravery' is characterised by the mental or moral strength to face danger or a difficulty (Matthews et al, 2006). 'Perseverance' is the ability to persist through obstacles and setbacks to achieve a goal (Duckworth, 2007). At the core of all these values, it is important for the individual to be *authentic* to themselves as we are then more likely to pursue goals that are intrinsically motivated (Lopez, et al 2010). People will pursue courageous acts because it is something that they believe in and that aligns with their values. Examples of this can be seen in fire fighters, nurses, doctors, and police who will risk harm to themselves to protect others.

In undertaking these roles, the impact on one's mental and physical wellbeing should also be acknowledged, as prolonged exposure to challenging experiences may result in burnout. In light of COVID-19, most (if not all) people have had to make adjustment to their plans, such as holidays, weddings, working, attending spiritual functions, or funerals. Stressors such as organisational change, personal stress, overloading of work, lack of social support, and emotional exhaustion (Jenkins, 2004) have been identified as factors that can contribute to burnout. In reviewing these factors, all of them would have been experienced by keyworkers at this time of COVID-19, and all intensified. The emotional exhaustion of holding a client's hand when they are dying, and knowing that they cannot be with their family, is something that is difficult to explain in words. Given that for some healthcare professionals this is a daily occurrence and happens several times in a day, it is unimaginable.

Fear and the demand to be 'brave' can make all of this so much harder. Services have changed rapidly and dramatically, which has seen hospitals and wards being closed and staff finding themselves working in new teams and in new environments. Many healthcare staff are working under extreme conditions with an absence of personal protective equipment (PPE), twelve hour shifts, while being away from their family and children – with some even living in hotels. Despite this, they continue to work, hoping for a better shift where they can help someone recover and get discharged.

This hope and drive will only work for a period of time, and so we should be taking care of ourselves and making sure that we take the time to do the things that we enjoy (Ser- & Sciences, 2011). I recently joined the 'video-calling' generation and now regularly meet with my family and friends for a catch-up and drink via WhatsApp and Zoom. The ability to see their faces, talk, and laugh about past experiences feeds my soul and through these interactions I am able to find the strength to continue with another week of lockdown. We have all seen the photographs of the grandmother dressed in full PPE so she could hug her grandson, people talking through windows, and families talking to their parents in care homes via Zoom and WhatsApp. These interactions demonstrate our resolve to be close to those we love and care about during times of challenge, and how the impact of a smile and hearing that they are alright will bring reassurance and comfort.

In one of the video calls, I explored what key workers thought about courage and fear. We have all heard of 'fear of the unknown', and this was an underlying theme in the discussion. COVID-19 was something new, and while guidance was being developed rapidly, there was a certain level of uncertainty; when would the schools re-open? Should everyone be wearing masks? How long would we need to social distance? How long would we need to work remotely? There was uncertainty, but this was mitigated by a sense of contributing to society. When the Nursing and Midwifery Council (2020) called out for retired nurses to return to the front line, this received a positive response of more than seven thousand nurses. Similarly, the National Health Service (NHS) request for volunteers was met with an overwhelmingly positive response, with over 400,000 people registering in one day (NHS, 2020). In certain situations, when things seem out of control, we can gain control and conquer our fear by focusing on the things that we can do.

In one video chat, we brainstormed the words 'courage' and 'fear' and this information was used to form a word cloud.

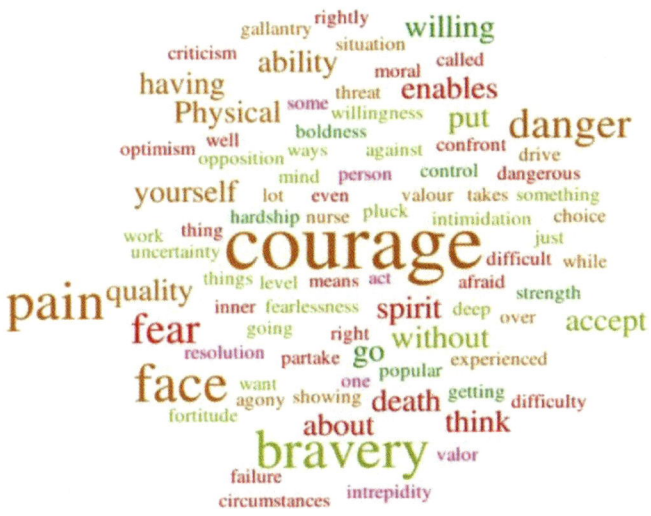

Listening to the conversations, I realised that we all used different words – bravery, confront, drive, willingness, boldness, gallantry – but we all meant essentially the same thing: we needed to push past our fears to experience something new. There was a sense that courage was something we did; it was an action – actions like going to work your shift, holding someone's hand as they were dying, clapping for those who had recovered and were being discharged, or simply smiling and hugging your partner as they walked out the door to go to work whilst underneath the smile praying that they were safe.

What was interesting about the discussion was that the 'action of courage' was motivated by the promise of a greater reward. For the nurses in the group, it was about helping patients to recover whether from COVID-19 or any other illness; this ability gave them fulfilment and pride. When asked to define courage they said:

> 'I think courage to me means willing to put yourself out there and accept criticism and drive something that your you're willing to partake

in. It takes courage to go and accept that you want to be a nurse and you're going to go for it.'

'I think that in a lot of ways, courage is about having experienced failure and about getting over it.'

'And just having inner strength as well. And some level of optimism is that things will work out. A very deep one and should not be afraid to put yourself out there.'

'Do the right thing against the circumstances.'

Those that were partners, family, and friends said that they had to offer reassurance and support so that their loved ones would find the comfort and strength to carry on with their work. They said that while they feared their partners would test positive for COVID-19, some of them purposely chose to not engage in media stories or online chat groups about tragic cases, as they wanted to keep their home and conversations a 'safe' place founded by love and hope.

Courage is associated with several synonyms (bravery, boldness, heroism, perseverance and endurance) (Lopez et al., 2010) and in reviewing the definition of these terms, it is apparent that courage can be the beacon of light when faced with the overwhelming need to run and hide. As human beings, we are born with the 'fight or flight' instinct. This means that when we face a perceived 'threat', we react by either standing and 'fighting' the threat or leaving the situation to avoid the 'threat'. If this is the case, perhaps courage is just a human response to a potential threat. Peterson and Seligman (2004) described courage as taking action when faced with internal and external opposition. This 'opposition' could be internal fear based on psychological thoughts and beliefs, and external fear based on the physical reaction to fear in the body (sweating, heart pacing, breathing quickly, shaking) (Rachman, 2010). Thus, overcoming opposition could be a true reflection of courage.

Courage is fluid, and there are varying perceptions of how courage is measured in society (Putman, 2001). This aligns with society's perception of rewarding certain professions with the title of being courageous, such as firefighters, soldiers, and – more recently – nurses and caretakers. Other key workers – school teachers, delivery drivers, bin collectors, shop staff, those in the transport industry, and other staff working in public health and other industries – are all working to support us, so that we may continue with our daily lives. These key workers should also be given the same status of being courageous as they are also risking their lives to continue working.

Are there people who are unaware of this opposition, though? If we take an example, like running into a burning building to rescue a child, is this individual being courageous or fearless? This raises questions over whether courage is about the result that has been achieved or about the person, their professional occupation, and the choices they have made in a particular situation.

For me, courage is about the person, the choices that they make and the action they take. Key workers are making the choice to go to work and keep all our essential services operating, and this says something about that person and their values. When I signed up to be a registered mental health nurse, I signed up to protect and uphold the professional values of protecting the patients and the public. While my focus is now on training the future generation of nurses in upholding these non-discriminatory values, my goal remains the same: to protect the public, my patients, and the students. Being a nursing student working on the front line during this time of COVID-19 is probably one of the greatest learning curves that our students will meet, but the experience will – I hope – help make them resilient and help them to find their true motivation being a nurse.

Gee (1931) explored 'bravery' in relation to American soldiers in World War I. He identified the different 'layers' of bravery and how it ranges from an individual level to a group consensus. A common theme was a sense of teamwork, and recognition that whilst the soldiers had a common cause, different members of the team would occasionally have to go 'above and beyond' the others to save the whole group. This was 'individual' bravery, where the individual worked alone; 'altruistic' bravery, where the individual would have to risk their life to save others; or 'bravery under physical duress', where the individual would proceed with their identified mission despite injuries (Pury, 2013).

All of these could be termed 'physical courage', and there is a sense of fulfilment that comes with this type of courage: the individual feels accomplishment from benefitting others (Putman, 2010). This concept of bravery is dependent on a person in the group being the 'hero', and could put pressure on certain individuals to perform their 'courageous' act, when in fact, they would not have made that decision had they been given a fair choice. I am sure we have all had that moment when we wondered if we should be going to work and if this was the right decision for our family and loved ones, particularly when they are in the shielding group. I think we have all had this moment, whether we acknowledge it openly or in private!

Shaffer's (1947) work explored courage from the angle of reducing fear and the motivations that would reduce the fear when soldiers were on the battlefield. The type of equipment, efficiency of the work, teamwork, and leaders in the team all contributed to increasing the courage of the soldiers. Interestingly, by following the government guidance on social distancing, handwashing, only going out the house for exercise or groceries, reading stories of those that have recovered from COVID-19, and talking to my family and friends has helped to reduce my fear. As I have learned more about COVID-19 and how to protect myself and my family, this has helped to reduce my fear and to find a 'new normal'.

Deutsch (1961) discussed moral courage and the idea that external and individual factors are influenced by the individual's internal conviction or instinct. Moral courage is about understanding the motivation for the courageous act and in this, there is a need to discuss the topic of a 'moral compass' and what that means to individuals. It could be argued that our morals are 'shaped' from birth by the influence of our caregivers. Bowlby's work (1969) was based on the notion of secure attachments and the importance of developing secure attachments, as these influence positive relationship developments in adulthood. Brendtro, Brokenleg, and Van Bockern (2005) discussed the 'circle of courage' in relation to courage in children and how it is developed through promoting the strengths of the children to influence growth and internal development of courage. While moral courage is influenced by 'internal conviction' (Putman, 2001), this can be shaped by others in certain individuals and situations.

We have seen an army of volunteers register to support the community and individuals in the community supporting their neighbours who were classed in the vulnerable group. My sister-in-law works in a high dependency unit in a general hospital and after her twelve-hour night shift, she comes homes to cook and deliver meals to her neighbours. Talking to her inspired me and made me realise that small things can make a big difference. A friend of mine is in the shielding group and is at home alone with two children. Knowing that she could not go out to do her shopping, I have been delivering her shopping when she could not book slots for home delivery. This is a small gesture, but it ensured that she had food and cleaning products.

Psychological courage is the ability to face one's unhelpful behaviours (Putman, 2010). This type of courage is mainly associated with negative emotions such as stress, sadness, and dysfunctional relationships. In these situations, the individual makes the conscious effort to confront challenges by restructuring core beliefs and systematically desensitizing oneself to the fear. Lopez et al. (2003) argued that psychological courage could be developed through training and became 'vital' courage. This was explained in the context of talking therapies such as Cognitive Behavioural Therapy, where professionals use their clinical expertise to educate and support individuals to identify the impact of their thoughts and feelings on behaviour (Stallman, Kavanagh, Arklay, & Bennett-Levy, 2016).

When compared to moral and physical courage, vital courage has a lower due to being based on the challenges that individuals encounter as part of daily decisions (Lopez et al., 2003). I feel that this vital courage is the most important type of courage because it focuses on the daily challenges that we experience. To build a puzzle, you need all the different pieces; to see the full story of our lives, we have to overcome the challenges that we meet along the journey. Going to work when you know that your colleagues have died takes vital courage and an inner strength, which no one can ever understand, apart from key workers, partners, and families.

All types of courage share the core idea of making authentic choices for oneself and others. In pursuing any form of courage, the person must be psychologically ready to tackle the challenge and open to what needs to happen as a result of the courageous act (Putman, 2010). The barriers to pursuing a courageous act can include choosing not to get the information needed to make the decision, or rationalization, which may involve hiding behind role, policies, or finances; the individual then relies on others to make the decision for them (Hannah, Sweeney, & Lester, 2007), often viewed as the path of least resistance. Nevertheless, making authentic choices is a true test of courage, as there will be risks and existential anxiety.

I enjoy watching television, and now I find myself often saying, 'this must have been before COVID-19…' as I watch people dancing on Strictly Come Dancing or attend weddings on Don't Tell the Bride. I wonder if I will ever hug my friends to say 'hello', or shake hands and not feel nervous about germs and COVID-19? At the end of this lockdown, I am uncertain about what will become the 'new normal' and the emotional, physical, social, and mental impact of COVID-19 on. We have seen companies and airlines going into administration, a rise in domestic violence, mental health problems, obesity, alcohol use, and poverty. While financial schemes such as furlough leave, business loans, or self-employment funding have been introduced by the government to combat some of this, the social and economic impact of COVID-19 is yet to be revealed. In questioning life post-outbreak, I choose to use the lessons learnt to dispel my fear, and realise that whilst the experience of lockdown has been challenging, I have made it through. If I can overcome this, then I can handle whatever life throws at me.

Are we heroes? A 'hero' is someone who comes in and saves the day – superhero characters such as Batman and Wonder Woman, or soldiers returning from war. When courage is viewed as 'heroism' it is seen as the only way forward to maintain one's integrity in the wider group (Kilburg, 2012). While it is important for us to know our limits and competency levels, during these times of challenge, where teams are under tremendous pressure, there is the risk that individuals may try to work outside their areas of expertise. It is important to know that we all have our part to play in the team and sometimes this is all that is required. Trying to do something that we have not been trained in, because we want to be the 'hero', may actually cause more detriment than good.

In conclusion, COVID-19 is something that we were not expecting to happen, but it has now taken centre stage in all our lives. The initial fear triggered panic-buying and long queues at the shops, but has now led to a world where people volunteer to care for the vulnerable groups in the community. COVID-19 has affected all of us, and while we have experienced fear, we have somehow found the strength to push past this and continue with our roles and define a new way of living and working. Our initial response was fear, but it is courage that has propelled us to survive and move forward with our lives. There are different types of courage – physical, moral, and psychological – but in talking to my friends and family, I realised that we actually have a shared language and understanding of courage. Courage can be internally or externally motivated, but it is my belief that through courage we drive past our fear, for the benefit of our own health and well-being as well as the wider community. We are all superheroes in the story of our lives, and through courage, all things are possible.

# Compassion, Care and COVID-19

*David Rawcliffe & Kathy Swanzy-Derben*

The coronavirus pandemic has resulted in fear, anxiety, and uncertainty across the globe (Ahorsum, Lin, Imani, Sefferigriffiths & Pakpour, 2020; Schimmenti, Billie & Starcevic, 2020; Smith, Ng & Li, 2020; Sonis, Kennedy, Aaronson, Baugh, Raja, Yun and Whte, 2020). Public awareness of the virus' infectious nature initially led to panic-buying and empty supermarket shelves. Daily reports of the morbidity and mortality rates associated with the pandemic has made many people acutely aware and fearful of their risk of getting the virus and potential death. Of course, levels of fear have varied, and as a consequence, there have even been tools developed specifically to measure COVID-19-related fear, such as the 'Fear of COVID-19 Scale' (Ahorsu et al, 2020).

As the virus spread across the United Kingdom (UK), the number of patients admitted to hospitals across the National Health Service (NHS) increased. The NHS was overwhelmed with the sheer volume of patients admitted with COVID-19. The UK government, like other governments around the world, responded to the situation with policies such as social distancing, self-isolation, stay-at-home orders, and 'lockdowns' in an attempt to reduce the spread of the virus and reduce its impact on health systems. In addition, large hospitals known as 'Nightingale Hospitals' were built within a short time frame, to help meet the demands associated with treatment of COVID-19 patients. The increased volume of infected patients led to a shortage of personal protective equipment (PPE), raising the risk of health and social care professionals and further exacerbating their fear of contracting the virus (Smith et al, 2020; Sonis et al, 2020).

## Defining Fear

Fear is a negative emotion characterised by extreme levels of avoidance in response to a perceived threat (Schimmenti, et al., 2020). Schimmenti, et al. (2020) suggest that fear associated with COVID-19 is psychologically structured around four interrelated domains, namely 'fear of the body/fear for the body', 'fear of significant others/fear for significant others', 'fear of not knowing/fear of knowing', and 'fear of taking action/fear of inaction' (Schimmenti, et al., 2020, p.41). They argue that these four domains depict the bodily, interpersonal, cognitive, and behavioural dimensions of fear elicited in response to COVID-19 as a way of coming to terms with the reality of the situation (Schimmenti et al, 2020). These domains of COVID-19-related fear are not linear or hierarchical, but portray the complex and multifaceted nature of fear experienced by people during the pandemic.

Despite the fear generated by the pandemic, there has been an equally unprecedented demonstration of humanity and compassion, such as communities pulling together to show kindness to each other, over half a million members of the public volunteering to work in the NHS, and companies working in collaboration with the NHS to manufacture essential equipment such as ventilators to meet the unprecedented demand. In this respect, it could be argued that the emergence of the pandemic and its associated fear has ignited a focus on compassion. Sonis et al. (2020) assert that the extreme fear and uncertainty that is associated with the pandemic has called – and continues to call – for compassion.

## Compassion, Meaning, and Fear

A common definition of compassion cited in literature is an awareness of the suffering, distress, or pain of another, accompanied by the willingness or desire to take action to remove, reduce, or alleviate the suffering (Chochinov, 2007). Morse, Bottorff & Anderson (2006) define compassion as 'a strong emotion or sentiment stimulated by the presence of suffering that evokes recognition and mutual sharing of the despair or pain of the sufferer. In sharing the other's suffering, the caregiver expresses compassion that strengthens and comforts the sufferer' (Morse, Bottorff & Anderson, 2006, p.80).

Kanov, Maitcas, Worline, Dutton, Frost, and Lilius (2004) describe compassion as a dynamic process, which includes the three interrelated elements of noticing, feeling, and responding to another's suffering. These definitions of compassion suggest that for compassion to be demonstrated, there needs to be the presence of *suffering*, attentiveness to *notice* the suffering, and the motivation to take the necessary *action* to ameliorate the suffering.

Egnew (2009) argues that people need help to find meaning in their personal suffering. Frankl (2011) argues that 'Suffering ceases to be suffering in some way, at the moment it finds a meaning'. What does it mean for them? For some, this meaning will include fear of dying, fear of leaving behind loved ones, fear of recovering well enough to be discharged from hospital and finding that loved one's are in hospital, fear of being a burden on their family and the professionals, and fear of passing on the virus to the very people caring for them.

These meanings of compassion suggest that compassion is relational and is demonstrated through connection and interaction with the person experiencing suffering or pain (Kanov et al., 2004). They argue that connectedness is the basis of compassion, and that without connection, suffering would not be acknowledged, and compassion could not be expressed.

The literature also postulates different attributes of compassion. Compassion is a 'multi-textured response to pain, sorrow, and anguish and includes attributes such as kindness, generosity, and acceptance' (Feldman & Kuyken, 2011, p.143). Crawford, Gilbert, Gilbert, Gale, and Harvey (2013) assert that the ability to show compassion is dependent on the individual's ability to develop a 'compassionate mentality'. The attributes associated with this 'compassionate mentality' include being kind, gentle, warm, caring, comforting, reassuring, supportive, and encouraging (Crawford et al., 2013).

These attributes demonstrate the complex nature of compassion. The Strengthscope (2019) confirms that some people are simply energised by compassion, as they 'demonstrate deep and genuine concern for the well-being and welfare of others', and Jazaieri, Lee, McGonigal, Jinpa, Doty, Gross, and Goldin (2016) found that compassionate attributes increases caring behaviours.

Although COVID-19 is highly infectious and has triggered fear globally, as well as challenged healthcare professionals about their own need for self-preservation from the disease, most have risen to the challenge and responded with compassion by continuing to deliver high-quality care to patients with the virus. Sonis et al. (2020) contend that communication, empathy, and compassion of healthcare professionals could even be enhanced by the COVID-19 crisis.

The pandemic provides numerous opportunities to demonstrate compassion, small acts of kindness and meaningful differences to improve patient and staff experience. Cunningham, Diaz, and Slawek (2020) assert that COVID-19 challenges healthcare professionals personally and professionally, and they have needed to rise to the challenge by looking for opportunities to show compassion in the midst of significant suffering and trauma.

**Compassion and the NHS**

Compassion is seen as the cornerstone of high-quality care by patients, families, healthcare professionals and policymakers (Department of Health (DH), 2008; 2009; 2012; Maben and Griffiths, 2008; Youngson 2008; Badger and Royse, 2012). The Willis Report (2012) confidentially declared that the future of nurse education should give and continue to develop 'compassion with care'. For years, the National Health Service has strived towards being a values-based organisation and delivering compassionate care, with former Chief Nursing Officer for England Jane Cummings declaring, 'I want to make sure we give our patients the very best care, with compassion and clinical skill, ensure pride in our professions, and build respect.' (Department of Health (DH), 2012) The document defines compassion as 'how care is given through relationships based on empathy, respect, and dignity – it can also be described as intelligent kindness, and is central to how people perceive their care." (DH, 2012, p.13). Health Education England and the Nursing and Midwifery Council (2015, p.12) set the direction needed to ensure 'compassionate care'. The NMC (2018) The Code requires nurses, midwives, and nursing associates to treat people with '1.1 kindness, respect and compassion'.

The importance of compassion is emphasized internationally in most professional codes of ethics in healthcare (American Psychiatric Association, 2001; Paterson, 2011) The American Psychiatric Association (2001) requires doctors to compassionately provide competent medical care, while in New Zealand there has been a campaign to make compassionate care a patient right (Youngson, 2008; Paterson, 2011).

**The Emerging COVID-19 Crisis**

There is, then, general agreement that compassion is a good thing – that is until it came to the COVID-19 crisis, when suddenly the Nursing and Midwifery Council and others began examining the need to increase staff to provide 'care' (NHS, Scottish Government, Department of Health, Welsh Government, Council of Deans of Health, NMC, RCN, Unison & Unity, 2020). The government agreed to changes in the regulations so student nurses could be placed on a temporary student register, which gave most students in their final six months of training three choices: join the new student register by becoming a student employee, suspend their training, or continue their training in the normal way. The last option is generally not a real option, as NHS Trusts and universities do not feel able to support the traditional forms of training. Effectively, it has felt to many that the NHS and the NMC demands compassion in their nurses, but are not actually treating their students with the same level of compassion; rather, they are responding to the perceived needs of patients presented in the emerging coronavirus crisis for more caretakers.

And yet, the picture is complex: we are hearing examples of Trust managers becoming increasingly visible and displaying the values of compassion and moving towards a more visible compassion-based leadership (see Observing the Leadership, in this book).

## Our Natural Tendency Towards Self-Criticism

The Oxford English Reference Dictionary (Oxford University Press, 1996) defines criticism as 'finding a fault, a statement or remark expressing this', something which involves an 'analytical evaluation'; it can be either a 'positive' or a 'negative' concept. When it is a positive concept, the individual learns from the experience of being critical, learns to problem-solve, and grow.

As an example of this positive criticism, David (one of the authors) remembers an incident from his practice:

> 'I made a drug error. I thought about ignoring it, but quickly decided to report it. She was reviewed by the medical team and we monitored her physical health as she slept, a little longer than normal. I learnt I was in an organisation that was compassionate and learnt to check and re-check when administering medication.'

Generally, self-criticism is viewed as a negative concept, because it is known to frequently stop growth and drain energy (Strengthscope, 2019; Linley, Willars & Biswas-Diener, 2010). Gilbert (2013) states self-criticism is the 'fear of compassion', relating this to feelings of frustration and anger. Neff (2003a, b & c) says self-criticism has three main sub-themes of self-judgement, including self-condemnation, social isolation, and intrusive thoughts. Gilbert (2013) relates this social isolation to 'avoidant behaviour patterns', 'fear of exposure', and considers the intrusive thoughts as people seeking new ways to self-condemn.

Health professionals, like most other people, often dismiss praise that they receive. A doctor who responded to an ex-patient commenting, 'You saved my life, thank you!' may well respond by saying, 'Well, that's my job!' Diminishing and possibly dismissing our own achievements can negatively impact on our self-esteem and self-efficacy levels. This 'modesty' is the negativity bias in action (Covert & Reeder, 1990; Rozin & Royman, 2001; Rashid, 2015, Fredrickson, 2012).

Hayes, Strosahl, and Wilson (2011) argue that one of the answers to negativity is to learn to accept it as part of the whole self. Fredrickson's (2012) research confirms that positivity includes the ability to counter the negative. Losada and Heapy (2004), Gottman (1994), and Jenner (1997) all argue that the individual and those around them need to try to address the imbalance of negative statements by applying more positive statements, and that there needs to be far more positive statements; our natural tendency is to focus on the negative. It could be argued, therefore, that the media emphasis on reporting deaths needs to be refocused instead on the numbers who are recovering from COVID-19.

Sometimes the self-esteem and self-efficacy is supported or compromised by self and social comparison (Festinger, 1954; Kanten & Tiegen, 2008; McInerney & Putwain, 2017). Gilbert (2013) says, "from school through to later life, we 're encourages to compare ourselves with others". For Neff (2011) also, self-comparison is something that we do naturally. The theory of *social* comparison was first proposed by Festinger (1954), when he suggested that individual behaviour is changed to allow them to fit in with other people, particularly those who are similar to themselves. Marsh & Parker (1984) and McInerney & Putwain (2017) both affirm that this comparison can, in fact, help to build our self-esteem, although Renick and Harter (1989) warn it could also help to tear down self-esteem.

Kanten and Tiegen's (2008) research shows that we often negatively compare ourselves to our earlier life. For staff going through the pandemic, this may mean that they compare their earlier performance to their current performance, where more people are dying than normal, and may begin to view their old self as successful and their present self as unsuccessful.

'I (David) was talking to a community mental health nurse, who was visiting Sam in order to administer his regular depot injection. He approached their door, then on the doorstep he "gowned up", put on gloves and a visor (his personal protective equipment), then rang the doorbell. He said the individual's paranoid feelings were increased by his appearance. He didn't say it, but I wondered if he was comparing this relationship with the previous one, and part of him was feeling guilt at causing increased anxiety and at the same time he was happy that he managed to give the injection and kept himself safe in the process.'

'Esteem' is to 'have a high regard for, greatly respect, and think favourably of' (Oxford University Press, 1996). Self-esteem is, effectively, respecting oneself. It is understanding who you currently are, and it is influenced by what we have done or achieved and what we believe and value. 'Efficacy', meanwhile, is defined as 'sure to produce the desired effect' (Oxford University Press, 1996); it can be seen that self-efficacy is to do with the 'I', choosing to know how to produce or do something, and then opting to do it.

Self-efficacy is associated with the ability to self-regulate (Wolters and Pintrich, 1998). The effective individual is able to 'analyse and evaluate their own behaviour thought and emotions …' choosing and pursuing their 'goals' (Maddux and Kleiman, 2016) and further includes the regulation or our emotional responses to events (Bong and Skaalvik, 2003).

Applying self-esteem and self-efficacy to the healthcare professional, they can say, for example, 'I am a good nurse' and 'I chose to provide compassionate care to a person or a group of people'.

The promotion of higher levels of self-esteem and self-efficacy leads to increased levels of success, which in turn leads to higher levels of self-esteem and self-efficacy (Zimmermann, 1995; Bong and Clark, 1999; Liu, Kaplan and Risser, 1992).

Both positive self-esteem and higher levels of self-efficacy, then, are protective factors for mental health (Rutter, 1997); Shoshani and Steinmetz, (2014) confirm that the level of self-esteem relates directly to the level of mental illness and mental health, so leaders and other professionals need to focus on promoting mental health in the workplace. This can be achieved by helping the individual teams and healthcare professionals to recognise where they are being successful during the COVID-19 crisis, and this can lead to 'compassion satisfaction'.

One of the dangers of adopting a self-critical approach is an increase in the likelihood of errors, leading to threats to the levels of mental health issue rising and the likelihood of suicide being increased (Neff, 2011).

> 'I (David) remember when I was in practice and Carol "successfully died by suicide", and how it made me feel both guilty and shamed, knowing "I could have done better for her". I was fortunate, as instead of self-medicating with alcohol to forget, which I was encouraged to do, I talked through the issues with my mentor and learnt that although the situation was sad, we did our best.'

This situation could easily have turned into destructive self-criticism and behaviours, negatively impacting self-esteem and self-efficacy, and directly leading to burn out and compassion fatigue. In the COVID-19 crisis, this set of arguments can be applied to where a nurse who does not know that they are ill goes into work and passes the virus on to others to be then diagnosed, and realises that she could have been the reason colleagues and patients were infected. Some work with a trusted and knowledgeable mentor may need to happen to help the nurse express their concerns and rationalise them.

**Burnout, Compassion Fatigue, and Compassion Satisfaction**

As we've seen, exposure to suffering and trauma such as that caused by COVID-19 could also have a detrimental impact on the well-being of healthcare professionals (Sprang, Clark and Whitt-Wosley, 2007; Perry, 2008;

Austin, Goble, Leier and Byrne, 2009; Young, Derr, Cicchillo and Bressler, 2011; Rossi, et al., 2012).

Under normal circumstances, between 16-85% of healthcare workforce are described as suffering from compassion fatigue (Slatten, David, Carson, and Carson, 2011; Potter Deshields and Rodriguez, 2013; Smart et al., 2014). Studies identify compassion fatigue and burnout as barriers to the delivery of compassionate care (Sprang, Clark and Whitt-Woosley, 2007; Perry, 2008; Austin et al., 2009; Young et al., 2011; Rossi et al., 2012).

Many of the theorists writing about burnout and compassion fatigue state that they are interchangeable concepts (Nimmo and Huggard, 2013; Jenkins and Warren, 2012; Sodeke-Gregson, Holttum, and Billings, 2013; Hegney, et al., 2014). However, it has equally been argued that compassion fatigue is a concept in two parts: the first being burnout and the second being the negative feelings related to this. These may be fear, intrusive thoughts, and avoidance, plus periods of hyper-vigilance (which is often related to Post-Traumatic Stress Disorder) (van Mol, Kompanje, Benoit, Bakker and Nijkamp, 2015; Cocker, 2016).

Burnout may develop through factors such as working excessive hours in stressful and unsupportive work environments impacting on individual's capacity to care (Rossi, et al., 2012; Schaufeli and Bakker, 2013). Compassion fatigue is something that develops over time (Zhang, Zhang, Xiao Rong Han, Wei, Ying-Lei Weung (2018). Hooper, et al. (2010) see it as the cost of caring for others in emotional distress. It has been referred to as the 'helper syndrome' (Figley, 1995) and simply 'caring too much' (Yoder, 2010). Circenis and Millere (2011) suggested the triggers were continual use of emotional energy and empathy, which may then be potentiated by some previous personal trauma and prolonged secondary trauma, all resulting in both objectifying and depersonalisation of the patient and their suffering. A qualitative study on compassion fatigue in Canada (Austin, et al., 2012), exploring the experiences of both adult and mental health nurses, found that participants were shielding and distancing themselves from the suffering of patients and their families, were emotionally detached from patients, and experienced feelings of irritability, anger and negativity which they tried to ignore in order to cope with their work. Participants reported feeling overwhelmed, disengaged, impotent, hopeless, and ineffective and felt they were not as competent and committed as they used to be. They spoke of trying to 'survive' and questioned their own professional identity and the kind of nurses they used to be. Hence, it can be argued that while healthcare professionals are encouraged to strive to towards achieving compassionate care, there needs to be effective supportive structures and systems to minimise the risk of compassion fatigue and burnout.

Compassion fatigue results in a diminished capacity to care, high levels of absenteeism, workforce drop-out and poor quality of care (Nimmo and Huggard, 2013); the individual feels both physical and mental exhaustion and does not cope well with their environment (Cocker and Joss, 2016). Matters become more complicated when one person who is suffering from burnout or compassion fatigue is on the team, and thus unable to fulfil their full clinical role: others on the team may have to compensate to provide good quality care, and soon this situation can lead to a whole team suffering from compassion fatigue.

Strengthscope (2019) warns that those who overuse their strength of compassion can become exhausted as they allow others to take advantage of them. For example, as students are expected to go into practice with increased responsibility and expectations, their new and often ill-defined or emerging roles may increase pressure, while at the same time students have to complete academic assignments and practice assessment documents. The pressure is on – and the danger of burnout is high. Careful management, which has elements of emotional and behavioural support, and raising positive achievements is clearly needed.

There needs to be effective supportive structures and systems to minimise the risk of compassion fatigue and burnout. What can be done to help prevent burnout and compassion fatigue in these times of COVID-19? There are two methods that are demonstrated to be effective: one is that of developing compassion satisfaction and the other is self-compassion (Neff, 2003a, b, and c; Gilbert 2013).

Compassion satisfaction is an 'expression of the positive aspects of caring' (Zhang, et al., 2018) (Table 1).

| Table 1: Compassion Satisfaction ||
| --- | --- |
| **Compassion Satisfaction Promoter** | **Reference** |
| Compassionate organisation, which is positive and effective work environments | (c), (d) |
| Building social supports at work | (a), (c) |
| Building work relationships | (a) |
| Effective support of leader who are seen and this includes a supportive supervisory element | (a), (e) |
| Effective support of managers | (e) |
| Effective mentoring | (a) |
| When the individual feels valued by others | (c), (d) |
| Finding space to look after oneself, so you need to take your breaks, eat healthy, sleep. | (a) |
| References: (a) Alkema, Linton and Davies, 2008. (b) Amin, Vankar, Nimbalkar and Phatak, 2017. (c) Ariapooran, 2014. (d) Slatten, David, Carson, and Carson, 2011. (e) Wu, Singh-Carlson, Odell, Reynolds, and Su, 2016. ||

An example: A student nurse who has gone to her student employee placement is greeted by the ward manager, who recognises that coming into her placement at this time might lead to burnout. They then proceed to explain how the student will be supported in the situation, demonstrating a compassionate organisation, a supportive environment, building a work relationship, and initiating an effective mentoring relationship.

## Self-Compassion

Men are more likely, it seems, to be self-compassionate than women (Neff, 2003a): in the NHS, which employs more women than men, self-compassion becomes even more important.

But what is it? Self-compassion is 'self-nurturing, looking after the self, teaching self, self-mentoring, self-soothing, self-protection, self-acceptance, and self-belonging' (adapted from Gilbert, 2013). Neff (2003a, b, and c) identifies three sub-themes of self-compassion: self-kindness, understanding common humanity, and adopting mindfulness techniques.

Those that are self-compassionate develop self-soothing and self-reassuring behaviours (Gilbert & Miles, 2000; Gilbert, 2005; Gilbert, Clarke, Hemple, Miles and Irons, 2004). These increase the person's ability to self-regulate (Terry & Leary, 2011) and to develop general coping skills (Neff, Hseih & Dejitthirat, 2004; Allen & Leary, 2000), such as asking for help (Neff, Rude and Kirkpatrick, 2007) and learning to be assertive.

Those that operate in self compassion will have higher levels of energy (Strengthscope, 2019; Linley, Willars, and Biswas-Diener, 2010). People can learn to be self-compassionate (Bluth, 2017; Germer, 2009) and it is a quality that can be modelled (why not think of someone you think is self-compassionate, then think about what they do to show this, before thinking how you can adopt some of these strategies).

## Self-Kindness

Those that are self-kind learn several key lessons, which recognise their own value and importance to society. Reynolds, Palmer, and Green (2019) highlight that this is about learning the lesson of being 'kinder to themselves, even in highly negative experiences'. The self-kind can be in positions where they feel out of control, but rather than crumble under the pressure they 'accept' the feelings, embrace the situation, and commit to some form of action (Craske and Hazett-Stevens, 2002; Robins, Schmidt III, and Lineham, 2011).

The self-kind develop positive relationships (Neff and Vonk, 2009), which is healthy because it leads to flourishing and well-being (Seligman, 2011). These positive relationships are based on mutual respect, and the knowledge that they are reciprocal in nature mean both sides can seek help from the other when this is needed. Warren, Smeets, and Neff, (2016) and Neff, Rude, and Kirkpatrick (2007) all record that those operating in self-kindness will ask for help and be happy to accept this.

The self-kind are not afraid to make mistakes (Hall and Fincham, 2005; Neely, Schallet, Mohammed, Roberts, and Chen, 2009) and know that they can learn from the situation, having what Dweck (2017) called a 'growth mindset'.

One element of self-kindness is the ability to self-forgive, which includes 'feelings, actions, and beliefs about self in relation to a perceived or a real transgression (Wohl, DeShea, and Wahkinney, 2008). When the individual takes responsibility for a mistake, they re-affirm their values and seek to make reparations (Fisher and Exline, 2010; Wenzel, Woodyatt, and Hedrick, 2012), effectively demonstrating their ability to learn from and to self-forgive (Bell, Davis, Griffin, Ashby, and Rice, 2017).

Strengthscope (2019) warns that the person who operates in compassion may put other people's needs before themselves, and this can become draining. Indeed, the NMC (2008) in their Code of Conduct used to tell us, 'Make the care of people your first concern, treating them with dignity and respect.' This was removed, as it misses the idea that sometimes our own needs have to be met so we can care for others. We need our breaks, space for us to reflect, to eat, drink, and hopefully socialise.

Another issue that can obstruct self-kindness is the need to operate in perfectionism. This can come from a genuine need, for example a surgeon needs to be perfect at what they do. However, we often do things to avoid being negatively judged and condemned. The perfectionist writer may write, edit, re-edit, and never submit their work because of the need to feel their work is perfect; their effort is all about getting that perfect score and ignores other needs. One lesson of self-kindness is that we need to decide when we have reached the 'good enough' stage.

Neff and Vonk (2009) remind us it is easier to be kind towards others than it is to be kind to self. They suggest that this could be a starting point for developing self-kindness. Imagine you are really upset after making an error. Pause a moment, then imagine this was your best friend in distress. Then hear yourself give them your best advice, listening carefully for responses so you can respond helpfully. Once all the advice is exhausted, switch positions and imagine your best friend giving you the same advice. Hear what is said, and as you hear, confirm to yourself you will take these lessons on.

**Common Humanity**

'Common humanity' is an important sub-theme of self-compassion (Neff 2003a, b, and c) and it is closely related to our need to belong one to another (Maslow, 2013). Common humanity is recognising that we are all part of humanity, that one needs to see 'one's experience as part of the human experience' (Neff, 2020).

Suffering is one of the factors of common humanity, and learning lessons from the suffering of those around us, seeing how they cope, and then copying these behaviours is one element (Neff, 2011; Reynolds, Palmer, and Green, 2019). Germer (2009) argues that common humanity is about learning how individuals face their adversities and dilemmas. Neff, Kirkpatrick, and Rude (2007a, b) and Frankl (2011) suggest that when individuals face suffering and adversities, they can find meaning, and in finding meaning they build hope.

Togashi and Kottler (2015) remind us that the individual yearns for connectedness to other human beings. Zimmermann, et al., (2019, p.6), commenting on the idea of 'being human amongst humans' (Kohut, 1981) (sometimes called twinning), suggest 'we look to find in the other an experience of likeness, a feeling of sameness that is shared, which results in the consolidation of self-experience'. We thus understand that 'all human beings are fallible...' (Neff, 2011, p.62), that we all make 'wrong choices', and that 'feelings of regret are inevitable'. This is reassuring, as it can mean that we begin to understand 'imperfection is part of being a human being' (Neff, 2017). So, rather than having to push people away because I am feeling different, ashamed, or guilty about something, I can choose to see that we are all the same. I can share my issues, with less likelihood of being condemned; it is more likely, then, that I will receive help.

## Mindfulness

Mindfulness is considered one of the key sub-themes of self compassion (Neff, 2003a, b, c). It teaches the mind to be flexible (Hsu & Langer, 2013). For Kabat-Zinn (2014) mindfulness is about knowing oneself better so that we learn to mobilize personal resources in problem solving. It involves both formal and informal exercises, the formal being to learn and practice the discipline, while the informal is adopting mindfulnessapproaches in different everyday situations (Shapiro, de Sousa & Hauck, 2016; Bluth, 17; Germer, 2009; Altman, 2011).

Mindfulness can be easily integrated into everyday life (Altman, 2011; Brown, Ryan, and Cresswell, 2007). It is used to help the individual to address issues of intrusive thoughts, including fear and rumination on fear (Neff, 2003a, b, c. Neff, Rude and Kirkpatrick, 2017a) and it intends to help the individual to balance their individual experiences (Arimitsu, 2016).

To become a non-attached, impartial witness and using all of their senses is the objective of mindfulness (Germer, 2009; Kabit-Zinn, 2014). The exercises should be non-judgemental (Orsillo, Roemer, Blocklerner, and Tull, 2011) and this allows this to be open to the emotional, logical and behavioural experiences (Altman, 2011; Shapiro, de Sousa, and Hauck, 2016).

There are many different exercises that can be completed to help us to learn the lessons of mindfulness, and to do these over a period of time to help them to become a habit is important (Altman, 2011; Kabit-Zinn, 2014). It is important to sometimes change the exercise, but not the habit, as this will help maintain the learning (Lyubomirsky, 2012).

Examples of exercise include meditations (Neff and Germer, 2018), loving-kindness meditations (Fredrickson, Cohn, Coffey, Pek, and Finkel, 2008; Zeng, Chiu, Wang, Oei, and Leung, 2015; Hoffman, Grossman, and Hinton, 2011) and body scanning (Akhtar, 2018). Further exercises can be found in Altman, 2011; Bluth, 2017; Germer, 2009; and Kabit-Zinn, 1994, 2014).

## Final Thoughts

'It's a very, very important time for all of us and it has changed us!' says Estelle Kabia-Caulker, a third stage mental health student (note this quote was used with permission from the student). She is so right about this, but the question remains: are we being changed negatively or positively? Are we shifting towards burnout and compassion fatigue or more positively towards compassion satisfaction and self-compassion? If we are to move towards the positive, it will partially involve factors external to self; for example, how governments, organisations, and teams are functioning and making decisions to support staff. In part, moving towards the positive is an internal process, and involves how we choose to view things (moving from a negativity bias to a positivity bias); learning about and choosing to operate in self compassionate ways, including self-kindness, self-forgiveness, understanding that we are all humans who make mistakes, and learning to be awake in the present moment.

# Solitude - Threat or Opportunity?

*Martin Weegmann*

The current crisis has forced a vocabulary upon us: lockdown, social distancing, shielding, isolating, quarantine. They might be necessary, but these and similar terms have powerful connotations. Solitary confinement is considered the worst sanction meted out in prisons, and for most people the idea living in (imposed) separation from family or friends for a long period would be a living hell.

On the other hand, to be *with* certain others at close quarters would be hellish for some people. Lockdown, curfew, and grounding are terms normally associated with punishment. Quarantine is a chilling word, first used to reference leprosy and subsequently applied to the Black Death and plagues. In the psychiatric and psychological literature, quarantine is associated with negative states- stress, stigma, fear, and grief (Brooks, et. Al., 2020). Isolation is even spoken of as a disease and societal curse, given what is known about its deleterious impact on health and well-being (Griffin, 2010). Even on a temporary basis, for some people, the prospect of even a few evenings alone would be a challenge, as if being torn asunder from the sustenance of social bonds.

What might the threat of confinement and of having more time in one's own company be? While I do not dispute the evidence and reality of the negative consequences of isolation and separation, I want to leave to one side what Kemp elsewhere in this book calls a 'rhetoric of fear' and explore the positive potential of solitude in particular. Solitude, whether practised far from or relatively close by to others (people can be 'alone together'), is a somewhat elusive notion, more a quality than a physical fact. I draw on a range of resources, from the spiritual and literary, before turning to clinical considerations.

## Monasticism: Spiritual Traditions

*Monasticism,* in ancient Greek connotations, is to do with being 'alone' and in Western and Near East monasticism it is associated with living a self-disciplined, devotional life in relative isolation from society, or at least with much-reduced interaction with others. Elsewhere, in Asia and the far East, whilst monasticism has different hues and tones, there are similarities with Western traditions, at least in form.

The image of a Lord, prophet, or some other holy man receiving insights and revelations in a secluded and bare environment- a desert, cave, wilderness, or from a height- separated from others but subsequently communicating their experience to followers, disciples, the uninitiated, and so on, is a common cultural template (Shapin, 1991). Spiritual journeys, from a point of departure, through a stage of privation and trial, and re-entry into to wider society, are ways of marking time and cultural rites of passage. According to Van Gennep (1960) and Turner (1969), rites of passage are about how a person or lead through a liminal, 'betwixt and between' phase (a threshold) which results in social graduation- a 'coming of age', ordination, consecration, naming, marriage, and so on. On the other side of the threshold, as it were, the person(s) gain admission into a community or fellowship of some kind. Holy men or women are different in that they lead rather than are led (at least not by human beings), and in this sense have an elevated spiritual status. They are 'spiritual virtuosos' who inspire others (Weber, 1963).

The Desert Fathers (and Mothers) and hermits of early Christian tradition sought refuge in the deserts of Egypt, Palestine, and Syria, and their examples led to the development of formal monasticism (Chadwick, 1993). Their acts of retreat were modelled on Christ's life, time in the desert, and Passion. Deserts, as emblematic places, were both frightening and heavenly (Enenkel and Göttler, 2018). For Anthony the Great (later St. Anthony), solitude, asceticism, and sacrifice were alternatives to becoming a martyr in a time prior to the legalisation of Christianity. Paradoxically, for solitary ventures, hermits attracted others; pilgrims came to visit and before long 'deserts became cities'. There were three main kinds of monastic model: (a) that of the hermit, living in complete separation and austerity; (b) the coenobitic life (from the Greek for 'common' and 'life'), consisting of communities of monks (over time hermits became monks) and nuns living a strict, devotional life; and (c) much smaller groups of monks and nuns gathered around a spiritual leader. Monasteries were formalised, each order devising its own complicated codes of eating, silence, prayer, recitation, stillness, rest, welfare, and housekeeping; the cultivation of 'solitude together'.

By the early medieval period, there were many monastic orders, both great and small. The proliferation of monasteries and hermits posed a threat to the authorities, evoking fears of heresy, so much so that by 1215, the Lateran council forbad the forming of new orders. With 'wilderness' and 'desert' a metaphor as much as a physical place, new spaces of retreat arose, like the small islands favoured by Celtic Christians (called 'deserts in the sea') and urban versions, with town hermits and recluses (Hill, 1993). Some towns in England, such as Norwich and York, had many such places and individuals who, acting as spiritual counsellors and arbiters, were much visited, including an interesting sub-type: the anchorite.

The anchorite or anchoress is a person (from the Greek *anachorein* — to retire or retreat) who voluntarily withdrew from society into a small physical space, a cell or anchor-hold, built usually beside a church (Dyas, et al., 2005). The decision to enter such spaces, duly consecrated, was a decisive 'separation from a previous world', using a phrase from Van Gennep (1960, p. 21). Whereas hermits travelled, anchorites, by definition, stayed put, sometimes to the ends of their lives, their solitude sealed by physical enclosure, their minimal needs met by means of a hole in the wall.

One famous anchoress- also the first-known female author of a book in England and a contemporary of Chaucer- was the mystic Julian of Norwich (Windeatt, 2015). Julian's remarkable *Revelations of Divine Love* (2015) are her reflections upon a series of visons (or 'showings') she experienced about Christ and God; other than her spiritual reflections, we know virtually nothing of her actual life. The notion of life modelled on 'divine example', and the literature of 'exempla', was influential in medieval times, including the physical imitation of Christ's suffering and asceticism, vows of poverty and other forms of self-privation.

The solitude sought by such persons for reasons of spiritual perfection was not so much that of an 'isolated person' alone with their thoughts, in the way in which we may see it nowadays; assorted mystics, monks, hermits, and anchoresses did not regard themselves as being alone, but as always in the presence of God, as they understood God. Julian used another medieval trope of 'un-making' herself, or of 'setting at naught', so as to invite openness to Divinity and the three wounds of 'compassion, contrition, and longing for God' (McNamer, 2010, p. 7). In one section, Julian describes a vision of God showing her a small object, like a hazelnut. She writes this up as a parable to demonstrate the fact that God created it (the nut representing the world), loves it, and cares for it; 'Truly the maker, the carer, and the lover' (Julian of Norwich, 2015, p. 45). With astonishing theological independence and striking self-expression through writing, Julian's solitude allows her to ensilage a God as all-enveloping, mother-like figure, who forever embraces us as his children (Windeatt, 2015); the 'simple soul should come to him in a bare, plain, and homely way' (op. cit., p. 46). Holed up, quite literally, Julian was never alone in this sense.

A survey of different spiritual traditions would require far more knowledge and more space than I have. Asian and far-Eastern spiritualities, or codes, or ways, have so much to teach us about the value of solitude; each has its own mystics, hermits, wandering wise-men, and versions of monastic living (Holm and Bowker, 1994). Early Buddhism regarded monastic calling and its various stages of retreat (including the avoidance of the 'talking life') as the royal road to liberation. While ordinary people may fear solitude, religious masters embrace it as the ultimate form of surrender, wonder, and connection with the whole; a sense of unification, calm, or enlightenment results.

Whilst being a whole other subject, it is interesting how much modern, particularly Western psychology and mindfulness practice, takes its cues and actively borrows from ancient, eastern spiritual traditions (Kuyken and Feldman, 2019). Not only this, but 'retreats' are everywhere, and so too is well-being tourism.

## Literary Solitudes

If the religious and spiritual have their special places of submission and purification, so too have the writers and poets with their garrets, libraries, 'rooms with views', hallowed interiors, huts, second homes in the country, and so on (Bergmann, 2017). Eugene O'Neil's plays are often inspired by his own family experiences, and yet he wrote them in rigorous, silent isolation, his writing rooms set high and away from the household (Gelb and Gelb, 1960). One can have mental retreats even if one does not have physical retreat, where the literary, scholarly, or religious self is cultivated. The mode and medium of writing itself shapes the outpourings of solitude, as in the case of the protestant spiritual diary, which acts like a 'disclosing enclosure' of self-examination and moral accounting (Botanaki, 1999; Windeatt, 2016). If not spiritually conceived, however, spaces and places of literary inspiration are endowed with a secular aura, hallowed inasmuch as they support or allow creative activity. Foucault's (1986) notion of heterotopias is useful, in that while such places exist in reality (unlike utopias), they are marked aside as being distinct from their surroundings (e.g. rural/urban, interior/exterior) just as distinctions like sacred/profane or divine/earthy apply to religious sites (Stenger, 2018). Non-disturbance, an important aspect of solitude, helps the aesthetic process — hence, Keats found inspiration 'by my solitary hearth' and Wordsworth 'wondered lonely as a cloud', to name but two of the Romantic writers, even if they were otherwise sociable people (quoted in Shapin, 1991).

In 19th century America, Emily Dickinson retreated into the interior of her father's house (although she still had visitors), famed as reclusive poet. If the language of 'privacy' and 'withdrawing rooms' and chambers was already there in the culture, Dickinson turned them into art forms, the 'company of one' and in so doing, 'fashioned a radical interior life by shunning a conventional exterior one' (Fuss, 1998, p. 3). Whether Dickinson's life of retreat is pathologised or romanticised, her withdrawal, and the astonishing uses to which she put solitude, is unquestioned. Dickinson (1994) is a poet who turned things on their head when she posed questions such as, 'It might be lonelier, without the Loneliness' and posited, 'That solar privacy, A soul admitted to itself'.

A near-contemporary of Dickinson, writer Henry David Thoreau (1817–1862) famously turned his back on town-life, built a hut in the woods, and in writing the book *Walden*, became a philosopher of solitude (Lovell, 2017). Thoreau regarded solitude as his companion and did not see himself as hermit — like Dickinson, he also had (some) visitors. A student of Emerson, Thoreau is celebrated as a philosopher of self-reliance and independence of spirit, both related to American values, and for forging a new relationship with nature, even if he was judged a loner and a crank by some contemporaries. Negative judgements of this sort are amongst the hazards that such individuals bear; there are plenty of other philosophers, and the religious, who opposed solitude as a 'monkish virtue', one more likely to inflate the ego than reduce it, even as encouraging sinful melancholia. Part of the transcendentalist movement, Emerson, Thoreau, and others turned to Nature rather than God. Thoreau was famed for his minute observations of his surroundings; finding beauty in the small things and tranquil participation in his surroundings mattered. It is argued that in the transcendentalist approach, 'nature becomes a field of exchange, even a kind of sociability for the receptive soul' (Lovell, 2017, p. 127). The ancient metaphor of the wilderness was reconfigured, as no longer being a place of privation or deformed chaos but one of fullness and wonder, just as it was for the Romantics or the 19th century landscape painters (Thomas, 1984). Prompting the modern conservationist movement, Thoreau's spot by the pond (made now a monument of stones) is a visiting place for secular pilgrims. In a memorable passage, Thoreau (2017, p. 132) connects the solitary to the social, when he wrote, 'I had three chairs in my house; one for solitude, two for friendship, and three for society.'

## Deconstructing the Clinic

Shifting to a different domain, I will briefly explore some clinical aspects of the situation in which psychotherapists and their patients are finding themselves, using my own practice (NHS community services and small independent practice) as a reference point.

The first thing to acknowledge is that within an incredibly short space of time our existing (previous) assumptions and usual 'frames' of how we work have gone. For example, we are accustomed to working from the vantage point of the consulting room — the territory of the clinic — with the patient who makes the journey to see us. By definition, the consulting room or clinic is away from the patient's home, which we do not see — that is their private domain and a separation of home/therapy is built into the arrangement. This is the same for the therapist, except for those who do private work from their own homes or who (far more, now) conduct online therapy from their homes.

Regarding the home/therapy distinction, I know of one patient who finds the act of attending a clinic to be a grounding experience, 'real' somehow, and that having online therapy at home undermines a separation they would prefer to maintain between the two. Another patient spoke of the positive structure that is provided by the practical act of getting ready for an appointment, leaving the house, and the train journey there and back. Environments matter, and much depends on material space and circumstance; home is not always safe. It must be asked, what does the patient return to?

I am impressed by the wide variety of responses my patients have shown to the national emergency. At the onset, I had rather assumed that most people would approach the prospect of lockdown and isolation with dread, and some *are* clearly struggling: 'it's come at the worst possible time' commented a depressed patient who abhors their own company. Others adapted quickly and some enjoy more time alone. Some seemed ahead of me, so to speak, and were relieved by my decision (slightly belated in their view) to suspend face-to-face therapy, intuiting that it was difficult for me or the service to accept (which it is).

Two long-term patients, both generally comfortable with their own company, are amongst those who have positively embraced the current situation. Both are creative and have found themselves with more time than they previously had to devote to such activities. Of this new time, one said something along the lines of, 'now I can actually have those conversations within myself that were mostly postponed'.

I often inquire of my patients, 'What sort of company do you keep with yourself'? Or variations upon, 'Do you have a friendly relationship with yourself?' and 'What is it like when you are alone?' I also like to know, 'How do you spend and enjoy time when away from others?' Our trainings place great premium upon relationality and the centrality of human attachments, the capacity to have close relationships, for obvious reasons. However, this can creep into a range of normative assumptions about human life and how it is meant to develop, as in the idea that 'interpersonal relationships of an intimate kind are the chief, if not the only, source of human happiness' (Storr, 1988, p. ix). Those who have not attained such a state, or at least experienced it at some point, are easily viewed as incomplete individuals who illustrate developmental deficits. If internalised by the person concerned, as they often are, they carry considerable shame for not measuring up to a societal standard. One patient complained that everything they watched on television was oriented towards couples and dating — and predominantly heterosexual couples at that — or towards families; 'It's not me!' they protested. Storr (op. cit.) incisively points out that these kinds of assumptions about the nature of 'true happiness' are relatively new in historical terms, and in acknowledgment of Winnicott, reminds us that the capacity to be alone is itself an important capacity. Winnicott (2018) noted that more had been written by previous psychoanalysts on the fear or the wish to be alone than on the *ability* to be alone.

There are some times of transition and particular distress, such as bereavement, loss of job, divorce, or receiving a serious medical diagnosis, in which some people (and this is hard to predict who) require and benefit from a period of withdrawal; their friends and therapists can find this a challenge and seek assurances that the person is 'okay'. Cohen (2017) suggest that such times and states invite or require a 'deep solitude' that is important for psychological restoration and may be a precondition for it. One might speculate that the person concerned needs time to 'regroup' themselves and find catharsis, even to dull the pain, for want of better descriptions. With such a societal and therapeutic emphasis on loneliness and the 'hole' that, say, a loss entails, we may miss the restorative aspects of solitude. Not only this, but times of significant change and transition are times 'when one's narrative of self-identity and relationships with others that may have been taken for granted for many years may need to be reframed, reinterpreted, and revised' (p. 163). Relative solitude may, like aesthetic retreat, help some people to 'stop' participation in life-as-usual and to take stock.

## Conclusion

Solitude proves difficult to define, being something more than simply being alone. A secluded activity, solitude is usually a choice and has an intentional quality — a person does something with the time they set aside, creating a mental clearing. But are reading, prayer, fishing, walking, and gardening necessarily expressions of solitude, or are they simply activities performed by oneself whilst (relatively) alone? Is solitude in everyday life a cultivated, mindful deed rather than an automatic activity? Mere withdrawal is not the same as solitude. Does solitude require special time to be set aside, and demand a particular space, even if that is mental space? However, solitude is defined, I suggest that we can learn a great deal about it from some of the religious, philosophical, and literary authors that I have made reference to.

Not everyone enjoys the current restrictions on our freedom of movement, and some actively hate it. Most are pragmatic and are adapting their lives accordingly. On the positive side, and where the right conditions are present, the current situation allows some time and space for people to develop a relationship with themselves, for which solitude is of great assistance. Might it even be that therapy, for those who attend, is a modern form of retreat, in the presence of another?

# Moral Injury and Rehabilitation in the COVID-19 World

*Dr Scott Galloway*

## The COVID-19 Context

On the 12th March 2020, the COVID-19 outbreak was declared a pandemic, with significantly higher mortality rates than other recent pandemics (Williamson, Murphy and Greenburg, 2020). Vulnerabilities were quickly identified, particularly in the elderly and those with pre-existing medical conditions. As the virus took hold across the UK, and the mortality rate in other countries mounted, the impacts on an already stretched NHS were expected, and have proved to be extreme, with a need to re-configure, suspend, or re-provide much of the health provision across the UK in order to manage isolation, infection, admission, Intensive Care Unit and death rates.

As the COVID-19 pandemic spreads, and as demand for medical resources outstrips supplies, healthcare professionals may have (had) to choose who among their patients receives the benefit of treatment – and in some cases, make an active choice knowing their decision will influence who lives and who dies. Being forced to make such painful decisions is deeply distressing for staff committed to providing the best possible care for all their patients, and for many staff this will be felt as a direct contradiction of the principle of 'do no harm', as they are forced to make 'least worst decisions' in their care provision.

Just as clinicians grapple with the painful realities of the appearance of COVID-19, the NHS is also having to prepare for a series of 'COVID waves' where successive outbreaks will place sustained strain on the care system and clinical staff. At the same time, across the world, economies are in shutdown and unable to produce the very resources upon which the NHS relies. 'COVID-19 is likely to affect a large proportion of the population ... it may last several years ... there is little or no surge capacity in the NHS, and it is possible that serious health needs may outstrip availability, and difficult decisions will be required about how to distribute scarce lifesaving resources' (Guidance Note BMA 2020).

Furthermore, the NHS has been subject to years of efficiency drives, accompanied by a population with greater lifespan, an increasing elderly population with more substantial healthcare needs, and the ability to treat ever more complex and life-threatening illnesses across the lifespan. And then came COVID-19 — an unknown challenge with expectations of substantially higher mortality rates than seasonal flu, an unknown disease progression, an unknown (but expected) series of waves of outbreak, the potential for mutation, and no proven vaccine available.

While the infection mortality rate is not yet fully understood, it appears to be considerably higher than that of other recent pandemics, and COVID-19 may therefore place a sustained and substantial demand on an already overstretched National Health Service (NHS), with three specific areas of concern (Williamson, Murphy and Greenburg, 2020):

1) A lack of specific resources

2) the impacts of self-quarantine at home for staff themselves, leading to lower staff numbers to treat ill patients, and potential loss of NHS staff to the disease

3) increased risk from having to perform already highly challenging duties in a more constrained manner.

The anticipated impacts on services have already been apparent, and if demand outstrips the capacity for clinicians to deliver best practice healthcare, they will be forced to make decisions that will deny some patients the care they would ordinarily have received outside of the pandemic. The psychological consequences of being responsible for having to make such painful decisions which contradict deeply held core beliefs as a caregiver might be considered a risk factor for the development of burnout, or even perhaps PTSD (post-traumatic stress disorder) - but a more recent and clinically appropriate concept is potentially at the heart of the inability to provide the best clinical care in the COVID-19 context — that of moral injury.

## Moral Development

The development of a sense of moral injury presupposes both the existence of a personal moral code and a transgression or damage to that code in order for the moral injury to be felt. The development of morality in an internalised moral code has been the subject of Piaget's (1965) defining works, who first described the development of rules of interpersonal behaviour and morality in girls and boys. Lawrence Kohlberg (1974) subsequently demonstrated a stage theory of morality, with the now well-established concept of progression through a succession of moral stages, each one more advanced, and a movement away from self-centredness and towards a morality of the many, where the individual is concerned with serving not their own selfish needs, but the needs of the greater good.

Carol Gilligan and colleagues (e.g. Gilligan and Attanucci, 1988; Gilligan 1993) further developed the conceptualisation of morality, setting out fundamental differences between boys and girls in how their moral codes developed – in essence, boys being more concerned to apply the strict rules of 'the game', and males therefore had a morality based on a defining principle of 'justice'. For girls however, sustaining and not damaging relationships was more important to governing social interaction and behaviour. Gilligan's work recognised a model of morality which for women is founded on a principle of caring for others. The huge body of moral development literature is also consistent in its support of the principle that moral awareness and reasoning increases with a combination of education and age – which also brings social experience, where the moral code underpinning human relationships and conduct is developed and established.

In the context of the impact on healthcare provision for COVID-19, it is easy to see how the clinician's core ideals and 'health care morality', with their strict and powerful ethical codes of 'do no harm', and providing the best clinical care at all times, are compromised. The pragmatic decisions clinicians are forced to make, where clinical need exceeds system capacity or resources sometimes have terrible consequences, and present fundamental challenges to these moral principles. These impacts are referred to as 'moral injury'.

## What Is Moral Injury?

Moral injury had its conceptual and research origins not in healthcare, but in the post-Vietnam War scrutiny of the impacts on veterans of that conflict, first recognised by Camillo Bica and Jonathan Shay, and further developed by Robert Lifton (Molendijk, Kramer & Verweij, 2018). At its core, moral injury is 'damage done to the soul of the individual' (The Moral Injury Project, Syracuse University, 2020) and which crucially 'locates the source of distress in a broken system, not a broken individual' (Dean, Talbot & Dean, 2019).

The term was coined by psychiatrist Jonathan Shay (1994) who viewed moral injury in veterans as having three components:

- Moral Injury appeared from a betrayal of what is morally right,
- by someone who holds legitimate authority,
- in a 'high-stakes situation'.

Moral injury arises from a context or events where there is a compulsion to act, or not act, which is so significantly at odds with one's beliefs and moral principles that it fundamentally undermines those core moral principles. These impacts are not just felt in some abstract code, but strike at the heart of who the clinician is as a caregiver and a person, and may leave them with fractured confidence, doubt their ability as a caregiver, and concerns about their capacity to manage similar circumstances in the future.

Such events are often referred to as 'potentially morally injurious events' and in a wartime context, Litz et al. (2009) described the long-term impacts of potentially morally injurious events, which arose in circumstances where soldiers perpetrated, failed to prevent, or bore witness to events that transcribed deeply-held moral beliefs. Soldiers may have had to watch or participate in acts of intense pain, suffering, and cruelty that shattered their core beliefs about humanity. The psychological, behavioural, spiritual, and social consequences of such events they called "moral injury".

Farnsworth et al (2017) offer a helpful model of moral injury, setting out definitions of three core concepts:

**Morally injurious events:**
Defined as a situation in a 'high-stakes' environment where an individual perceives that an important moral has been violated by the actions of self or others.

**Moral pain:**
The experience of painful and distressing emotions and cognitions with a moral 'content' in response to a morally injurious event.

**Moral injury:**
Moral injury is the damaging consequences of being unable to address or resolve the moral pain precipitated by morally injurious events.

Mollendijk, Kramer, and Verweij (2018) add an important additional dimension to the conceptualisation of moral injury – that of the dynamic interaction between personal attributes, moral codes, and context. Their well-reasoned proposition is that previous models of moral injury imply an application of a rigid and inflexible moral code, and that the appropriate model is one based on a more fluid interplay between moral code, situational context and self-perceptions. The experience of morally injurious events, their impacts and outcomes are therefore different for different people. Beliefs and expectations, values and norms, beliefs, and cognitions are all applied to a specific situation, but are all, in turn, shaped by the individual's experience of that situation, and the overarching context in which s/he is placed.

In healthcare, moral injury has been described as the consequence of 'knowing what patients need and being unable to get it for them' (Dean & Talbot 2020), and which leaves the clinician questioning their own ability, ethics, and morality. As an internal experience, these consequences leave the clinician feeling guilty, angry, depressed, and disgusted (Williamson, Stevelink & Greenberg 2018), and with significant impacts on clinician mental health — a clinician suicide rate has been reported in some countries as being twice that of the general population (Talbot & Dean, 2019).

Williamson, Murphy, and Greenburg (2020 p1) define moral injury as 'the profound psychological distress which results from actions, or lack of actions, and violates one's moral or ethical code' and which leads to negative self-perceptions and profound feelings of shame – that most powerful of painful and self-destructive emotions. These authors set out a number of moral injury risk factors for frontline key workers, particularly germane to the COVID-19 context:

- If there is loss of life to a vulnerable person

- If leaders are not perceived to take responsibility for the damaging event

- If leaders are unsupportive of staff

- If staff are unprepared for the emotional and psychological consequences of the decisions they must make

- If the potentially morally-injurious event(s) occur concurrently with exposure to other traumatic events (e.g. death of a loved one)

- If there is a lack of moral support following the morally traumatic events

**Why Moral Injury? Why Not Burnout or PTSD?**
Why is this 'condition' not burnout, or 'just an extension of burnout'? For many years, clinician burnout has been a painful but frequent consequence of a commitment to providing the best possible healthcare in a context which is

often experienced as unhelpful, or actively disabling, with a disconnect between 'the administrators' and the realities of frontline care. A conflict can emerge between the core belief of providing the patient with the best care and the contextual demands of the NHS, which all too often are felt to detract from the ideal. The long-standing frustrations of a career in this environment can lead to dissatisfaction, demoralization, and burnout.

However, burnout often implies a lack of resilience or some failure of coping in individuals (Dean & Talbot, 2020), but it is not an appropriate attribution to make of the clinician's response to a context of healthcare demand exceeding the care system's capacity to cope. A more relevant concept is that of 'moral distress' — the consequences of a conflict between knowing the right thing to do and not being able to do it, due to the institutional or situational context.

One might argue that moral distress is but an extension of burnout; that may be a supportable position in conceptualising the consequences of the day in, day out process of having to compromise between health care ethical ideals and systemic realities. Yet what happens when the context compels a real and powerful challenge to one's moral code? Moral injury is the result of the profound psychological distress generated from the consequences of one's actions, or the lack of them, which violate a core moral or ethical code.

And why not PTSD? PTSD (Post-Traumatic Stress Disorder) can develop in any situation where a person feels extreme fear, horror, or helplessness and is usually considered to be an understandable consequence of being exposed to horrific or life-threatening experiences – such as motor accidents, being caught in natural disasters, being subjected to assaults, or witnessing violent deaths.

PTSD as described above therefore typically arises from events where the person is either subjected to, or witnesses, events which are deeply traumatic, but which are not usually the consequence of an active choice to commit such acts or to behave in a particular way. Rather, these are events which happen to the individual, and are not done by the individual, and often entail a threat to one's own life.

While experiences of fear or helplessness, or witnessing horrific events may occur in healthcare, and there is certainly a degree of overlap between PTSD and Moral injury — trauma severe enough to cause PTSD may well also cause moral injury. There are, however, key differences in this COVID world that make the causes, contexts, and treatment of moral injury distinct from PTSD. Being forced to make active decisions to treat one patient and withhold care from another is traumatic, and may lead to symptoms of PTSD appearing, but it is also *morally* challenging, and compels the clinician to violate a core, self-defining moral code. It becomes a choice not so much of what is the best treatment I can provide to this patient, but being aware of the consequences for other patients of that choice. The moral injury associated with the consequences to one's professional, personal, and moral beliefs must be addressed as a different construct, with different causes and different treatments.

**Discussion**

The constraints of providing healthcare in the context of the COVID -19 pandemic, challenge the clinician's deepest-held beliefs about what is right and good, self-efficacy and competence, self-esteem and core morality. The inability to provide care, and having to make active decisions to provide care to one person and withhold it from someone in the next bed, is in direct conflict with a caregiver's fundamental beliefs about their role and themselves as a person.

The impacts on the ability to fulfil the clinician role consistent with personal beliefs, training, ethical and experiential learning are significant. While professional, organisational, and situational guidance provides a framework to legitimise a morally injurious decision, it is the consequences of the personal implementation of that decision that must be understood and acknowledged by the senior service leaders.

Evidence has indicated that PTSD sufferers have experienced a threat to their mortality, while moral injury sufferers have 'suffered repeated insults to their morality' (Dean, Talbot, and Dean 2019), and it is this risk in the COVID-19 context that most threatens a legacy of moral injury for overstretched and under-resourced clinicians.

## Protecting Staff from Moral Injury

The implications of moral injury being a manifestation of a 'broken system' are that the responsibility lies not with clinicians needing to develop greater resilience and more effective coping mechanisms, but in the 'system' acknowledging and remediating its shortcomings, acknowledge and support the clinicians who feel the consequences and who make the life and death decisions brought upon them by the institutional shortcomings and overwhelming challenges posed by the pandemic.

Williamson, Murphy, and Greenburg (2020) offer some recommendations of protective factors which organisations should implement to mitigate some of these impacts:

1. Frontline staff should be briefed about the potential for morally-injurious events, and the thoughts, feelings, and behaviours that may result.
2. Have these briefing discussions led by high-level supervisory staff (to ensure the service leadership acknowledges and 'owns' the challenges and the context in which staff will have to work).
3. Managers should encourage staff to seek early appropriate support (and ensure that the offer of such support is not associated with a failure of coping or resilience on the clinician's part).
4. If informal help does not work (i.e. difficulties are not resolved and persist) – provide access to professional help as soon as possible (and ensure that such support is provided in the longer term)
5. Ensure these resources are available, well-advertised, and that professionals providing support are briefed about and understand Moral Injury (induct clinicians who may not have had experience of moral injury in the important similarities but differences in clinical approaches between PTSD and moral injury)

6. Leaders should proactively check in with teams, be empathic, and encourage help-seeking (and sustain this empathic exploration well beyond the duration of the pandemic).
7. Psychological screening and debriefing techniques are ineffective – healthcare organisations must:
   a. (Continue to) monitor staff exposed to potentially morally-injurious events
   b. Facilitate effective team cohesion (acknowledge and reflect different coping styles, individually different emotional and psychological consequences, and identify and establish organisational, and personal support processes)
   c. Provide readily available informal and formal psychological support

And for those staff *providing* such support:

1. Ensure the care is prioritised and accessible to front line staff (this will require organisational and leadership commitment in the face of systemic resource challenges).
2. Clinicians must be aware of the reticence of moral injury sufferers to disclose and address deep feelings of guilt and shame, and sensitively explore these issues (and must sustain the empathic exploration of these issues in therapy, from within an informed treatment model).
3. Ensure supportive treatment continues to be available in the long term.
4. Clinical staff must maintain contact with (other) vulnerable patient groups and ensure they too can continue to access care, remotely if needs be (service leads may need to establish and sustain new, flexible ways of working to enable access to treatment for these groups)
5. Clinicians should encourage patients to seek and use coping mechanisms and resources, and limit viewing of COVID-related news and information.

Professional bodies also have an important responsibility in developing ethical guidelines which clarify changed expectations, processes, and clinical practice in the face of impacts on care-provision capacity. Many professional bodies such as the British Medical Association (2020), the Royal College of Physicians (2020), and the British Psychological Society (2020) have been quick to produce such guidance which is essential to clarify what, and to what extent, best practice rules have been adapted in the face of the pandemic challenges. Such guidance can afford some reassurance where personal morality is challenged by situational context, with authoritative 'permission' to behave in ways which would not ordinarily be professionally acceptable.

Much has been written about ethics and clinical decision-making, and long-held guidance has had to be rapidly re-framed. For example, the Royal College of Physicians (2020) has produced an ethical framework to support decision-making during the pandemic, with specific guidance on expected clinical and resource decision-making underpinned by a set of core values:

- Accountability
- Inclusivity
- Transparency
- Reasonableness
- Responsiveness

The intention of this guidance is to 'promote action and decisions that are fair, reciprocal, respectful, and equitable' and to support clinicians as they cope with increasing demand.

While such guidance may offer support in the heat of the COVID-19 battle, it cannot be assumed to provide a longer-term 'inoculation' against the development of moral injury-related consequences as the world transitions into 'the new normal'. Evidence from the experience of wartime trauma suggests that as veterans return to and re-engage with a 'normal' world and a peacetime moral code re-asserts itself, they reflect on and judge themselves and their wartime actions – sometimes harshly. As Molendijk, Kramer, and Verweij (2018) note, 'undeniably, guilt can also be appropriate' (p.38) and as the morally-injured person reconnects with a non-conflict (or non-COVID) world, retrospective personal judgements about actions in the heat of battle are often stained with shame and guilt. The thoughts 'I should have done better' or 'I could have done better' mean that moral injury may emerge when clinicians have had time to reflect on and judge themselves against their ethical and moral codes.

Senior leaders in healthcare must therefore continue to observe, identify, and support clinicians who may develop Moral Injury some way into the future as they have time to reflect on and re-experience those morally-injurious events. When these emerge, senior leaders must allow and encourage sustained ethical, practical, emotional, and psychological support to their staff.

**Treatment of Moral Injury**

Much of the research in moral injury to date has been carried out with military personnel and veterans, although the emergence of the concept of moral injury in healthcare will no doubt foster debate in the context of this wave of this wave of COVID-19 — and the expected future waves of the pandemic. However, there are helpful guidance documents being produced at pace to provide advisory principles targeted at identifying, addressing, and remediating the root causes of moral injury.

In order to reduce the potential for development of Moral Injury, Greenburg et al. (2020) discuss the importance of providing early support to clinicians — through preparing workers for the moral dilemmas they will face during the pandemic; by providing information on the potential for moral injury and enabling ward-level discussions to provide forums for staff sharing in a safe and supportive space. They note the importance of being sensitive to those staff who may be avoiding moral injury-related discussions (and who may need it most), and the importance of providing both immediate and long-term help.

There is now a wide range of online resource material available (e.g. Psychologytools.com/psychological-resources-for-coronavirus-COVID-19) addressing the challenges facing healthcare workers, the impacts of quarantine, coping with the COVID-19 illness, how to maintain health and well-being, and how to manage trauma. In addition, specific guidance has been offered for staff care (e.g. Williams, Murray, Neal, and Kemp, 2020) which makes practical personal and organisational recommendations for managing the stresses and impacts of COVID-19.

Once this wave of COVID crisis abates, it will be all too easy for healthcare leads to seek a return to 'normal', but service leads would do well to ensure they offer and follow up on the monitoring and identification of vulnerable staff, and the implementation of appropriate treatment processes in both short and longer term.

Providing social support before and after the morally-injurious events can reduce the impact of the powerful damaging emotions of guilt and shame (Litz et al., 2009). While their work has been in the context of moral injury and repair in war veterans, their model has relevance for the potential consequences of potentially morally-injurious events clinicians experience in the COVID-19 context. They propose that there are two core routes to "moral repair and renewal" – psychological and emotional processing of the morally-transgressive act(s), and exposure to 'corrective life experience'. This rehabilitation process requires fully disclosed and shared re-living of the experience, increasing exposure to good deeds, eliciting positive evaluation and feedback from others, and the giving and receiving of care and love.

Translating a model developed for war veterans to a healthcare context would also suggest the importance of:

- Providing and encouraging the safe, non-judgemental disclosure and exploration of the caregiver's role-based experience; the nature of the morally-injurious decisions and events they have experienced, and their emotional and cognitive and intrapersonal responses to the morally-injurious acts.

- The importance of supporting and enabling the caregiver to re-engage with positive caregiving, where they can re-assert a sense of personal and professional competence, ownership, and authority for their role and their moral principles.
- Organisational and peer support to enable or re-enable clinical work and care delivery, which fosters a re-building of trust and faith in one's ability to deliver the best care within a 'normal' context.

The implications of these findings are that moral injury can only be addressed through a process of empowering the sufferer to voice their experience and distress, and to be supported by healthcare leaders and patient counsellors in the expression of that experience. Currently, there are no manualized approaches to treat moral injury-related mental health difficulties. In fact, some standardized treatments for PTSD (e.g. prolonged exposure) may potentially be harmful and worsen patient feelings of guilt and shame. Some emerging US evidence suggests that adaptive disclosure (where forgiveness is received from a benevolent moral authority) and acceptance and commitment therapy may be helpful (Borges, 2019). UK clinicians also report using an amalgamation of validated treatments (e.g. compassion-focused therapy and schema therapy) to treat patients affected by moral injury.

The 'Molendijk model' (Molendijk et al., 2018) described earlier also reminds us of the importance of not assuming a standard or predictable set of responses and outcomes to moral injury. There is a complex dynamic inter-relationship between experience, cognitions, self-perceptions, personal moral code, the context, and the morally-injurious event. This will mean that (as in any clinical condition) individual-specific manifestations of moral injury must be explored and respected within those broader presenting themes typically associated with moral injury.

A core component of successful moral injury treatment, as with all psychological interventions, is therefore a commitment on the therapist's part to sensitively explore the patient's experience. The therapist must enable a therapeutic process which fully recognises the patient's thoughts, self-perceptions, and responses to their moral injury. As a core component of treatment, the therapist must understand and acknowledge the unique interaction between personal experience, personal moral code and morally-injurious context, and then enable and legitimise the expression of the patient's thoughts and beliefs, guilt and shame through an informed, safe, and non-judgemental process.

**In summary:**

|  | Burnout | PTSD | Moral Injury |
|---|---|---|---|
| **Cause** | Extended period of providing care in an unsupportive, under-resourced environment.<br><br>Threat to Coping | Personal exposure to life threatening events<br><br>Threat to Mortality | Personal exposure to events which severely challenge core personal moral code<br><br>Threat to Morality |
| **Symptoms** | Malaise<br><br>Fatigue<br><br>Frustration<br><br>Cynicism<br><br>Inefficacy<br><br>Reduced ability to perform<br><br>Lack of accomplishment<br><br>Passivity<br><br>Emotional exhaustion<br><br>Detachment | Anxiety<br><br>Fear<br><br>Depression<br><br>Avoidance of the events or reminders of the events<br><br>Withdrawal<br><br>Chronic hypervigilance<br><br>Flashbacks<br><br>Guilt<br><br>Shame<br><br>Outbursts of | Guilt<br><br>Anger<br><br>Shame<br><br>Disgust<br><br>Depression<br><br>Social isolation<br><br>Loss of trust in self and others<br><br>Loss of meaning in life<br><br>Negative self-attributions<br><br>Cognitive avoidance<br><br>Avoidance of engagement with therapeutic help |

|  |  | panic or anger |  |
|---|---|---|---|
| **Core fear** | Being overwhelmed | Dying | Doing the unthinkable |
| **Core cognitions** | I can't cope | I am going to die | I am a terrible person |
| **Core defence** | Avoid stress & pressure | Avoid fear | Avoid shame |
| **Treatment** | Mindfulness<br><br>Rest & Relaxation<br><br>Identification of unhelpful coping strategies<br><br>Development of greater role-based competencies<br><br>Development of occupational and personal resilience<br><br>Role re-negotiation<br><br>Compensatory activities | Trauma-focussed Cognitive Behaviour Therapy (CBT)<br><br>Eye Movement Desensitisation and Reprocessing (EMDR)<br><br>Sensitive and trusting therapeutic relationship and support | Organisational/Leadership ownership of responsibility<br><br>Educate staff in advance of the expected situation<br><br>Acknowledge the power of the systemic, cultural, and situational contexts<br><br>Sustain engagement with and support from staff by senior leaders<br><br>Offer, legitimize, and enable help e.g. Adaptive Disclosure, compassion-focussed therapy, schema –focused therapy<br><br>Always - Facilitate therapeutic exploration of guilt and shame in safe, non-judgmental ways<br><br>Actively monitor at risk individuals over longer periods<br><br>Support and re-enable<br><br>Re-establish and live personal values |

Although it has been identified for some time in the impacts on war veterans, moral injury is a relatively new concept in healthcare and may risk being confused with the more familiar concepts of burnout or PTSD. There are indeed overlaps between PTSD and moral injury, but the core difference is in the distinction between a threat to life (PTSD) and the threat or insult to morality which can lead to moral injury.

The importance for clinicians working (and struggling) in the pandemic context is a distinction between what many will label as (a conflation of) burnout/ PTSD, and what may more appropriately be labelled as moral injury. While both conditions require acknowledgement, support, and treatment, the key distinction is that while PTSD sufferers may have some symptoms overlap with those experiencing moral injury, moral injury has shame and guilt at its core. In addition to individual treatment, moral injury prevention and treatment also requires proactive and ongoing acknowledgement by organisational leaders of the damaging context in which the clinician has been working.

The locus of responsibility for these impacts must be clearly laid at the door of a health system overwhelmed by the demands of the disease, and not as an attribution of poor coping and resilience in individual clinicians.

Finally, in acknowledgement of the trauma that our healthcare staff will experience, and the need to understand and support them in managing the impact of COVID-19 on their souls, this is an excerpt from a song acknowledging the pain of war in veterans:

*'Carry on my wayward son*
*For there'll be peace when you are done*
*Lay your weary head to rest*
*Don't you cry no more'*

**-Kansas, *Leftoverture***

# Creating Safety in Uncertain Times

*Dr Sara Northey*

*"The first task of recovery is to establish the survivor's safety. This task takes precedence over all others, for no other therapeutic work can possibly succeed if safety has not been adequately secured."*

Judith Herman (1997)

Psychological research tells us that promoting a sense of safety is an essential element in supporting people and communities during periods of crisis and disaster (for example, Hobfoll et al., 2007). However, the coronavirus pandemic has had a seismic effect upon the world, and at the time of writing, the future trajectory of the illness and the extent of its future impact remains unknown. Many key workers find themselves in situations where they may be supporting people who are feeling overwhelming fear, whilst also feeling afraid for themselves and their loved ones. They may feel unsafe and uncertain about what the future may hold, both personally and professionally. This chapter will explore how psychological techniques can help people to create a sense of safety, empowerment, and hope, even amid fear and uncertainty.

## COVID-19 Through the Lens of Trauma

A recent blog post in the British Medical Journal (Simpkin, 2020) describes COVID-19 as being *'defined by uncertainty'* in relation to myriad factors, including the trajectory of the pandemic, the risk of harm to loved ones, the accuracy of mortality figures, the availability of medical equipment, and the impact of the pandemic upon the global economy. Uncertainty can leave people feeling understandably anxious and unsafe, triggering a response in the sympathetic nervous system (often referred to as the 'fight, flight, or freeze' response). This may exacerbate existing difficulties with psychological wellbeing, as well as triggering the development of new difficulties, for instance with generalised anxiety or low mood. The systemic therapist Barry Mason coined the term 'unsafe uncertainty' (Mason, 1993) to describe the experience of fear, powerlessness, and hopelessness people can experience when encountering a problem with no clear solution.

Some clinicians (Horesh & Brown, 2020) have argued that it may be useful to understand the COVID crisis through the lens of trauma, as it shares many characteristics with other mass traumatic events, in terms of its scope and the degree of fear and threat many people are experiencing. The impact of the event upon different individuals is likely to depend upon a number of factors, including the degree to which they or their loved ones have been directly affected by COVID-19, but also numerous contextual factors, such as whether or not they have experienced prior traumatic events and the amount of social support available to them (Adams & Boscorino, 2006).

At the time of writing, it is too early to say whether significant numbers of people will develop COVID-related post-traumatic stress disorder (PTSD), or other common reactions to trauma such as anxiety and depression (Mason & Birch, 2018). It is standard clinical practice to delay diagnosis of PTSD until at least a month after a traumatic event has occurred (National Institute for Health and Care Excellence, 2018). This is in recognition of the fact that distress is entirely normal during and in the immediate aftermath of a traumatic event, and most people will naturally recover without the need for any therapeutic intervention.

Research suggests that, following a traumatic event, approximately 15% people may go on to develop PTSD, which includes intrusive memories of the traumatic event, including nightmares and sometimes 'flashbacks'; avoidance of anything that reminds them of the trauma; and hyperarousal symptoms including sleep difficulties, irritability, and poor attention and concentration

(Breslau et al., 2005). However, in the case of a mass event such as COVID-19, if even a small minority of individuals present with ongoing post-traumatic symptoms, this would constitute a huge number of people.

Moreover, in the case of COVID-19, it is also a crisis where the end point is currently unclear, and the trauma is therefore continuous. Most research and guidance about how to help people after a traumatic event has focused on what to do after a crisis or trauma has passed and the evidence-base is less clear regarding how best to support people in the midst of a crisis (Billings et al., 2020). However, previous research into continuous traumatic stress suggests that where there is a constant sense of threat, people can remain in a continuous state of 'high alert' and hyperarousal, which can lead to difficulties with sleep, concentration, irritability, and constantly feeling 'on edge' (Lahad & Leykin, 2010). Alternatively, some people may get into a chronic state of immobility or inertia (Levine, 2008). People may attempt to cope with these feelings through avoidance strategies, such as social withdrawal, or avoidance of reminders of the trauma. Or they may attempt to numb their feelings using alcohol, drugs, overeating, or even overwork.

It has been suggested that trauma is characterised by a 'shattering of assumptions', whereby a traumatic event damages a person's previously held beliefs and assumptions, including their assumption of being safe in the world (Janoff-Bulman, 1992). For families, there can be a disruption of the 'protective shield' which parents strive to provide for their children, to keep them safe (Pynoos, Steinberg, & Wraith, 1995). This can leave people in a state of intense anxiety, confusion, and despair, which can give rise to the symptoms of PTSD.

A group of psychological trauma experts came together in 2007 to delineate the evidence regarding the most helpful approaches to take in the immediate and mid-term aftermath of disaster and mass trauma (Hobfoll et al., 2007). They proposed five principles to guide and inform best practice:

1) Promote a sense of safety
2) Promote calming
3) Promote sense of self and collective efficacy
4) Promote connectedness
5) Promote hope

Although the five elements are not ordered in terms of importance and are all essential, this chapter focuses primarily upon the first principle of promoting a sense of safety, as it can be argued that safety is the foundation upon which recovery is based (Herman, 1997) and is essential in reducing the physiological arousal associated with fear and anxiety (Bryant, 2006). Research suggests that even in the case of continuous, ongoing threat, people who are able to establish even a limited sense of safety have a significantly lower risk of developing ongoing difficulties, including PTSD (Bleich, Gelkopf, & Solomon, 2003).

## Creating Safety at Multiple Levels

It has long been recognised that a staged approach to therapeutic work is crucial in assisting recovery after disaster and trauma. As far back as the work of Pierre Janet in the late 1800s, it has been proposed that stabilisation must occur before the therapist and client do any uncovering or processing of traumatic memories. Judith Herman, in her seminal work *Trauma and Recovery* (1997), described a three-stage model of recovery:

> 'The central task of the first stage is the establishment of safety. The central task of the second stage is remembrance and mourning. The central task of the third stage is reconnection with ordinary life.' (p. 155)

Herman emphasised that progress through these stages is not linear, and that the path of the recovery is inherently turbulent and complex, but for most people, the course of recovery will be marked by a gradual shift 'from unpredictable danger to reliable safety'. She proposed that the establishment of safety needs to occur across a number of domains, including the individual's sense of safety in their own body and mind, their sense of safety in relationships, and their safety in the external world.

In considering how to help people to feel safe both during and following the COVID crisis, it is important to recognise that an individual's sense of safety in their own body and mind is inextricably linked to the broader social and political context in which a person lives (Burgess, 2020).

The psychologist Urie Bronfenbrenner (1979) formulated his Ecological Systems Theory to explain how an individual's development is influenced by how they interact with the world around them, at multiple levels, from their personal relationships to the broader social context, and how this may shift and change over time. Bronfenbrenner's model can be adapted to illustrate how we may consider the creation of safety, both internally and at multiple layers of the systems around a person.

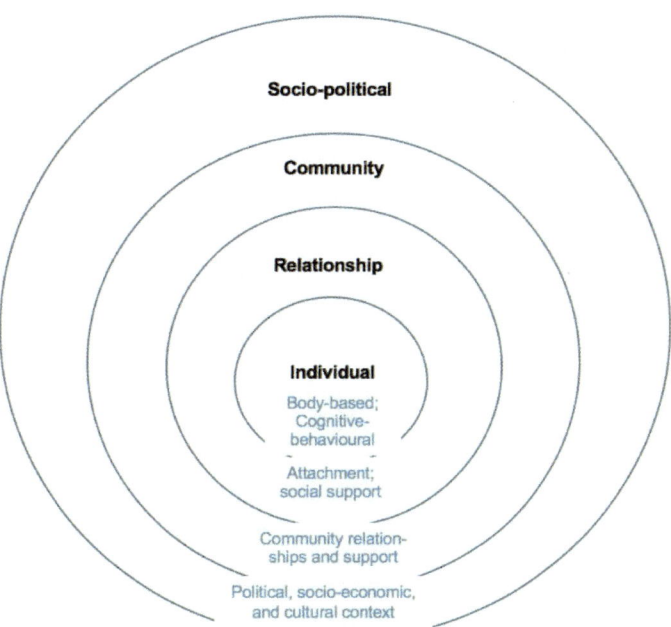

**Diagram 1: Eco-systemic approach to creating safety**

## Individual-Based Safety

### Body-Based Approaches

A crucial step in creating an internal sense of safety both during and following a crisis is to ensure that people's basic physical needs are met. Guidance drawn up by a group of UK trauma specialists focusing on support-planning for hospital staff working with COVID-19 recommends that priority is given to ensuring that the physical needs of healthcare workers are met, including their needs for rest, sleep, food, and safety, including appropriate access to personal protective equipment (Billings et al., 2020). In the long term, body-focused approaches can be essential in helping people to down-regulate the high levels of physiological arousal associated with chronic anxiety and post-traumatic stress (Mason & Birch, 2018).

Bessel Van Der Kolk (2014) in his book *The Body Keeps the Score: Mind Body and Brain in the Transformation of Trauma* suggests that body-based approaches can help people to have experiences that 'deeply and viscerally contradict the helplessness, rage, or collapse that result from trauma'. Recent research into the function and effects of the vagus nerve, which is a nerve connecting the brain to several internal organs, suggests that body-based approaches can have a direct 'bottom-up' impact from the body to the brain, by modulating arousal and stimulating the social engagement system, which helps people to feel safe and socially connected with others (Porges, 2009). Van Der Kolk suggests that several body-based approaches, including martial arts, dance, and massage could be potentially effective, but one of the most widely research body-based practices is yoga.

Yoga is a set of practices originating in India several thousand years ago. Although there are numerous subtypes of yoga, all yogic practices consist of varying degrees of focus upon breath practices (pranayama), stretches or postures (asana), and meditation, or mindful awareness, with the aim of creating a sense of 'union' or integration between these areas (Mason & Birch, 2018). Research has shown that numerous components of yoga including conscious breathing, meditation, physical activity, relaxation, chanting, and safe social interaction within class settings are associated with regulation of the autonomic nervous system (Yackle et al., 2017). It has been suggested that regular yoga practice can provide tools for helping people to come back to a physical 'baseline' more rapidly after a distressing experience (Streeter et al., 2012). Van Der Kolk (2014) found that ten weeks of yoga practice significantly reduced PTSD symptoms in a group of patients who had not responses to medication of any other form of psychological treatment.

However, not everyone will feel comfortable or willing to begin a yoga practice, and it is likely that other body-based practices are likely to be effective in reducing physiological arousal and increasing an internal sense of safety. For instance, simple breath practices, including diaphragmatic breathing and lengthening of the out-breath, have been found to decrease arousal and anxiety (Mason & Birch, 2018).

*Cognitive-Behavioural Approaches*
A number of individual psychological therapies incorporate breath and body-based practices, in addition to cognitive — or thinking-based — techniques, including 'third wave' cognitive behavioural therapies such as Mindfulness Based Cognitive Therapy (MBCT: Teasdale et al., 2000), Compassion Focused Therapy (CFT: Gilbert, 2010) and Acceptance & Commitment Therapy (ACT: Hayes, Luomo, Bond, Masuada, & Lillis, 2006).

Mindfulness-based approaches involve guiding people through a set of practices aimed at improving their awareness of the present moment, often through sustained attention upon body sensations, or the breath. This can help people to become more aware of the ebb and flow of their thoughts and feelings, and less caught up in them, a technique Hayes, et al. (2006) terms 'defusion'. Research suggests that mindfulness can calm down the sympathetic nervous system, enabling people to feel more in control of their emotions and less likely to be thrown into a state of 'fight, flight or freeze' (Van Der Kolk, 2014).

Russ Harris (2020) produced a recent guide for coping with emotional distress during the COVID crisis, based upon core principles from Acceptance and Commitment Therapy (ACT). The guide is based around the acronym 'FACE COVID', with each letter standing for a particular strategy:

*F – Focus on what's in your control*

*A – Acknowledge your thoughts and feelings*

*C – Come back into your body*

*E – Engage in what you're doing*

*C – Committed Action*

*O – Opening up*

*V – Values*

*I – Identify resources*

*D – Disinfect and distance*

Harris emphasises that although it is not possible for people to control what happens with the coronavirus on a medical or societal level, and it is also not possible to eliminate feelings of worry and anxiety, it is possible for people to focus on what is in their control: their actions.

As part of this he recommends an Acceptance & Commitment Therapy exercise called 'Dropping Anchor' (Harris, 2019). The idea of the exercise is that much like when a boat drops anchor to steady itself during a storm, this exercise can help people to create a sense of stability during times of emotional distress and uncertainty. The exercise does not involve pushing away or 'getting rid' of unwanted thoughts or feelings but enables people to 'hold steady' while the feelings pass. Harris recommends a three-step approach of 1) acknowledging emotions and bodily sensations; 2) coming into the present moment, for instance by noticing the breath and pressing the feet into the floor; and 3) engaging with the world, by noticing sounds and items in the room, and engaging in intentional action guided by one's core values.

Compassion-focused exercises form a core part of ACT, as well as other therapeutic models such as Compassion Focused Therapy (Gilbert, 2010). This is based on the idea that self-compassion activities, such as directing kind, non-judgmental awareness toward feelings of discomfort, can help to activate the soothing and calming system, and thus deactivate fear and threat-based systems, thereby increasing feelings of safety.

*The Safe Place Exercise*

Creation of an imaginal 'safe place' is a core part of initial stabilisation work within a number of evidence-based, trauma-focused therapies, including Trauma-Focused Cognitive Behavioural Therapy (TF-CBT: Cohen. Mannarino & Deblinger, 2017) and Eye Movement Desensitisation & Reprocessing (EMDR: Shapiro, 1995). This involves bringing to mind a real or imaginary place which brings about a feeling of safety and calm. It can be helpful to visualise this place with considerable detail, including sensory details such as sounds, smells, and textures. Both TF-CBT and EMDR therapy involves repeated rehearsal of the safe place, so that people can return to it as a place of refuge when trauma memories are activated. For some individuals who have experienced severe or complex interpersonal trauma, it can be difficult to bring to mind a 'safe place', so instead it can be helpful to bring to mind an image or memory that they associate with feeling calm or pleasant feelings.

**Relationship-Based Safety**

There is a large body of evidence to suggest that social support and sustained attachment are a crucial element in enhancing safety in the aftermath of crisis and disaster (Hobfoll et al., 2007). As Bessel Van Der Kolk (2014) points out:

> 'Study after study shows that having a good support network constitutes the single most powerful protection against becoming traumatised. Safety and terror are incompatible. When we are terrified, nothing calms us down like the reassuring voice or the firm embrace of someone we trust... It is critical to communicate with loved ones close and far and to reunite as soon as possible with

family and friends in a place that feels safe. Our attachment bonds are our greatest protection against threat.'

However, social support is not always easily available or perceived as a source of safety. The 'secure base' afforded by attachment with an attuned and available caregiver in infancy is the bedrock of many people's sense of safety within the world. However, inconsistent caregiving or interpersonal trauma within childhood can have a significant impact upon people's sense of safety within relationships, which can have a significant impact upon their broader psychological wellbeing and can make it more difficult for them to make use of social support in the aftermath of a crisis (Herman, 1997). For people who find it difficult to trust others for these reasons, attachment-focused approaches to therapy can be helpful (Hughes, 2007).

Hobfoll et al. (2007) also warn that another potential negative impact of social support following mass trauma is if rumours and 'horror stories' about traumatic events are shared without a balancing emphasis upon mutual support and recovery. This can also be exacerbated by media reports following disaster, which can inadvertently increase feelings of being unsafe.

In the context of COVID-19, social isolation and shielding of those most vulnerable is likely to have reduced the ease of access to social support for many, particularly those who are not able to contact loved ones by phone, video calling or social media. It is important that alternative means of maintaining social support are found for people without access to technology.

For healthcare staff, team relationships can be a crucial source of social support, particularly for staff members who may be working long hours or may be separated from loved ones. Billings et al. (2020) advise that team cohesion is associated with positive mental health of team members, and that informal peer support and camaraderie in the face of a shared experience of trauma are more helpful than having specific individuals trained in trauma approaches.

## Community-Based Safety

As an extension of social support provided by people's personal relationships, support provided both informally and formally within local communities can also be an importance source of safety and security following disaster. Community-level outreach interventions providing practical support, monitoring of well-being, and psychoeducation about post-disaster reactions can be valuable both during and following a crisis (Hobfoll et al., 2007).

Harris (2020) includes a community-focused approach within his Acceptance and Commitment Therapy (ACT) based 'FACE COVID' guidance. He suggests that people consider what they can do to improve life for themselves or other people in their community during the COVID crisis. This is guided by ACT principles and research which suggests that values-based action can increase people's sense of purpose, meaning, and psychological well-being (Hayes et al. 2010).

## Socio-Political Context

Social, cultural, political, and economic factors have a huge and undeniable impact upon the sense of safety and psychological wellbeing experienced by individuals, families, and communities, especially during times of crisis. All forms of adversity are more common and the impact of adversity more severe within contexts of social inequality, marginalisation, deprivation, and discrimination (Johnstone & Boyle, 2018).

This is essential to consider within the context of the current COVID-19 crisis. There is a growing body of evidence to suggest that COVID-19 is having a disproportionate impact upon poorer and more marginalised communities (Pidd et al., 2020), and upon healthcare workers from ethnic minority groups (Rimmer, 2020). Devakumar, Shannon, Bhopal, & Abubamar (2020) suggest that governmental policy responses to COVID-19 have disproportionately affected people from ethnic minorities and migrants, as these people are often over-represented in socioeconomic groups, have limited healthcare access, or unstable jobs. In relation to psychological support and increasing feelings of safety, it is essential to recognise that no amount of individual body-based, self-help, or therapeutic approaches are likely to make a significant difference for people unless attention is also paid to these social, political and economic realities. As Burgess (2020) points out, 'A woman who has lost her job and cannot feed her family will find little relief from a meditation app'.

It is arguably essential for everyone, including healthcare workers, to be aware of and hold in mind the socio-political factors that affect people's sense of safety and wellbeing during the COVID crisis. If we can engage with the realities that shape people's experience of adversity, we will be in a better position to help to create meaningful change (Johnstone & Boyle, 2018).

In considering approaches to creating safety during the current time of 'unsafe uncertainty' characterising the COVID-19 crisis, it is clear that the different layers of the system, from the individual, through the relational, community, and broader socio-economic context, each have a mutual and interactive impact upon one another. It is arguably important to attend to each layer of the system to establish a sense of safety, and create the foundation needed to move towards recovery and well-being.

# A Time of Fear and Hope

*David Rawcliffe*

In the current climate of pandemic, we are experiencing daily reports of more and more intensive care beds being needed, with daily briefings from the government announcing the latest death toll. As this chapter is being written, the number of mortalities are reaching their first peak, and this raises the levels of fear in the general population. Fear has become a major factor of life for all; however, for nursing and other healthcare professionals, individual fears can grow and grow. Fear is often raised even further by hearing of friends and colleagues becoming ill; there is fear when they go home, thinking that they could have this virus in the non-symptomatic phase and be passing it on to their spouse, children, or parents. Already we have heard of one nurse who got the symptoms in Italy; her fear level was high, and rather than take this home to her family, she committed suicide (Steinbuch, 2020). Sadly, the number of staff suicides seem to be rising (Watkins, Rothfeld, Rashbaum, & Rosenthal, 2020; Mitchell, 2020).

One of my own personal tutor groups has recently had several posts about a mental health nurse, a matron on a dementia ward, who recently died from COVID-19. About six months ago, Boris Johnson described her as an inspiration, and the group all remarked about how knowledgeable, caring, and compassionate she was. Their emotional response was moving and hopefully productive as they remembered and celebrated the life of this influential and inspirational nurse.

I recently had a couple of online classes with the same mental-health student nurses. In the first class, I discovered that two of them had been tested positive for coronavirus, another had a family member at home with the condition, and all knew another nurse (or several) who had the virus. Many knew nurses that had died because of the virus. In the second class, two weeks later, those that had been sick were getting better, but another member of the group was ill. All remained worried about the virus, knowing the possible consequences. Some were choosing not to go back into practice, but most decided to help provide care and hope in a time of fear.

At the same time, students and healthcare professionals are going into the workplace knowing that their interventions can and do make a difference, finding hope and ways that this hope can be passed onto others. They're exploring new ways to help sick and dying people to contact their families via technology such as iPads, or by celebrating when they manage to discharge people home.

Fear and hope go hand in hand, and the fear of coronavirus is currently weighed against the hope and the truth that the virus will be beaten, using various strategies such as lockdown, the use of testing, and vaccines (in time).

This chapter will be considering these issues in the context of trauma and multiple traumas (Kinchin, 2005, 2007) leading to three possible outcomes: post-traumatic stress disorder (World Health Organization, 2013), post-traumatic growth (Joseph, 2015, 2012; Tedeschi, Shakespeare-Finch, Taku, & Calhoun, 2018) and **post-traumatic success** (Bannink, 2014). Protective factors will be identified, drawing on aspects of the PERMA Wellbeing Model (Seligman, 2011) such as positive emotion, engagement, relationship, meaning. and achievement. These will be discussed alongside **learned helplessness** (Peterson, Meier, & Seligman, 1995) and self-compassion (Neff, 2003a, b, 2017). The way forward identifies the role of the locus of control (Deci & Ryan, 1985; Layard & Clark, 2015) and how to help health professionals move towards hope in post-traumatic success (Bannink, 2014).

## Learning from Trauma Research

Trauma has been defined by the World Health Organization (2018) as an 'event which is exceptionally threatening and causes pervasive distress in almost anyone'. Blackmore and Troscainko (2015) suggest that trauma often feels 'overwhelming, unbelievable, and unbearable', which sounds like how most of us feel about the coronavirus pandemic.

The National Institute for Health and Care Excellence (NICE) (2005) established that most people suffer from at least one trauma in their lives. Grieve and Staudinger (2006) declared that 60% of adults have faced a major crisis (trauma). Although, as we will see later, most find ways to deal with the temporary setbacks and distress quickly, and only around a quarter of those who go through traumatic events will suffer from post-traumatic stress disorder (NICE 2005).

Rowntree et al. (2015) record that two-thirds of emergency personnel suffer from intrusive and distressing memories at any one time. The big question is whether this number will be echoed in healthcare professionals as a consequence of the things they will see, experience, and think during the coronavirus pandemic.

Health professionals care for individuals and these individuals can die, but as soon as one body leaves the bed another is being admitted. This can leave the health professional feeling overwhelmed, whilst having no physical or emotional space to resolve these feelings — an additional stress which may increase the fears and hopes in listening to one another, which can cause 'vicarious trauma' (Dworznik 2006), adding to their own intensity of fear. However, when individuals share these experiences, they may also be sharing their hopes.

The negative impact of trauma is increased where there are multiple traumatic events, when the individual feels that they have no control over the situation (Robinson & Rose, 2013; Solomon, Mikulincer, & Benbenishty, 1989; Werdel & Wicks, 2012), and when the event can be seen as life threatening (Kinchin, 2005, 2007), all of which can be seen happening in the rapid reorganisation of the health service so that coronavirus can be more easily treated. There is further a massive increase in mortuaries during this period, and these are being occupied more.

## The Impact of Trauma and Multiple Traumas on Memory

Memory following trauma is not an easy concept to understand. It involves notions demanding attention toward neurodevelopmental processes, such as 'sensory stimulus', 'working memory', 'short-term memory', and 'long-term memory'. In these, you have sensory stimulus, fore-brain neurotransmitters, such as adrenaline and acetylcholine and the hippocampus; these processes decide if the memories should be stored in the short or long-term memory. There are further processes around emotions which can be found in the limbic region and the brain stem (Van der Kolk, 2014) which affect memory.

Working memory is about what we do with information once we receive it in the brain (Baddeley, 1986). Martin (2006) states the working of the 'phonological loop' and the 'visuo-spatial scratchpad' are the most important aspects of working memory, and together they comprise the 'central executive'. The phonological loop hears sounds, which mainly come into the brain into the cortex of the fore-brain, whilst the visuo-spatial scratchpad is processed in other parts of the brain. The executive functioning then decides if the memory is worth storing or not, before it is sent to the limbic region/amygdala, where short-term memory is usually stored.

The functioning of the pre-frontal cortex is known to be divided into 'multiple memory domains', where each aspect is responsible for a different dimension of memory (Goldman-Rakic, 1992). This pre-frontal cortex is known to be responsible for handling working memory (Martin, 2006). However, following a period of trauma, the pre-frontal cortex will frequently have decreased functioning (Francati, Vermetten, & Bremner, 2007; Patel, Spreng, Shin, & Girard, 2012). The other area we need to consider is the role of neurotransmitters, for example, adrenaline and acetylcholine, which increase the acuity of visuo-processing and the ability to store memories (Martin, 2006).

274

In trauma, adrenaline may be released into the system, which prepares the body for 'fight or flight' (Van der Klok, 2014), this helps to engrave the memory into the mind. Acetylcholine may also be released, which is involved in cognitive processes such as attention and memory (Tranel, Nikolas, & Markin, 2020).

Attention and memory are closely related (Blackmore & Troscainko, 2015). Attention makes memories more fully accessible, and involves both functional and phenomena aspects (Smithies, 2011). The functional aspect is how the brain, its structures, and its neurons work, and the phenomena aspect is how the individual interprets their memories through logical and emotional responses, such as emotional decompression (Kinchin, 2007; Tronick, 2009).

Another two systems which work together are the rational and the emotional, which normally collaborate to form memories. However, in traumatic situations and their aftermath, they may not work as effectively together (Van der Klok, 2014). The memories become fragmented and are stored in disorganised ways (Baddeley & Logic, 1992; NICE, 2005). There are strong arguments that memories can be repressed (American Psychiatric Association, 2013) or dissociated (Ozer, Best, Lipsey, & Weiss, 2003); in the process, they cease to be available on a conscious level for the individual.

Working memory is converted into short-term memory if the brain considers it to be important. Alternatively, it may simply be forgotten, or in the case of major trauma, repressed, or in more 'acceptable' traumas, denied. The *repressed* trauma is not accessible to the conscious mind (Van der Klok, 2014), whilst the *denied* trauma can be accessed, albeit with difficulty. This move from working memory into short-term memory involves signals being sent from the pre-frontal cortex to the limbic region and the amygadla, whose functioning is increased when trauma is in the memory (Francati, Vermetten, & Bremner, 2007; Patel, Spreng, Shin, & Girard, 2012). This area of the brain is involved in emotional regulation (Marieb & Hoehn, 2016; Blows, 2010), and in deciding if the short-term memory should be stored in long-term memory, a decision made unconsciously (Blackmore & Troscianko, 2018). Later, the memory is sent to the hippocampus, where the storage and retrieval of long-term memories happens (Martin, 2006; Marieb & Hoehn, 2016).

## Trauma, Memory, and Recall

Understanding the way that memory works is important when considering trauma, but especially where there are multiple traumas. The individual may have fragmented and disorganised memories of the first trauma; effectively, the narrative story may not be consciously accessible to them. However, while the individual will not be consciously aware that the repression has worked for them, this could become embedded as a pattern for future traumatic memories, making it even more difficult to consciously access these memories (Van der Klok, 2014).

## The Three Responses to Trauma

It should be recognised that individuals will respond to trauma in different ways. This is dependent upon their own personal history, the intensity of the trauma, the number of traumas, and any protective factors such as meaning and the types of support they utilise, for example. As stated earlier, there are three main responses to trauma: post-traumatic growth (PTG), post-traumatic stress disorder (PTSD) and post-traumatic success (PTS).

Post-traumatic growth (PTG) is where the individual adapts and manages their response to the traumatic events by finding meaning in it and allowing it to strengthen their lives in significant ways (Ivtzan, Lomas, Hefferon, & Worth, 2016; Hefferon, 2013; Joseph, 2012). The majority of those that go through traumatic events will fall into this category by moving towards growth, with new understanding and life paths (Dekel, Ein-Dor, & Solomon, 2012; Elderton, Berry, & Chan, 2017).

Others will develop post-traumatic stress disorder (PTSD), where they suffer from disabling thought patterns following the trauma (NICE, 2005; Brewin, 2014). These thoughts may be intrusive and include flashbacks or being forced into rumination about some aspects of the event and distressing emotions (Kinchin, 2005, 2007; Nishi, Matsuoka, & Kim, 2010).

Michel et al. (2010) and Anderson et al. (2019) believe that PTG and PTSD should be viewed as one mechanism.

Post-traumatic success (PTS) has been defined as a combination of PTG and PTSD (Bannik, 2014; Dekel, Ein-Dor, & Solomon, 2012; Kashdan & Kane, 2011; O'Hanlon & Bertolino, 2012; Nishi, Matsuoka, & Kim, 2010).

Most people quickly learn from the traumas they face, yet may still be hampered by them for a while. Grieve & Staudinger (2006) argue for the need to assimilate and accommodate; that is assimilate new ways of thinking and where these are destructive in order to make accommodations in their individual behavioural patterns and how they think and feel about these and other events.

Effective PTS happens once the individual has worked through the issues of the traumatic events; for some it can be their immediate response. A key point about PTS is that the individual's 'story' about themselves changes as they develop, accommodate, and assimilate.

## SIGNS AND SYMPTOMS OF PTG AND PTSD

Traumatic event (or events) 'which are exceptionally threatening and would cause pervasive distress in almost anyone' (NICE, 2005).

| AREA | PTG | PTSD |
|------|-----|------|
| THINKING | Recognises the personal development, including changed priorities and new life path, because of the distress of trauma.<br><br>Recognises their own strengths.<br><br>Finding meaning / purpose from the situation.<br><br>"Benefit finding".<br><br>"Strength perception of self" | Repetitive and intrusive recollections.<br><br>Ruminations.<br><br>Heightened awareness.<br><br>Hypervigilence.<br><br>Hyperarousal.<br><br>Flashbacks.<br><br>Suicidal thoughts.<br><br>Compulsion. |
| EMOTION | Able to promote the positive, whilst minimising the negative. | Emotional blunting.<br><br>Numbness.<br><br>Loss of joy.<br><br>Depression.<br><br>Anxiety. |
| BEHAVIOUR | More able to face the next distressing situation.<br><br>Able to be more compassionate and empathetic towards others. | Avoidance behaviours.<br><br>Insomnia.<br><br>Addictive behaviours.<br><br>Inflexibility.<br><br>Sensation bound. |

| | | |
|---|---|---|
| **SOCIOLOGICAL** | Relationships become warmer.<br><br>New Social Bonds.<br><br>Adversarial growth | Social isolation. |
| **References** | Ackroyd, Fortune, Price, Howell, Sharrack, & Isaac, 2011; Bostock, Sheikh, & Barton, 2009; Gracey, Kinsell, Muldoon, & Fortune, 2015; Kangas, Williams, & Smee, 2011; Kashdan & Kane, 2011; Linley & Joseph, 2014; | American Psychiatric Association, 2013; Dekel, Ein-Dor, & Solomon, 2012; Ehlers & Clark, 2000; Kinchin, 2005, 2007; NICE, 2005. |

## Post-Traumatic Disorder or Post-Traumatic Growth?

*Protective Factors*

In the coronavirus pandemic, health professionals are being faced with an unprecedented level of illness and death, with the possibility and expectation of not being able to care for, treat, or cure as many of their patients.

Protective factors are important when considering the possible consequences of facing these devastating events. They may help the person learn and adapt their thinking, feeling, and behaviour, and thus move towards positive traumatic success; where these factors are not as present or effective, then the individual may need to work through either a positive traumatic growth process and/or through post-traumatic stress disorder.

The protective factors discussed here are what Seligman (2011) sees as the foundations of well-being: positive emotion, engagement, relationships, meaning, and accomplishment (PERMA). Intermingled with PERMA are aspects of learned helplessness (Miller & Seligman, 1975) and the elements of self-compassion (Neff, 2003a, b, 2017) which include self-kindness (self-forgiveness and gratitude), common humanity, and mindfulness.

Frankl (1988) argues that man has the 'unique ability to detach himself from even the worst condition'. It is recognised that many health professionals are good at compartmentalising different aspects of their life; what they are feeling when they are in their 'professional' setting may be different to what they are feeling on the way home, where yet another set of feelings may be present.

We know that where trauma happens, there is often emotional blunting, a general feeling of numbness (Kinchin, 2007; NICE, 2005). Miller and Seligman (1975) suggest that if a person felt trapped and could not escape a distressing situation, they would at some point, in essence, give up trying (learned helplessness), particularly when the person feels that they are not in control of the situation and distressing events are repeated, such as frequent deaths. Peterson, Meier, and Seligman (1995) attest that the individual could become 'inappropriately passive', and the healthcare professional would thus need to observe their own behaviours and that of their colleagues for signs of passivity.

This passivity can be seen in non-engagement or reduced input or snappiness. Those with an external locus of control (Deci & Ryan, 1985; Gross & Kinnison, 2014) and those who are unrealistically optimistic or pessimistic (Seligman, 1995) are more susceptible to these feelings of learned helplessness.

Michel et al. (2010) established that those who are 'in touch with their emotions' are most likely to go into post-traumatic growth, but one of the major issues health professionals may face, during and after trauma, is the fear that if they allow their emotions to emerge, these emotions may not be controllable in their professional setting. However, many writers would agree with Seligman that keeping feelings to oneself is bad for both one's mental and physical health (Grieve & Staudinger, 2006; Van der Kolk, 2015). Pennebaker and Seagel (1994) noted that efforts to control or repress negative emotions are counterproductive, and demonstrated that sharing these negative emotions improved the long-term future for the individual.

Therefore, 'negative' emotions can be defined as those emotions which either stop growth or reverse it (Fredrickson, 2001).

An example of a negative emotion which health professionals may currently feel is that of guilt, when they have not been able to give their best (maybe because they are simply exhausted or distracted). Rajakaruna et al (2017) established this condition may spread to others in the hospital, especially where personal protective equipment or procedures were inadequate in either quantity or quality.

Learned helplessness and disengaging can be on cognitive, emotional, or behavioural levels (Shoshani & Aviv, 2012; Fredricks, 2014). On the cognitive level, it means the person may turn up, but not apply skills and learning in practice. Emotionally, it may mean the person's emotions blunt, and they become numb and deny feeling. On a behavioural level, people could be absent for whatever reason, arriving late or trying to leave early or focusing on mundane things away from the emotional 'front line'.

Neff (2003a, b) showed that those who feel guilty may need to learn to operate in self-kindness, which includes the ability to self-forgive. A technique to help with self-forgiveness is to consider what we are feeling guilty about, then to imagine that we are talking to a junior health professional and ask them 'what advice would you give me?'

Understanding what Neff (2003a, b) calls our 'common humanity' can also be vital in moving us toward growth.

Common humanity involves embracing how the individual faces adversities and dilemmas in life (Germer, 2009; Neff, Kirkpatrick, & Rude, 2007a, b). It recognises that no one is perfect, and that being imperfect is part of our humanity (Reynolds, Palmer, & Green, 2019; Germer, 2009; Neff, 2017). To accept this can be reassuring and help us understand that if we're flawed, struggle, and make mistakes, we are not alone.

Trauma can induce social isolation or avoidance of other people (Kinchin, 2007; NICE, 2005; Ozer et al., 2003). In PTG, social support is seen as a major factor in the individual's ability to adapt and adopt new behaviours (Bostock, Sheikh, & Barton, 1989; Tedeschi & Calhoun, 1996). Adopting and promoting positive relationships is a major way forward for developing well-being for the individual (Seligman, 2011).

Lyubomirsky (2010) and Fredrickson (2001) both argue strongly that there is a major advantage in focusing on the 'positive' emotions too, in seeing them as protective factors. Once again, the health professional can look at what they are doing and recognise times when, for example, patients have smiled and said, 'thank you' and remember how they responded to this. Emmons and Stern's (2013) research confirmed the need for us to give and receive kindness and gratitude, recognising that these would raise the individual's level of positive emotion. Furthermore, kindness and gratitude can broaden and build other positive emotions and help them become an even greater protective factor (Fredrickson, 2001). Pennebaker and Seagel (1997) encouraged people who have gone through are going through trauma to write a journal expressing their emotions. They confirmed this raised their ability to deal with their negative emotions and to raise their positive ones at the same time.

There are broader societal influences that may help us toward PTG. People all over the country are demonstrating their appreciation of health and social care staff by clapping in the streets at 8pm on Thursday, putting rainbows in their windows, and by opening shops a little earlier for these staffing groups. And indeed, when Prime Minister Boris Johnson was discharged from hospital after his bout of coronavirus, he paid tribute to two nurses in particular. About a week later, they both responded with how valued they felt because he had named them. One minute's silence for the country to remember the fallen health professionals shows how valued health professionals are seen, bringing with it a sense of relationship and meaning.

Meaning is the basic motivation in man' said Frank (1988, p.162), and comes from 'our thoughts, bodies and emotions' (Thompson, 2019, p.2) and from our behaviour (Piaget, 1929). Frankl (1979) observed that man is always 'setting out' on his search for meaning, and most health professional will in some way be asking themselves about the meaning of their experiences. Abe (2016) believes that finding meaning in these experiences becomes one of our major motivators for either change or stagnation. Finding positive meaning is seen by Seligman (2011) as one of the major factors for the individual to move towards flourishing and well-being.

Van der Kolk (2014, p.175) says the impact of the trauma is dependent on 'how personally meaningful it was … at the time'. Tronick (2009); Michel et al. (2010); and Sears, Stanton, and Danoff-Burg (2003) argues that trauma is rooted in meaning-making. Gracey, et al. (2008) proposed that a meaning centred therapy is needed after a traumatic event. There is a strong argument that finding the meaning in trauma will impact on the pervasiveness of symptoms in PTSD (Kinchin, 2005. 2007), if positive meaning is found, post-trauma responses can move more quickly to PTG (Kashdan & Kane, 2011; Triplett, Tedeschi, Cann, Calhoun, & Reeve, 2020).

In defining meaning, Seligman (2011) and Baumeister, Vobs, Aaker, and Garbinsky.

(2013) state it is relating to something greater than themselves, so nurses may find meaning in helping the 3.4% who are dying (Semple & Cherrie, 2020), come to terms with their impending death, and communicate with their relatives via Skype or other available technology. They may further find meaning in the fact that the majority (96.6%) of those treated for coronavirus will recover. It can be viewed that these acts are altruistic in nature, which Yalom (1980, p.433) argued 'constitutes an important source of meaning'.

One of the ways forward is suggested by Frankl (1979, p.19) when he records that 'a literal translation of the term "logotherapy" is "therapy through meaning"'. Pennebaker, Kiecolt-Glaser, and Glaser (1988) demonstrated that writing for fifteen minutes about finding meaning in traumatic situations was useful.

In identifying both the meaning and the hope in a situation, the individual is beginning to identify their achievements, which Seligman (2011) records brings well-being and flourishment to the individual. Health professionals often face traumatic events and can record many successes in their professional lives, thus raising their own ability to face and process the traumas and observe their growth.

**The Way Forward**

Seery, Holma, and Silver (2010) demonstrate that those who have a history of 'handling moderate adversity' are more likely to be resilient and be able to work through a trauma. Most health staff will have dealt with distressing situations and learnt, through reflective practices, to deal with these. Some do this by finding a more experienced colleague in what Gopee (2018), Feeney, and Everett (2019) call an 'informal supervisory role' and talking through the issues with them, where they can explore the meaning of their experiences in a safe place.

Post-raumatic success may either be an immediate reaction, or something that happens after PTG and/or PTSD work has taken place.

Rotter (1966) developed a 'locus of control' scale which helped people recognise their level of internal or external locus of control. *Internal locus of control* was defined as believing that you are largely in control of your own life, whilst *external locus of control* was believing that you had little or no control over what happens to you. Most health professionals have high levels of professional efficacy, knowing their efforts have helped and can continue to help others, and thus have a situational internal locus of control, a protective factor for those who can develop post-traumatic stress (Solomon, Mikulincer, & Benbensishty, 1989).

Layard and Clark (2015) found and confirmed that those who are most likely to benefit from the 'positive psychology' approach are those who have this internal locus of control, whilst those who are most likely to benefit from a cognitive-behavioural approach have an external locus of control.

Some people may need to just 'work through' their emotions and give themselves and their colleagues permission to express the good (hope) and the bad (fear) emotions. This may be helpful in maintaining and developing positive relationships.

What we know from the research is that most health professionals will be able to face their fears and develop hope, through both compartmentalising and recognising that they and the health service have done a good job. They have saved lives and reduced suffering, bringing hope to others in difficult situations.

Some health professionals may feel overwhelmed before, during, and after their experiences — especially those who have faced multiple traumas, such as repeated deaths. These may need help in expressing themselves, some of which can be achieved using simple exercises, such as learning to journal, or through clinical supervision and establishing or re-establishing positive relationships.

This is all worth considering if you are experiencing the after-effects of trauma, whether you are someone with an internal or external locus of control; whether you have benefited or lost out by not discussing things with others; and whether you are currently experiencing elements of post-traumatic growth, post-traumatic stress disorder, or post-traumatic success. And it's worth reflecting on the good you've done, on common humanity, and on the fact that we all live with both fear and hope.

# At Any Instant:
# Fear, Hope, and Love in a Time of Fragmentation

*Kevin Acott*

"No-one ever told me that grief felt so much like fear. I am not afraid, but the sensation is like being afraid. The same fluttering in my stomach, the same restlessness…"

*CS Lewis (1961, p.5)*

---

**How hopeful do you feel at the moment?**

**How scared do you feel?**

---

I'm writing this for other people, but I'm also writing it for myself. I'm scared right now, yet hopeful. As a nurse and as an educator, I've always been scared, always been hopeful, but in the last few months one seems to have overtaken the other.

Two thousand years ago, Seneca suggested that 'we are more often frightened than hurt; and we suffer more from imagination than from reality' (2004, Letter XIII). Sitting here in 2020, self-isolating, I'm scared for my daughter, who's a doctor on the 'front line', and I'm scared for my other daughter who lives and works in a place that is still trying to wish the virus away. I'm sitting here, scared for my partner, my friends and family, my colleagues and students, and myself. I'm struggling with past grief and present grief and future grief. I'm scared, and I'm struggling, and I'm not really sure Seneca was right.

To be honest, I don't actually feel Seneca was right at all, though I think perhaps he was — at least partially. That old tension between what we feel and what we think is something we all seem to be grappling with, now more than ever. Somehow, we need to bring the two together, the emotional and the rational; I think we need to apply a 'dialectical' approach to coping with it all, an approach (as we'll see later) that blends the two without negating either. We need to see truth as shifting and nuanced; we need to recognise opposites as each containing some truth; we need to see the way we think and feel our way through this crisis as both reality *and* our imagination.

In this chapter, I will suggest that right now, the hurt *and* fear are real, *and* my imagination is making them worse. I feel frightened, with good reason. And a lot of the things I'm frightened about may not happen. 'There is no hope unmingled with fear, and no fear unmingled with hope,' said Spinoza (2017, XIII), fifteen hundred years after Seneca, and five hundred years before us. He was right, and to help us make sense of our present-day 'mingling', perhaps we need to try to extract more from the struggles of our shared histories?

Viktor Frankl is supposed to have said (though actually didn't), 'Between stimulus and response, there is a space. In that space is our power to choose our response. In our response lies our growth and our freedom.' Finding that place of mindful liberation, finding freedom from the virus and the fear it brings with it, can feel overwhelming — impossible, even. Yet some kind of middle way — temporary, perhaps, and partial — between wild optimism and dark resignation is possible, whatever we think of Frankl and his ideas, or of a statement that might seem a little crude and oversimplifying. When re-reading Frankl's work and discovering some of the unethical things he was supposed to have done as a doctor, and then discovering in passing that he never even used the phrase that's so often attributed to him, I found myself feeling irrationally and inappropriately angry. I realised anger burns through everything that's happening at the moment — both just, righteous anger, and anger that belongs somewhere else altogether. Anger and fear are always mingled, it seems.

Finding that space of freedom, free from fear, might in part be dependent on whether we see ourselves and the world in what Galen Strawson (2008) terms 'diachronic' or 'episodic' ways, in part on how we approach uncertainty, hope and hopelessness, and in part, most of all, on how we deal with what Irvin Yalom (1980) calls 'human givens'. This chapter will explore these ideas and offer questions, thoughts, and prompts that I hope help move you and me closer to this middle way. These will straddle the boundaries between psychiatry, psychology, and philosophy, and have sprung, in part, from a philosophical tradition that emerged from both secular and religious Judaism and was, so often, responding to persecution, terror, and hopelessness. I really hope a word, sentence, or paragraph here can help you find your middle path — that something may trigger some hope, help lessen your fear, and, perhaps help you deal with the losses and pain that have come – and may continue to come – with this terrible pandemic.

There are, of course, no easy solutions to the awful emotional, cognitive, social, political, economic, and spiritual dilemmas we find ourselves facing. I certainly don't think we should merely be looking for opportunities, seeing this crisis as a way of resetting the world, or building the utopia we always dreamed of, nor do I think we should be entirely giving in to some kind of nihilistic despair. Brennecke and Amick's seductive hedonistic phrase, 'Life is a gift. Take it, unwrap it, appreciate it, use it, and enjoy it,' is cited by Yalom (1980, p.437), disapprovingly. My own response to it, as I write it while drowning in fear and uncertainty, is one of irritation. And yet, maybe there is something useful we can draw from it.

Frankl (1977), who survived Auschwitz, talked about a 'tragic triad', the three struggles of guilt, suffering, and death, which we all inevitably face at some point in our lives. Right now, for a lot of us, it seems each of these is both all around and swimming wildly within us. Whatever we've previously done to try and mitigate the effects of the triad, to push them away, to pretend they don't exist, or to turn them into something else is being massively tested. How can we do what Frankl asks us to? How can we engage fully with these experiences and begin to affirm ourselves and our reality? How can we turn suffering into a catalyst for personal progress, build opportunity from guilt, and derive from the certainty of our own death the drive to act more compassionately toward ourselves and toward others? And how can we do this without disappearing back into the pretence that what we've seen, felt, and fought —and continue to see, feel, and fight — hasn't really happened and might not happen again?

'Man's search for meaning,' says Frankl (2006, p.57), 'is the primary motivation in his life and not a "secondary rationalisation" of instinctual drives. This meaning is unique and specific in that it must and can be fulfilled by him alone.' I believe that search is what we need to be talking about as we try and find the 'middle way'. We *can* find meaning and purpose while staring straight at the truth; it doesn't sit and breathe in the world, outside us, or in heaven, it sits and breathes within each of us, though the journey can involve lonely, frightening, angry confrontations.

The former rabbi, David Cordis (2016), suggests there are three balancing acts nations, communities, and individuals need to carry out in order to thrive: we need to find ways to balance the logical and the rational with the affective and the emotional, to balance, in other words, what he calls 'the assertion with the question'; we need to explore ourselves at the same time as looking clearly out at the world; and we need to look to the past for answers, warnings, and inspiration while developing both an individual and a shared vision for a transformed, brighter future. We need, in other words, to scream our fear of the virus, contextualise it, and approach it with logic; to acknowledge and work on our own suffering while seeing ourselves as intimately connected to — and needing to reach out to — a world of eight billion people. We must draw on our own and our culture's strengths, victories, and learning while carving together a living sculpture of a better life for all of us.

Marrying these things — accepting each side of Cordis' three strands as two twisting, ultimately indivisible ways we can make sense of our fear and anger

— can be made easier by thinking about them in, as I said previously, a 'dialectical' way.

What do we mean by 'dialectical'? Marsha Linehan (2019), the developer of Dialectical Behaviour Therapy, has drawn on this ancient philosophical — and more modern, overtly *political* — concept in an attempt to help us understand self-harm; face our contradictions; and understand how we are unable to regulate our emotions, be interpersonally effective, or tolerate distress. 'Dialectics,' she says, 'allows opposites to coexist; you can be weak and you can be strong; you can be happy and you can be sad. In the dialectical worldview, everything is in a constant state of change. There is no absolute truth, and no relative truth, either: no absolute right or wrong. Truth evolves. Values that were held in the past might not be held in the present. Dialectics is the process of seeking the truth in the moment, drawing on a synthesis of opposites.'

'Change,' Linehan (2019) goes on to say, 'is the only constant. Meaning and truth evolve over time. Each moment is new; reality itself changes with each moment.' From a Marxist perspective, dialectics 'at its simplest … starts from an awareness that nothing is eternally fixed or static … The way things change is not just due to external forces but also to the often opposing (or contradictory) consequence of internal processes.' (Marxist Memorial Library, 2019). Lenin (Kolakowski, 2005, p.727) talks, similarly, about a 'perpetual interplay' between cause and effect, the political and the personal, the universal and the individual, the conflict and the unity of opposites. This interplay can lead to distress, confusion, and alienation; it can also lead — as we become more conscious and aware — to positive, empowering change, for ourselves and for society as a whole.

I would suggest that, if we think about things in a more dialectical way, it can help us find the courage to tiptoe towards Frankl's space of growth, and try to bridge Cordis' gaps between the rational and the emotional, between self and others, and between past and future.

This more dialectical understanding of how we live, work, and love in this new world could help us also try ways of dealing with the fundamental 'existential' questions Yalom (and others before him) have posed. These questions have been dumped on us at birth, and are questions that, overlapping with Frankl's 'triad', we all must avoid, confront or answer – regardless of our situation – every single day. They come and go, but they're always there, lurking. Right now, they've abruptly re-entered our lives and intensified with the arrival of COVID-19. The questions are, essentially:

---

**How can I make sense of death?**

**How can I make sense of isolation?**

**How can I make sense of freedom?**

**How can I make sense of meaninglessness?**

---

Right now, as we struggle individually and collectively with these questions, it may start to become clear that there are two levels to each of them, and that these levels intersect. We're dealing with death as a real, material fact *and* with its meaning for us, in terms of loss, grief, and pain. We're dealing with isolation from each other as a real, material fact *and* with its meaning for us. We're dealing with 'freedom' as a real, material fact — we have choices, choices, for example, to 'go out' or 'stay in', to lockdown or not lockdown — *and* we have to engage with the meaning of our decisions. We're dealing with meaning itself *and* a fear of/knowledge of an ultimate, inherent meaninglessness — the apparent pointless, unjust, random, Godless carnage caused by the virus.

Let's take a deep breath and look at death first…

In Yalom's view (1980, p.27), we each have an instinctive, inherent terror of it: 'The fear of death plays a major role in our internal experience; it haunts as nothing else does; it rumbles continuously under the surface; it is a dark, unsettling presence at the rim of consciousness'. Ansell-Pearson (2013, p.8) cites DH Lawrence: 'Death, beautiful death searches us out, even in our armour of insulated will. Death is within us, while we tighten our will to keep him out.' Pema Chodron (2007, p.57) suggests, 'most of the time, warding off death is our biggest motivation … time is passing and it's as natural as the seasons changing. But getting old, sick, losing love – we don't see those events as natural. We want to ward them off, no matter what.' In *normal* times, all this is true. Then a virus comes along, and death is no longer just rumbling at the outskirts of our lives, and we stop being so willing to let the sand slip through our fingers…

Choron (1964), cited in Yalom (1980, p.43), identified three different species of fear and anxiety in relation to death and dying:
1) What comes after death (a fear that is partly the legacy of our religious and cultural upbringings).
2) The 'event' of dying itself (physical pain and the awareness of forthcoming death).
3) Ceasing to be, to exist at all, becoming nothing.

A potentially painful, difficult — but perhaps liberating — exercise you might want to try out right now (or after you've read this) is to consider which of these three things most frightens you, which you can maybe do something about, and which you're best placed to help others with. For me, the ceasing to be feels the most frightening; for you, it may be different.

As I write this, Pink Floyd's 'Wish You Were Here' has just come on the radio. It unexpectedly made me want to cry in its sadness, its yearning, and its beauty. I don't even particularly like Pink Floyd… but I think it somehow sums up in a few minutes what I'm trying to say in thousands of words. If you don't know it, have a listen. If you do, maybe have a listen anyway.

Hannah Arendt (1998i, p.11) writes: 'In their fear of death, those living fear life itself, a life that is doomed to die … Even if we should assume that there is nothing to fear, that death is no evil, the fact of fear (that all living things shun death) remains.' Maybe there's an opportunity here for us to use the confrontation with death to somehow reduce our fear? 'We flee from death through all the everyday things that we do, and fail to notice that death is our greatest potential,' says Van Deurzen-Smith (1997, p.41). Yalom (1980, p.40) argues the recognition and acceptance of death can contribute a sense of helpful poignancy to life and provide a radical shift of perspective. This new perspective can 'transport one from a mode of living characterised by diversions, tranquilisation, and petty anxieties to a more authentic mode'. He talks about 'urgent experiences' that stop us fleeing from death. This pandemic is the very definition of an urgent experience, and it seems to me that facing up to death and using this period to work towards accepting the truth, however it's forced on us, could help us face up to something else: our innate capacity to live fully and richly.

Yet nothing is that simple.


Yalom's second 'human given' is 'freedom.' While we dread death, he says, we usually consider freedom to be something desirable, something positive. Whatever political or ideological stance we take, the concept of 'freedom' is almost certainly at the core of it, desirable and necessary for happiness. There are those who have consistently refused to obey government instructions to lockdown because of the fear of losing their 'freedom'. And yet, freedom in the sense Yalom means it is much more obviously and intimately connected to anxiety, and more negative in its connotations. Being 'free' to make decisions, as Sartre suggests, we're faced with the choice of being 'authentic' — with all the anxieties that provokes — or settling into a kind of deluded, denying comfort, one which pretends we're not going to die, that we're not separate and isolated individuals, that life has real meaning to be found if we open ourselves up to God, the Universe, or whatever. The choice to be truly ourselves is what Yalom means by 'freedom' — a choice in which there is no God to guide us, nor earth beneath our feet. We're here, alone; we're free, alone; and we're responsible for our own actions, alone. 'It is easy in the world to live after the world's opinion; it is easy in solitude to live after our own; but the great man is he who in the midst of the crowd keeps with perfect sweetness the independence of solitude.' (Emerson 2018, p.5). Right now, as the virus seems to do whatever it wants, that clash is accentuated. From a dialectical point of view, we must choose to resolve the tensions between feeling falsely safe and grounded and being real, true, and flying without wings. Or we can choose not to...

Yalom's third 'given' is isolation. Charlotte Wolff, cited in Berry-Smith (2012, p.26), tells us that 'The greater part of our lives is spent with ourselves, no matter where or with what other people we may live . . . our imagination is the only companion chained to us for the whole of existence'.

Yalom suggests there are three types of isolation – interpersonal, intrapersonal and existential isolation.

## a) Interpersonal Isolation

Interpersonal isolation is generally experienced as loneliness and refers to our isolation from other people. It can come from our own fears, worries, and inabilities to connect with others; our lack of skill; the parenting we received; our genes. It can also come from physical, geographical separation, such being locked down, imprisoned, or in a mental health unit. Dowrick, cited by Berry-Smith (2012, p.26), says loneliness is one of the great dreads of our time and that most of us fear it intensely. She writes, 'being alone for protracted or involuntary periods is likely to be tolerable only for someone of relative maturity, whose sense of self is reasonably reliable — someone who can comfortably hold onto feelings of connection, even when there is nobody else there'. Over the last couple months, I've been starting to think that I'm not 'someone of relative maturity'. How about you?

## b) Intrapersonal Isolation

'Intrapersonal isolation,' says Yalom (1980, p.354), 'results whenever one stifles one's own feelings or desires and accepts "oughts" or "shoulds" as one's own wishes, distrusts one's own judgement or buries one's own potential'. How much are we all doing this now? How much did we do it before? I think I've been starting to realise more and more that this too is somewhere I could 'improve' as a person.

## c) **Existential** Isolation

Yalom's (1980, p.360) key focus is on 'existential isolation', which he describes as an unbridgeable gap between two people, and, even more fundamentally, a separation between oneself and the world. Existential isolation cuts beneath all other isolation. No matter how close I get to you, or to my partner, or to my children, there remains a final unbridgeable gap; each of us enters life alone and must depart from it alone. This is a 'nothing' at the core of being, and that 'in the face of nothing, no thing and no being, can help us; it is at that moment when we experience existential isolation in its fullest'.

Yalom's fourth 'given' is **meaninglessness.** In the television series *Mad Men (Smoke Gets in Your Eyes, 2017)*, the character Don Draper says, 'Love doesn't exist. You're born alone and you die alone, and this world just drops a bunch of rules on top of you to make you forget those facts.' It's hard not to feel like that at times, but I would argue his bleakness ignores our capacity to forge meaning. And I desperately want to prove him wrong.

What, Yalom (1980, p.422) believes we have no option but to ask, is the meaning of life? Why are we alive? Why were we put here? If we're inevitably going to die, and if nothing endures, then what sense does anything make? 'The human being seems to require meaning. To live without meaning, goals, values, or ideals, seems to provoke considerable distress. In severe form, it may lead to the decision to end one's life'. Frankl (1977, p.141) similarly suggests that a lack of meaning creates a sort of existential sickness. 'Those who survived the camps,' he said, 'were more likely to be those who could create meaning from the horror'.

The virus threatens to change the meanings of all our lives. I'm no longer going to do what I thought I was going to do. The way I hoped things would turn out has shifted dramatically.

I think we could benefit from trying to apply the four 'givens' to these cold, hard days; applying the challenges of Frankl and Yalom to our struggles, but in new ways. Yalom (2000, p.31) talks about Heidegger's idea of 'authenticity' and about mindfulness. When we're 'inauthentic', we just float through life, unaware of the 'authorship of our life'; it seems to just happen to us. There are times, though, where being 'inauthentic' helps me cope, and maybe helps us all cope. If I'm honest, my inauthenticity, my avoidance, and denial of what's going on has kept me going at times. There have been times writing this piece where I've felt a fraud: word after word masking my real desperation, the actual confusion and rage I feel. As I write, I'm trying to embrace both the value in doing so and the seeming pointlessness.

I know a dialectical approach here — allowing the truth in authenticity *and* the truth in inauthenticity — can spare us some of this struggle. But it's hard: emotion can almost entirely suffocate thought.

One further point about tackling death, freedom, isolation, and meaninglessness: so much of how we deal with all of these in times of crisis depends on our assumptions and beliefs about ourselves, the world, and other people. And this, in part, depends on whether we adopt a 'narrative' approach to life. There are those of us (Strawson, 2008, calls them 'episodic'), who tend to make sense of our lives as a series of disconnected scenes, here-and-now's that are not necessarily part of any coherent story. I think they are the people who are less likely to worry, suffer, and fear the past or the future, and are more able, perhaps, to be authentic. Others — me, maybe you? – are people Strawson calls 'diachronic'. They tend to see themselves as the main character in a narrative, a character who has a past, a present and a future: the star of a film in which the self remains constant, survives, and endures.

Which do you think you are, diachronic or episodic? At times, I realise my current struggles are at least in part because I make those linear connections, rather than sitting with what's happening now. Maybe we each need to develop the episodic side of our nature and stop telling those stories for a bit?

We could start talking about something 'trilectic' here, about the relationships between our past, our present, and our future. The virus has changed our views of each of these, whether we're 'episodic' or 'diachronic'. Nothing in the past, present, or future will ever be the same. Whether that changes our story depends on who we were before and on the choices we make.

Everything seems uncertain. Ultimately, the pandemic is demanding we face up to that uncertainty, those competing demands on us, and all the confusions that Yalom's 'givens' push us into. At times we try to ignore them, deny them, and get on with watching Netflix and dreaming of Spurs getting into Europe.

Keats used an odd phrase: 'negative capability'. He said we achieve negative capability (a positive thing, in his eyes) 'when a man is capable of being in uncertainties, mysteries, doubts, without any irritable reaching after fact and reason'. Hope can sometimes involve that irritable reaching, can itself be damaging. So, what if we allowed ourselves to experience hopelessness? 'Giving up all hope of alternatives to the present moment,' as Chodron says (2007, p.45), 'we can have a joyful relationship with our lives; an honest, direct relationship that no longer ignores the reality of impermanence and death.' She adds, brutally, 'there's no babysitter that you can count on. The whole of life is like that. That is the truth, and the truth is inconvenient.' Yalom's 'givens' are there, whether we want to face up to them or not.

I don't have a nice, neat conclusion to all this. I do want to take one final leap, though: I think it's okay to want a babysitter sometimes and — more importantly, perhaps — to want love, connection, or to be looked after. 'Love,' Arendt (1998i, p.242) says, 'by reason of its passion, destroys the in-between which relates us to and separates us from others.' And love is beyond the givens, babysitting, or dialectics. Love — whatever it means for each of us (and it may or may not involve a God), can be compassion, friendship, sex, familial love, romantic love, a generic and universal love, the love of duty and pragmatism, self-love… or any combination of these. It's something that's at the very root of health and social care, at the root of our existence. It isn't everything, but it's a *something* that can help us acknowledge and transcend the fear and the rage.

'Fearlessness,' says Arendt (1998ii, p.13), 'exists only in the complete calm that can no longer be shaken by events expected of the future.' I don't know how we find the love that leads to that temporary calm; I don't know whether it's within us, outside us, or both; and I know the virus seems to threaten it. I think facing up to death, freedom, isolation, or meaninglessness *and* allowing ourselves to avoid them, deny them, and run away from them can release us a little. As long as we make that struggle together and our versions of love can, in some way, connect with other people's, our stories or non-stories with other people's, our hope and hopelessness with other people's, our good and our bad with other people's; as long as our guilt and our pride, our joy and our pain, our certainties and uncertainties, all connect with other people's, then we can survive and change. We can go on living and dying, as well as we can. And we can prove Don Draper wrong.

One last thing: can I ask you those two questions again? And a third?

---

**How hopeful do you feel right now?**

**How scared do you feel right now?**

**How could you love more?**

---

# Part 4

## Life after fear

# A Change of View

*Dr James Turner*

I'm sitting at home admiring the view
Am thinking to myself - so are you
We're working from home the government said,
If you don't, you're likely to end up dead

Oh crikey, I thought without a pause
And gently shut all my external doors
I've spent weeks on my bum, in front of a screen
And hardly a touch in the world has there been

The weeks have passed and too many have died
Though our colleagues have strived and have tried and have tried
I cried when I learned of colleagues who'd gone
Their care and compassion was second to none

On Thursday's we clap for those on the line
Carers and nurses, doctors and mine
I hope they pass through for the stats are disturbing
In fact, I would say they are really unnerving

I hear in the care homes
Some staff have stayed put
To seal off the virus and pay it due heed
When this is all over some recognition they need

I look out of my window on sun dappled streets
And think it's not long till we all get to meet
In the meantime, we ponder and work through the day
And hope that the virus just bloody goes away

So, my friends in your homes and workplaces the same
Let's continue the fight and more of the same
This thing won't deter us, we'll flourish a new
With a different perspective and hopefully…. a change of view!

# COVID-19 At the Front Line: Interpretations, Emotions and Behaviours

*Dr Sanj Nathoo & Dr David Shaw*

Healthcare workers are trained to keep patients safe by providing fundamental care and assisting people to die with dignity. This remains unchanged with the current COVID-19 pandemic, despite the fact that it has already consumed thousands of lives (Qun Li *et al.,* 2020) and is a real threat to healthcare workers. There has been much media focus on the heroic and selfless behaviour of healthcare workers. However, the implications for staff, including the fear of becoming infected when looking after patients infected with COVID-19 and the fear of taking that infection home to the family has yet to be investigated. This chapter explores the experience of the fear among the general population, among those infected with COVID-19, and among health care workers. The justification for choosing fear as the focus of this chapter is that there is good evidence that both the general public and health care workers are fearful of contracting infectious diseases like COVID-19 (Delobelle *et al.,* 2009; Msiska *et al.,* 2014 & Steimer, 2002). The chapter draws upon the extant literature: COVID-19 statistics; the grey literature; and research into other infectious diseases.

**The Nature of The Beast**

On the 30th January 2020, the World Health Organisation (WHO) declared the present coronavirus disease (COVID-19) a public health emergency. Subsequently, on the 11th of March 2020, it was upgraded to a pandemic (WHO, 2020a). This was due to the alarming rate of transmission, and the fact that COVID-19 has become a real problem throughout much of the world, affecting a huge quantity of people.

It is known that the outbreak first started in the city of Wuhan, China, but rapidly extended to 192 countries, infecting nearly three million people and killing nearly 200,000 (WHO, 2020b) at the time of writing. Indeed, research suggests that the real size of the pandemic is much bigger than what has been reported in the media (Park *et al.,* 2020). Thus, this pandemic poses a global threat to lives that is unparalleled in modern times. Whilst most people seem to suffer from mild symptoms such as high temperature, shortness of breath, and upper respiratory tract signs, in the more serious cases (one in five), people develop severe lung infections, pneumonia, organ failure and death (Chen *et al.,* 2020).

COVID-19 is a novel virus and little is known about it. Thus, extensive research is underway in an effort to learn more about the disease; how it spreads, how it might be prevented, and treated (Mehta *et al.,* 2020). In the meantime, this lack of information means that epidemiologists, public health strategists, and front-line health workers are, according to an expert from Imperial College, "flying blind" (Altmann 2020, cited by Hawker 2020). This clearly provides the potential for fear arousal among all concerned. The beast has many unknown properties, but it is viewed by all as being malign and to be feared.

**Fear in The General Population**

Between the end of February to the middle of March 2020, many countries began imposing various degrees of 'lockdown' with the WHO advising people to stay mainly at home and minimise physical contact with others in order to reduce spread of the disease and to protect the healthcare system (WHO, 2020c).

In an attempt to curb the spread of the COVID-19 virus, WHO (2019) recommended a combination of actions including prompt diagnosis thorough testing, the practice of tracking confirmed cases and self-isolation. These actions have proven effective in countries such as South Korea and China (Anderson et al., 2020). It is also suggested that these actions can protect already overstretched health care systems globally (Santini et al., 2020). For older people, and those considered otherwise vulnerable, social isolation is considered to be a form of protection because of the serious threat of autoimmune, neurocognitive, cardiovascular and mental health problems (Santini et al., 2020). Older people are defined as being over 70 years of age and 50 years in specific susceptible categories (Haffower, 2020). In the UK, there is an appallingly ageist discourse with some suggesting that older people are abandoned to their fate in care homes (Keeley, 2020).

There are a number of reasons that people around the world feel fearful of COVID-19. First, there is the obvious fear of contracting the disease, suffering and perhaps being one of the significant minorities who require admission to hospital. Fuelled by government instructions to "stay at home", this leads to anxiety about sharing any physical space, even though social distancing from other people reduces the risk of infection. This is known to prevent some people from leaving home, even to seek help or to get fundamental supplies such as food (Greenstone & Nigam, 2020). Some people, perhaps with significant non-COVID-19 illness, avoid visits to their general practitioners or the Accident and Emergency Department due to fear of contracting the disease from other patients (National Health Service [NHS] England, 2020).

Another source of fear is financial uncertainty since, despite government support, lockdown can impact on daily living, job security and the survival of businesses (Maital & Barzani, 2020). The prospective economic implications of lockdown and self-isolation are extensive, so much so that much of the world is in or heading towards recession (Maital & Barzani, 2020). The world's economy shows a downward trend as every part of the economy, from manufacturing and tourism to education and healthcare, struggle with containing the virus, whilst managing the associated economic threats (French & Monahan, 2020).

Another source of fear is lack of information: the unknown. Since there is not yet a vaccine or cure for COVID-19, no-one knows when this pandemic will be brought under control (Carleton, 2016 & Öhman, 2000). This might be heightened if there is a loss of faith in national leaders due to perceived shortcomings in the management of the pandemic, for example through lack of testing, insufficient personal protection equipment or inconsistent messages (WHO, 2020d). Whilst unsubstantiated, press reports indicate a fear in government that this could trigger social unrest. Some countries have already seen a wave of panic buying, food stocking, price inflation and other behaviours, which only serve to heighten the problem (French & Monahan, 2020).

Social relationships have become an essential component of our genetic make-up, an evolutionary necessity through protection, reproduction and survival (Cacioppo & Hawkley, 2009). For most people, social relationships provide personal security so the experience of isolation can be a cause of anxiety, though this will differ according to individual circumstances. For some people, especially those who work away from home or who previously struggled to maintain an acceptable work, life or family balance, lockdown could be seen as an opportunity to enjoy more quality time with their loved ones (WHO, 2020e). This is particularly true in homes where there is spacious accommodation and a garden. For others, especially those living alone, isolation and separateness may be feared and have adverse emotional consequences. Isolation can impact on mental health or aggravate existing mental health problems (Bradbury-Jones & Isham, 2020). Ever since the pioneering work of Cobb (1976), social support has been shown to act as a buffer against stress and is associated with better mental and physical health. More recent studies by Haines and Hurlbert (1993) show that people with reduced network support tend to have poorer mental health outcomes, and Cacioppo et al. (2006) found that isolation amongst older people is a significant predictor of depression.

The elderly are likely to be at particular risk of social isolation and fear since they are more likely to live alone and are constantly told by the government that they are at high risk of dying should they contract COVID-19. It is also the case that the elderly might be living far from any family or close friends and would be deprived of social contact normally provided by day care centres and places of worship (Santini et al., 2020). Since isolation limits physical contact and face-to-face communication (Curtis 2014), many people turn to online technologies during the lockdown. Newman & Zainal (2020) argue that this should be encouraged in order to enhance social and family support. Platforms such as Zoom have enjoyed great popularity since the lockdown (Guardian, 2020) but, although the use of the internet is growing among the elderly, there are still 4.2 million people aged 65+ who have never used the internet (Age UK, 2016). Thus, the elderly are likely to be an isolated and fearful group during the lockdown.

The importance of social contact has long been evidenced. Health and other care workers currently have to relate to many individuals from a distance. Without close proximity, important components of communication, such as touch and non-verbal communication, are compromised. Active listening is a major means of conveying compassion and, according to Jonas-Simpson et al. (2006), is the basis of all interpersonal relationships and an indispensable ingredient of providing quality care. Health care workers face the challenge of conveying a sense of being valued and connected over the telephone or, in clinical settings, from behind a visor (Bray et al., 2014, Jonas-Simpson et al., 2006 & Nathoo, 2017). These trivial acts of delivering care with compassion can help both patients and their families (Sanghavi, 2006). There is clear evidence in the literature that effective communication is the foundation of and is fundamental in the provision of good compassionate care (Bramley & Matiti, 2014 & Curtis, 2014). There are implications for education since health care workers now need to adapt their communication skills to meet these new challenges. It has been reported that compassion among nurses is at least a partly learnt trait (Nathoo, 2017).

Thus, there are many sources of fear among healthy people, but the problem is likely to be even worse among those with underlying mental health problems, whose symptoms may be exacerbated (Shigemura et al., 2020).

This is apparent from previous viral epidemics such as Ebola, which has a high mortality rate but a low level of infectivity, where lasting mental health implications have been documented; COVID-19 could have even worse consequences (Shigemura et al., 2020). Over 10,000 people have died due to the Ebola breakout, particularly in West Africa (WHO, 2014), whereas COVID-19 has taken the lives of hundreds of thousands, and has affected almost of the entire world (WHO, 2020c).

Another, and perhaps unexpected, source of fear during the lockdown is associated with a significant increase in domestic violence (UK Home Office, 2020 & Townsend, 2020), defined by Bradbury-Jones & Isham (2020) as an array of maltreatments that take place within domestic premises. The British Broadcasting Association (2020a) reports that there was a 25% spike in calls to the Domestic Violence Helpline in the first week of lockdown alone. It is often assumed that home is a safe place (Hearn & Whitehead, 2006) but for many people, mostly women and children, it can be the place of abuse (Bradbury-Jones & Isham, 2020). This is partly due to the pressures of social containment, and it is noted that victims' avenues of escape are greatly reduced during lockdown (Refuge, 2020). Lockdown can be a time of fear for those who were already experiencing toxic domestic relationships. Inadvertently, the COVID-19 lockdown measures seem to have granted perpetrators more freedom to exercise power and abuse their victims.

**Fear in Health Care Workers**

Healthcare workers such as nurses and doctors, who are classed as frontline workers or key workers, are also afraid of contracting the virus, falling ill and possibly dying of the disease. This is borne out by many televised and audio-recorded interviews with health care workers (for instance, Tempesta, 2020). Whatever their fears, all health professionals have an ethical duty to care for patients and their families. For example, the Nursing and Midwifery Council (NMC) Code (2018, p. 10) suggests that nurses 'should work with colleagues to preserve the safety of those receiving care' and the General Medical Council (GMC) (2013, p.2) stipulates that doctors should 'make the care of your patient your first concern'. Despite the professional imperative to continue working, some health care workers are in self-isolation as a result of symptoms or family members with symptoms. This, of course, leads to staff shortages and more pressure on those who remain at the bedside.

Fear of becoming infected is hardly surprising among those healthcare workers who are perpetually placed in high risk situations (Panagioti et al., 2018). Brooks et al. (2020) compared five research studies that examined the psychological implications of quarantined people who were infected with Severe Acute Respiratory Syndrome (SARS) and Ebola between 2009 and 2010. They found that many healthcare workers who were in contact with infected patients started developing symptoms of acute stress as quickly as nine days after contact. In another similar study, Bai et al. (2004) reported that some of the healthcare workers who were quarantined for a period of time were left feeling extremely tired, irritable, having reduced concentration and poor performance, possibly caused by lack of sleep.

Various research studies feature health care workers who were quarantined during the SARS epidemic and showed that they were fearful not only becoming infected, but were particularly worried about passing the infection on to their loved ones (Braunack-Mayer et al., 2013; Bai, et al., 2004). Nearly 25% of the United Kingdom's population fall into a high-risk category by virtue of age or underlying pathology, (Jordan et al., 2020), so it seems certain that many health care workers will be in the high-risk category. In many cases, they will also have partners, young children and older parents. Research in Wuhan by Chen et al. (2020) supports this claim by making comparisons between staff characteristics and those of people who had died of COVID-19. Their study concluded that the deaths were mainly in the category of people who were above sixty years of age, with comorbidities such as respiratory and cardiovascular disease. Albeit, to a much lesser extent, other studies show that COVID-19 can take the lives of much younger people too (Wang et al., 2020). Therefore, COVID-19 warrants concern among young people and pregnant women, who have also expressed fear of infection (Wang et al., 2020). However, all research studies suggest that COVID-19 deaths are mainly concentrated in the older population (Chen et al., 2020 & Wang et al., 2020).

Data from the UK government reveals that COVID-19 affects healthcare workers from the BAME (Black, Asian and Minority Ethnic) groups disproportionately (Rimmer, 2020). Accounts suggest that most health care workers who died of COVID-19 were from BAME groups, but it is worth noting that nearly one third of doctors fall into that category, (BBC, 2020b) and a similar situation exists among other health care workers.

Studies by Delobelle et al. (2009) and by Msiska et al. (2014) revealed that healthcare workers working with HIV were fearful of becoming infected with the virus, but were also concerned about acquiring other types of occupational infections when caring for HIV positive patients. One of the arguments made in the Delobelle et al. (2009, p.8) study was that, whilst the overwhelming response from nursing staff was that of compassion and empathy, they also asserted that "nobody volunteered to be infected". In regards to working with HIV, it has been evidenced that with the protection of universal precautions there should be no risk at all to the health care workers (Welch & Bunin, 2010). When practising universal precautions, healthcare workers have to avoid contact with patients' bodily fluids by using protective equipment, such as gloves, masks and aprons (WHO, 2007). Therefore, education of all healthcare workers and adherence to universal precautions is paramount. The same principles apply to COVID-19, though the mode of transmission is different.

COVID-19 predominantly spreads through droplets via the mouth or the nose, which can happen during coughing, sneezing or speaking (WHO, 2020b). Unequivocally, personal hygiene practices are crucial, including frequent hand washing with soap and water for a minimum of 20 seconds (WHO, 2020d). WHO (2020b) advise that people should stay at home and maintain social distancing, keeping at least one metre from other persons. Those health care workers anticipating contact with COVID-19 sufferers or carriers must also wear personal protective equipment (PPE) as appropriate, for example;

masks and visors. In the UK and elsewhere there have been difficulties meeting the suddenly increased demand for PPE (WHO, 2020f & Ranney, Griffiths and Jha, 2020) and this has been the cause of great anxiety among health care workers (ITN, 2020). Failure to provide this key equipment to health care workers can compromise care delivery to very sick patients with COVID-19, but could also put the employee's lives at risk.

It has been reported that a substantial number of COVID-19 infections cases are work-related (Koh, 2020). Koh (2020, p. 3) extends his claim by stating that out 'of 138 patients treated in a Wuhan hospital, 40 patients (29% of cases) were healthcare workers'. Whilst many hundreds of care workers have unfortunately succumbed to COVID 19, it is highly likely that the fatalities could have been prevented, had there been adequate PPE available. As a result, some workers have threatened to leave the profession. (Newman, 2020). Alongside the fear of personal infection, some health care workers report being avoided, disconcerted and hassled by members of the public who have felt fearful due to the nature of their work (Koh, 2020).

In order for NHS hospitals to prepare for the expected surge of admissions, a number of measures were instituted to increase bed availability and minimise infection risk. These measures included cancelling elective surgery and deterring the non-emergency cases from visiting hospitals (Burki, 2020). As noted above, this might have contributed to (non-COVID-19) sick people's reluctance to visit hospital due to fear of infection or a reluctance to add to the burden on the NHS. The result was that people suffering from serious medical problems, perhaps cancer or cardiac disease, avoided seeking medical assistance (Kutikov *et al.,* 2020). Of course; the risks of delaying treatment for many health conditions can have serious adverse effects (Kutikov *et al.,* 2020) and these add to the death toll resulting from the pandemic.

**Easing Restrictions; tuning down the fear**

COVID-19 was unknown to the world just a few months ago but is now considered a major pandemic, with rising number of cases and deaths internationally. Everyone's life has been unsettled and changes have been made, whether staying at home or avoiding others through social distancing. We have seen that there are various costs to this crisis: physical, emotional and economic. But fear has permeated all levels of society including health care workers, who are the vanguard of this crisis.

In all countries that have passed the initial peak, the debate has turned to how and when the lockdown restrictions can be eased or lifted. Speculation exists as to whether society and the NHS can ever get back to 'normal', or whether it is a matter of adjusting to a new normal. The main fear among policy-makers is of course the danger of a second wave of infection should restrictions be lifted too early. This would lead to more hospital admissions, more loss of life and more economic burden for individuals and the country (Prem *et al.*, 2020). For instance; one research study suggests that lifting the social distancing intervention at once could inflate the rate of infection (Kissler *et al.*, 2020), whilst another study recommends the maintaining of lockdown, with episodic easing (Singh & Adhikari, 2020).

Easing restrictions in some Asian countries such as Taiwan, Singapore and Hong Kong have resulted in a second wave of infection, compelling the respective governments to impose harsher measures than were formally in place (White et al., 2020). It is worth noting that as nations pursue a way forward to relax the lockdown, their main aim remains to strike a balance between maintaining the public health and mitigating the financial impact (White et al., 2020). However, as yet, there does seem to be any agreement or framework on the way to lift the lockdown. Instead some Asian countries, such as Hong Kong, have implemented a gradual easing and suppressing approach (White et al., 2020 & Mason and Stewart, 2020). It appears that the fears of policy-makers are shared by the public as polls show that the general population would be fearful about resuming 'normal' life even after restrictions are lifted (Dixon, 2020).

As Kang et al. (2019) argue, this pandemic is a new form of stress that does not compare with previous calamities, such as natural disasters or war, which are often localised to a region and offer the possibility of escape or avoidance (Morganstein & Ursano, 2020). Anyone can become infected anywhere and the outlook is unknown. It's no wonder fear is widespread among policy-makers, health care workers and the general public alike.

# My COVID Experience

*Nicola Jhumat*

I can remember the day the fear started. I was awaiting news of the birth of my nephew. It was Friday 13th March 2020. I decided that I needed to come into work during my annual leave as I'd been told, "we need to prepare for COVID: it's going to hit us hard!". At the time, I recall thinking it seemed a little "over the top" and surely it wasn't going to affect us as much as China? I got into work and I remember ordering PPE and making plans for the isolation of patients. I felt excited, but a little fearful. I got a text from my sister later that afternoon that my nephew had arrived. As I was driving to Wolverhampton from work, I remember thinking I felt a bit run down: strange for me as I normally have bags of energy!

I got to Wolverhampton, met my family, and everyone was so excited to find out when my nephew might be returning from hospital. I noticed through the evening that my throat had started to hurt, and I felt tired and lethargic. I got a text from my colleagues later saying we now had a stock of PPE for the wards and they had finalised the isolation plans for each ward. I remember thinking that they must have worked overtime but at least we would be prepared; I had no idea how imminently it would hit!

Sunday morning, we had news that my nephew would not be coming home straight away and had been taken into intensive care as one of his lungs had collapsed. The family were devastated: As he was the first grandchild in the family, we were all scared and anxious.  We were informed that we could not go to the hospital, as there had been a ban on all hospital visits. We were desperate to support our sister and my nephew.

I was feeling so low in mood and scared, praying and hoping that my nephew would be fine. I was feeling incredibly tired and experienced horrible headaches. I was taking naps throughout the day: I thought this was maybe my way of coping with the sad news. But, as always, I couldn't switch off from work and checked my emails. I saw that my supervisor had emailed me to say she had COVID 19 symptoms and that she would be off work for seven days. I started feeling even more worried about things.

Later on, I began a shift for the 'Single Point of Access Team' and as I was answering the calls my throat and voice were getting progressively worse. I had answered at least 30 calls, so I presumed that it was because I had been talking so much! I then took a call from a frequent caller who I have good rapport with. I answered with, "Hello Single Point of Access Nicola speaking," …which was received with "Oh my god, you sound awful, like you have Corona!" It was at that point the penny dropped… I had caught the virus! As I read and watched the news through the night, I realised that I had most of the symptoms.

In the morning, I told my family I needed to go back to London as I thought I had COVID symptoms. My Mum was laughing, telling me not to be silly, that I needed to stay to see the baby. But I didn't want to risk infecting people and was becoming increasingly more worried. I was gutted to be leaving without seeing my nephew. I thought to myself, 'He will probably have teeth by the time I see him!'

I got to London, texted my colleagues and told them that I thought I had COVID-19 symptoms. They were supportive: one asked me not to come anywhere near him! I was to isolate for seven days. I started to feel worse and worse - headaches, night sweats, feeling absolutely exhausted! On day four, I lost my sense of taste and smell and I started to feel I had no idea what was going on! I wanted to come back to work to help one of the senior colleagues because he was on his own dealing with the beginning of lockdown. We were not given priority for testing as health workers at the time. However, despite all of this, I believed it was best I self-isolate for the next seven days because I did not want to infect my patients or colleagues.

I spent every day at home during isolation absorbing the news and becoming more and more anxious. The restrictions were getting stricter and the death rates were rising. I started to realise the real level of threat to our nation. Day nine of being isolated and it was time to go back to work. I was feeling scared and anxious about what I was going back to. I came in to work and learned straight away I should go to a 'bronze meeting'. I had no idea what it was but was told to attend. I sat in the meeting and with all teams in our area were on the conference call. Colleagues were listing the staff that were off sick and patients that were positive.

That was only the beginning. We immediately realised that staffing was going to be a huge issue: there had been approximately ten people who were sick with symptoms. We then had three patients on one of the wards who were being isolated in their rooms after reading high temperatures. I knew that this would cause ward staff a lot of anxiety. The three patients later tested positive and I was asked to go and inform them that they had already caught the virus. I remember feeling pretty scared and I could feel the anxiety of all the staff in the room adding to my own fears. I agreed to go and inform each patient about their positive result.

I told all three patients about their positive results. There was one in particular who was quite tearful, and asked me if he was going to die. He said, "I don't have much family, will you be there for me?" I felt so upset for him at that point and reassured him. I told him that I had suffered with the symptoms and that I was now back at work. I told him that I would do my best to visit him as much as I could in his room, and we would provide him with some entertainment. He was given a DVD player and a radio, which seemed to help him settle down. I tried to visit him as much as I could, which he told me he really appreciated.

Looking back, I feel like every day there was a new challenge to face, each one tougher than the next. The numbers of staff going off sick seemed to increase day by day. I was calling agencies to cover. However, they had heard that the ward had COVID19 patients, so were refusing to send staff to our Trust site. Staff were deployed from other areas of the Trust, but the majority were unable to start immediately.

The Trust created a process of fast-track recruitment for healthcare support workers. I knew several people who expressed an interest in working for the NHS. I contacted them and the next day, I interviewed nine people for a health care assistant role for the bank. We needed those staff desperately and I knew it was very important to get them recruited and up and running as soon as possible. The interviews were fitted in in between conference calls and daily discharge meetings. I felt like I was constantly working at a 100 miles per hour.

We were told in one of our morning conference call that we were going to close a ward and reopen it as a mental health COVID ward. I remember the room falling into silence as we absorbed the news. The unit was already struggling with staff and we were all afraid what would happen if we had a whole ward of COVID patients.

The new COVID mental health ward meant that we needed to close beds. I had a good oversight of the patients on the units and who we could discharge easily and safely, so I immediately started to work with the Consultants and ward managers on discharging patients. The more I worked on this, the more I found myself enjoying the work. For periods, some of the fear dissipated. I was proud of myself when I was achieving results and supporting the ward to discharge numerous patients within a short period of time. It was a hugely difficult task, but it gave me insight into a new, or latent, skill I may have. As a team, we discovered that putting more emphasis on community care allows patients to be discharged efficiently and shortened inpatient admissions.

We are a mental health unit and we are required to deal with high risk patients who are a risk to themselves or others. During this time, we had a patient from the Psychiatric Intensive Care Unit who was placed in seclusion. The patient was very unwell and aggressive towards staff when they entered the seclusion room. Every time the patient required food or medication, he needed at least 12 staff to restrain him due to his level of risk of physical violence. He was a well-built man over six feet tall. As managers, we needed to support staff and be a part of the seclusion reviews. We found it difficult to get enough staff every time to go into seclusion. It proved to be a frightening and taxing experience for all involved.

The patient was not recovering quickly, and we needed to perform a restraint roughly twice a day for two weeks. I was heartbroken for staff who had to enter an environment which could prove risky. The restraints were difficult and traumatic, and four staff were injured during this time. I remember feeling that we could never repay them enough for what they face and for being so hardworking, resilient and caring.

During the peak of COVID we found out that three of our long service colleagues had died due to COVID. This obviously affected staff in a major way. I spent so much time consoling staff and sharing their pain. For each of their funerals, we arranged a special tribute; staff really appreciated this as it was a way to say goodbye to their colleagues. It was a surreal time for me as I felt that I was organising funerals every week. There was so much grief and fear around.

During all of these experiences, there were many days my peers and I cried together, acknowledging how much pressure we were dealing with. Without the support of my peers I do not think I would have coped during the peak period. We supported each other, we laughed and cried together. There were times where I did not think we would cope but as managers, we continued to put a brave face on for staff and tried to maintain a positive attitude in order to support and energise our fearful, grieving, workforce.

Life has been stressful, full of fear, and grief and confusion. But we've maintained our hope. My hopes for the 'new normal' are that our relationships with other bodies and organisations, such as the housing department in the local council, will continue to strengthen. During the peak period; we had direct links with the head of housing and funding panel members. We had a daily call with housing, and felt cases were thus dealt with more efficiently. Funding was now being approved both rapidly and fairly, in the form of care packages and supported accommodation. We managed to discharge a number of patients during these calls, a true reflection of how integrated care should work.

We've been able to recruit a number of bank staff which reduced reliance on agency staff. There was a speedy response to employment checks and the Human Resources Department have been responsive to our service needs. Trust Executive team members will continue to spend time in the local sites. I appreciated the trust health and safety team supporting us actively with a seclusion review. I feel that it was of huge benefit to both parties. I think there was learning on both parts from this experience.

The infection control team will keep visiting our site and providing training to staff around PPE and COVID advice. Recruitment has become far more efficient which I hope will continue.

As managers, staff wellbeing was the most crucial thing we needed to do to be able to help them cope with what they were facing. They had lost their colleagues and were dealing with isolating COVID patients. I personally felt that direct formal and informal support was needed every single day and we needed to provide several different approaches to let people know they were supported. I felt great waves of compassion for our staff at times and was determined to show them that management wanted to support them and acknowledge that they were dealing with extreme pressure.

We organised several different approaches to support our staff:

- We set up a wellbeing room for staff with relaxation and mindfulness activities
- The psychologist offered 1:1 sessions
- We ran relaxation groups every day for staff
- There was a remembrance room where staff could go to pay their respects for their colleagues that had passed away

- We initiated a 'Return to Work' group
- We organised hot meals to be served to staff every day from a local charity

The COVID experience, I can only describe as being a frightening rollercoaster, waiting for it to slow down and eventually stop. We are in the phase where it seems to be slowing down and we have been told to "stay alert." I only hope that the rollercoaster does not start again.

There are unique challenges to working in mental health. Even without COVID-19, our work in mental health units is extremely stressful, full of fears, uncertainty and sadness, as well as laughter, growth and optimism. We need to continue with the good practices we identified during COVID-19 that have made our work more efficient and enhanced quality. We will always look after and cherish the staff that work for our beloved NHS. Oh – and my nephew is now two and half months old and doing really well!

# Your Money or Your Life: The Dilemmas of Unlocking the Lockdown

*Ade Odunlade & Ryan Kemp*

Stand and deliver your money or your life!
Try and use a mirror no bullet or a knife!

And even though you fool your soul
Your conscience will be mine
All mine

Lyrics of Stand and Deliver! By Adam and the Ants (1981)
Songwriters: Marco Pirroni / Adam Ant

Across the world a number of countries are now, as of late May 2020, in the process of unlocking the lockdown. The main question is how to unlock, and in what manner should the journey back to 'normal' be approached? Indeed, will there ever be a return to normal or to some sort of steady-state 'new normal' as it is now generally being referred to.

We have witnessed the unprecedented situation of a world-wide lockdown and the massive economic impact is beginning to cause uneasiness. It is now time for politicians to get back to the centre stage as the virus starts to threaten the economic prowess that has been the boast of leaders like Donald Trump. Has the time now come for scientists and health care leaders to get back into their labs and wards and influence from there? Who will occupy the centre stage of decision making in this emergency?

In the UK, the government responded with money to support businesses, workers and different sectors of the economy. The initial support level offered by Government was to Furlough staff by paying up to 80% of their salary subject to a maximum of £2,500 a month. At the time of writing, the number of people getting the support was approximately 7.5 million of the working population. The government borrowed 64 billion pounds in April 2020, more than it forecast for the entire calendar year. This is a huge economic burden for any government; attention thus shifted to easing the lockdown.

Easing lockdown was never going to be an easy set of decisions. The battle is between fear and economic revival. Across the world, the number of unemployed is rising at an alarming rate and comparisons to the great depression are being made. So how safe should it be before people can go back to work? The government has indicated that the R rate (measuring the rate of transmission of the virus) should be significantly below 1 (thus the infection rate is declining) before any significant unlocking can be undertaken. At the time of writing, the indication is that the R rate going in that direction, but people are still dying at a daily rate in the hundreds. No vaccine or significant medical breakthrough is anywhere in sight.

**Releasing the Lockdown is deadly; Not releasing the Lockdown is deadly**

This political dilemma, of how quickly to ease the lockdown, seems on the surface obvious. If the lockdown is kept in place, we save lives. This will result in fewer infections and therefore fewer deaths. This is undeniable, as the various lockdowns around the world have proved. So why the dilemma? Clearly in the UK, where the death toll in late May was heading towards 40 000 deaths, the government must choose to protect lives? Surely it can't be any other way.

We would suggest it is far from that simple. If lockdown persists, the following is also very likely: continued economic stimulus; higher government debt and possibly currency devaluation; higher personal debt levels; higher business failures (especially in certain sectors); higher unemployment, possibly affecting the youth more significantly. All this this adds up to a significant economic shock to the UK economy, but also to the world economy. These sorts of shocks do not play out or become resolved very quickly. It would probably take a generation to repay these debts, as it did after the Second World War. The economy will take several years to regain the GDP (Gross Domestic Product) lost during the lockdown. Individuals will become less wealthy and more indebted. All of this adds up to more poverty and economic hardship across a wider ambit of society.

Poverty, however, is not just buying and owning things. It has wide scale effects, some of which are often ignored. For example; it is likely that this economic shock will again widen the gap between rich and poor and this in turn will have significant effects, even if households cope with the day to day effects. Income inequality has been shown to increase mental health issues, increase physical health issues, result in higher crime and lower life satisfaction (Fiscella & Williams, 2004). It has been shown to result in lower life expectancy. Inequality is deadly. Children brought up in poverty have significantly more health problems immediately and over a life-time than those brought up outside poverty (AAP COUNCIL ON COMMUNITY PEDIATRICS, 2016). Poverty has significant effect on mental health, with the mechanisms likely to complex and multiple (see Burns, 2015). In addition, and perhaps it is not surprising that the same effects are seen with physical health and longevity (Fiscella & Williams, 2004). Ultimately, this means economic problems become quality of life and health problems. And the effects are literally deadly. People die from the poverty. To ignore economics is to ignore the fact that people will die from financial hardship.

While I travel to work during the COVID-19 period, I see signs which read "stay apart". We are told to "keep a distance", to "socially isolate" and avoid human contact. Others are dangerous and we should not, outside our family, touch, hug or shake each other's hands. Rightfully, we are being driven apart to avoid the spread of the virus, but how long can we sustain this separation. A second major issue which will persist if the lockdown is delayed, is loneliness. Many people now live alone, 7.7 million (almost 12%) in the UK in 2017 (Guardian, 2019) and this is made more complex if these individuals are in high risk groups. Loneliness was a significant issue in the UK before lockdown (Conclin et al., 2014), so the social distancing and isolation strictures of the lockdown have added to these concerns. It should be noted that being alone is not the same as loneliness (see Martin Weegmann's chapter in this volume) and some can benefit from alone time. But many suffer from isolation and it affects both our mental and physical health. A recent review of 128 papers, all but 2 found loneliness and social isolation to be detrimental to health. Depression and cardiovascular disease were the most common adverse health outcomes. In summary we can see that loneliness is another significant risk factor which could be ignored in our attempts to determine when and how to unlock the lockdown.

It is clearly difficult to estimate what the effects of poverty and loneliness will have on the population if lockdown is continued. Would it be as large as the effect of a mass infection of the COVID-19 virus? Impossible to predict some would say. However, it does point to the complexity of the decisions facing the government in making unlocking decisions. Continue lockdown and the virus is contained, but poverty and loneliness have their pernicious effects. Unlock and the virus will continue its spread across the population with its unique ruthless efficiency. Now modelling can have some part of this decision making, but ultimately these amount to clever guesses. With multiple variables, it is near impossible to model such scenarios very accurately. At the end of the day, politicians will have to make decisions. Either option is deadly and this where the ultimate responsibility of leadership is borne.

## Battle between Science and Politics

United States have become a particular battleground of Scientists versus Politicians, perhaps soon to be a tasteless game we will all play on our smartphones. The leaders of Science, such as Dr Anthony Fauci, head of the National Institute of Allergy and Infectious Diseases (NIAID) produce evidence, create models and weight up strategies. The Politicians, led by Donald J. Trump, populist president and lover of conspiracy theories, insist on unlocking immediately and set dates they invariably have to change. Brazil is another country struggling with such a standoff.

It appears as though Dr Fauci wants a careful and prolonged unlocking, while Donald Trump seems to be focussed on his political standing considering that the November election is close. Economic disaster is never an election winner.

In the United Kingdom, the government has started with unlocking what is deemed a calculated approach, although the four nations of the United Kingdom all appear to be taking different routes out of lockdown. What is it that the Prime Minister could see that informed process of unlocking the country that the politicians in all other four nations of Scotland, Wales and Northern Ireland couldn't see? Are we now in the territory of politics deciding on unlocking the country rather than the facts evidenced by science? It's a new type of fear driving the decision making – political fear! It is interesting to watch each nation making their arguments, despite the indication that for each the situation is more or less similar. It is even more interesting if you live just across the border and you can't drive yourself across it. You may like to exercise and work, being vigilant of course and maintaining social distance, but if you cross the border you risk being arrested.

Even more interesting is the plea in England to drive to work and avoid overcrowding on the trains and tube lines. Days after the announcement, Transport for London announced the reintroduction of the congestion charge, which was suspended due to COVID-19. As if that is not sufficient, the price will be going up from £11.50 to £15. Welcome to the post-COVID world. The reality is beginning to become apparent - all of us will be paying back the costly price of fighting this pandemic.

Teaching Unions are not feeling amused by the prospect of unlocking of schools. These unions are now openly opposing the unlocking. Even Premier Division footballers are expressing doubts and reservations. The British Medical Association has declared support for the teacher's union. Our society may be getting back to some sort of normal and another battle has started. An attempt by the government to convince the unions by arranging a meeting with scientific advisers ended with no conclusion. The scientists are now appearing to be falling down the pecking order of utility, previously being used to provide assurance to the public. While the unions are standing in opposition to the government, a number of councils across England – Liverpool, Gateshead, Hartlepool, Newcastle and Sunderland have joined in raising concerns about reopening schools.

According to the BBC, Gateshead Council leader Martin Gannon, said his town would be sticking to the 'stay at home' message that was enforced in England before the new announcement to 'stay alert'. 'Stay at Home' is still being used in Scotland, Wales, and Northern Ireland. Quoting the interview, he said; "I think we are beginning to unlock too early and there are going to be consequences. We do not have the same legislative powers as Scotland, Wales, and Northern Ireland in the North East. But if we did, I would be doing exactly the same as what they are doing and staying with the lockdown."

The UK Government has run a daily press conference since the start of the emergency. Latterly, we note that they field politicians who are advocating more and more for the need to open the country. They talk of a delicate balance, yet of the need to protect the economy which has suffered a severe battering and also the need to prevent a second wave of infections. Unlocking the lockdown may be a process of trial and error with some elements of science woven into it. It does not appear to be only a scientific process. Certainly not 'led by the science', a much-repeated mantra until this point by UK government ministers.

## Ultimate Choices

When all is said and done, ending the lockdown and managing the transition back to the new normal is a national decision. It is really is a planetary choice, but at this point in time we are unable to cooperate on that scale. As a national question, it falls to government and to them alone. No matter what subject experts might say, the decisions are complex, and opinion is unlikely to be at the level of consensus. The public are unlikely to be unified in their opinion. Therefore, difficult decisions are needed; leadership is needed. Any politician may claim to be "led by the science" or to be making "evidence based" decisions, but the truth is the evidence will not be sufficient. Beyond science and facts, this will require wisdom and integrity. It will require leaders who can look deep into their souls, consult with their God and find the time to contemplate the future. Almost forty thousand people have dead already. How many more can we take? These are questions of ultimate importance.

As the world unlocks, various businesses are now making big decisions about the future of work and how services are delivered. Quite clearly, we are not all going to be working from offices as before, people are now going to think differently about how they provide their services, and we now know we can do more with reduced workforce, and at last welcome to the digital world! What will the world be with social distancing becoming a new norm, face masks now becoming fashion accessories – we all used to think Michael Jackson was freaky wearing masks everywhere he went, but now we all are in the same boat.

**Welcome to the new world.**

# Biographies

## Kevin Acott

Kevin is an experienced educator, clinician, coach, inspector and manager in mental health and social care. His clinical, educational and research interests are in self-harm, mindfulness and the arts, empathy, and the impact of trauma. He currently works at Buckinghamshire New University as a Senior Lecturer.

## Prince Ade-Odunlade

Managing Director, Jameson Division in Central and North West London NHS Foundation Trust

Ade is a mental health professional with extensive experience in clinical leadership, clinical transformation, workforce development, learning and development, and senior management roles gained over the last 25 years.

He has a wide range of qualifications and experience as a professional in Medical Sociology, Sex & Couple Therapy, Mental Health, Economics, Communications, Project Management, Coaching, Medication Management, Medical Law, Epidemiology & Statistics, Business Administration, Computing and Healthcare Leadership.

## Laura Cavill

My Contribution in a nutshell: I have "suffered" from poor Mental Health for about 30 years now. I never imagined, through all the crises, chaos, homelessness and symptoms of my ill health, I would ever have opportunity to write poetry again, share it, enjoy it and feel proud. One Community scooped me up in its safety net and continues to carry us all in our recovery.
Thank you. X

*Robyn Doran*

Robyn is Chief Operating Officer for CNWL NHS TRUST, which is a large community-based organisation with a £500 million turnover and 7000 staff spread over 160 sites.

She has worked in the Trust for over 30 years. Robyn has worked as a non-exec in the private sector as well as many voluntary sector organisations. Robyn qualified as a registered psychiatric nurse in New Zealand in 1983. She has held a number of positions in management in various mental health, addiction, offender care, learning disabilities and community services in New Zealand, Australia and England.

In 2005, she completed her MSc in Change Agent Skills at Surrey University. She has an interest in maximising individual's potential and building dynamic and effective teams working within in complex environments.

In July 2017 Robyn led the NHS provider response to the Grenfell disaster. She describes this as a privilege and one of the most challenging and rewarding assignments she has worked on in her 37 years in health care.

Robyn has recently completed a Diploma in coaching as she feels it will be invaluable in her role as a leader in the NHS and also working alongside the Grenfell community.

*Dr Ian Ewing*

Dr Iain Ewing MRCP graduated in Medicine with Distinction in Clinical Practice from the University of London in 2006. He was appointed as a Consultant Physician and Hepatologist to an NHS Foundation Trust in 2015. He has published original research on the molecular basis of tumourigenesis, and review articles on gastrointestinal cancers and novel endoscopic findings. Dr Ewing is a specialty Clinical Lead and Divisional Governance Lead, and continues to see acute general medical patients, alongside his specialty and managerial interests.

### Dr Scott Galloway

Dr Scott Galloway is a Consultant Clinical Psychologist and now Chief Clinical Information Officer with extensive experience of both NHS and private practice in mental health, learning disabilities and offending. His doctoral thesis examined the development of morality in offenders and non-offenders with learning disabilities, and his personal experiences of wartime conflict and their impacts on a moral code inform this chapter.

### Neil Gardner

Neil Gardner is an Artist/Illustrator, who has work in private and public collections in the UK, Europe and the USA. His preferred medium is watercolour, pen and ink.

The design depicted is based on the idea of the world at war, struggling to come to terms with an invisible enemy, COVID 19. The people who are tasked to fight and tame the enemy are frontline Health Care Professionals. They tirelessly and unselfishly throw their heart and souls in to the daily battle.

The virus is an indiscriminate killer, that does not respect gender, colour, creed or seemingly age. The crisis has highlighted even more than before, our need to love and respect our HCP.

### Nicola Jhumat

Nicola is a Practice development Manager/Lead Occupational Therapist and senior research practitioner for Park Royal centre for mental health.

Qualified in 2008 at Brunel university and has worked in mental health for the entirety of her career. Nicola has worked in mental health for 12 years and has clinical experience and expertise in acute and forensic mental health settings. Nicola has working experience in acute mental health, forensic inpatient, community, rehabilitation, home treatment team, health-based place of safety, single point of access and outreach OT.

Nicola's current role is to lead a therapy team and provide therapeutic program to a large mental Health hospital. She has a passion for working in mental health and part of her role is to research and demonstrate the effectiveness of occupational therapy in acute mental health.

### Dr Ryan Kemp

Ryan Kemp PhD, is a Consultant Clinical Psychologist and currently Director of Therapies in Central & North West London NHS Foundation Trust. He is Honorary Professor of Clinical Practice at Brunel University London and associate fellow of the British Psychological Society. His first book, *Transcending Addiction*, was published by Routledge in 2018.

### Dr Anna Maratos

Anna Maratos is a recently qualified Group Analyst working in the NHS. Her first degree at Oxford sparked her interest in the psychology behind UK politics and the interpersonal challenges that often seem to accompany power and privilege.

### Ntsoaki Mary Mosoeunyane

Ntsoaki Mary Mosoeunyane is a senior lecturer in biopsychosocial sciences for health studies. Currently holding a position for Black and Ethnic Minority (BAME) Lead for student issues, a writer/blogger for Positive Psychology People (PPP) and author of My Life in England. She has research interests around narratives of how racial bias impact well-being amongst BAME groups. An active participant in BAME forums and keen on collaborative work to develop strategies on 'race-dialogue' beyond COVID-19.

### Claire Murdoch, CBE

Claire Murdoch CBE is Chief Executive of Central and North West London NHS Foundation Trust, appointed in 2007 and overseeing CNWL's expansion into community and out of hospital healthcare, sexual health and offender care in London, Surrey and Milton Keynes, as well as mental health and psychological therapies in North West London and Milton Keynes. In April 2016, she was also appointed National Director for Mental Health, at NHS England. She has been a registered mental health nurse for 36 years. Claire has extensive clinical and leadership experience in mental health and community care, the NHS's middle pillar between GPs and Acute hospitals.

***Dr Sanj Nathoo*** (DProf, MSc, FHEA, Dip. Nurs, Ed. & Health & Safety)
Sanj qualified as a nurse in 1996 and was promoted to a charge nurse after two years. He joined Higher Education as a Senior Lecturer at the Buckinghamshire New University 2002, where he has been teaching on many nursing courses at both pre and post graduate levels. He has experience in curriculum development and programme coordination. His research interests and written articles are mostly based on 'compassion and caring in nursing, the older person, safety and quality of care in nursing'.

***Dr Sara Northey***
Dr Sara Northey is a Clinical Psychologist who has worked in the NHS for 20 years. Sara has a special interest in child and family trauma, and currently works as clinical lead for children and young people in the Grenfell Health & Wellbeing Service. Sara is also a qualified yoga teacher and is particularly interested in the integration of body-based and psychological therapies for post-traumatic stress.

***Margaret Pratt***
Margaret is an adult nurse lecturer at Bucks New University but has enjoyed a varied nursing career, from Trauma and Orthopaedics to working at the world-famous Dean Street Sexual Health Clinic, London. She's been a police officer, private detective and postwoman. From gaining a 1st Class Honours Degree at Bucks University she's finally found her calling. Margaret is married with two children, has two German Shepherds and loves riding her motorbike.

***Dr Pras Ramluggun***
Dr Pras Ramluggun is a Senior Lecturer in Mental Health at Oxford Brookes University. He is a Senior Fellow of the Health Education Academy. In his teaching he encourages a culture of collaborative enquiry with students.

His clinical expertise is in forensic psychiatry and is a former Clinical Lead for the Prison Primary Mental Health Services. His pedagogic research is on the enhancement of teaching processes and student experience with a focus on promoting students' emotional resilience and mental wellbeing.

### David Rawcliffe

David Rawcliffe is a Professional Lead for Mental Health at Buckinghamshire New University. He started mental health nursing in 1977. He holds degrees in Mental Health, Education and Applied Positive Psychology. He has three times won the award for most inspirational tutor. Presented at the European Applied Positive Psychology Conference, National Research conferences and International Nurse Research Conferences. He is published on nursing students, mentors and autism.

### Margaret Rioga

RMHN, FHEA, MA (Education), BSc (Substance Use and Misuse) MSc Applied Positive Psychology

Margaret is an Associate Professor of Education and Professional Practice. She has extensive experience of working in Forensic Mental Health services and in academia working in pre-registration nursing. Margaret's specialist area of research is recovery, service user and carer involvement. Her recent work has been exploring the interrelationship between mental health recovery models and positive psychology interventions.

### Dr David G. Shaw (DGS) (MA, MSc CSci, PhD)

David is semi-retired academic in health psychology working independently.

### Brian Sheppard

Brian has been Qualified as a Registered Mental Nurse for the past 20 years. During this time, he worked as a Community Mental Health Nurse, Dual Diagnosis Specialist Nurse and then later as the Clinical Lead for Dual Diagnosis. Brian started his career as a lecturer/ senior lecturer 7 years ago, where he taught mental health nursing to post reg community health nurses. He now teaches Mental Health nursing to pre reg nursing students at Bucks New University. Brian's main interest and research was Cannabis and Mental Health, and Transgender Mental Health.

### Nolene Sheppard

For over 20 years, Nolene Sheppard, a holder of an Executive MBA, has worked within the healthcare industry. She held upper management positions, as well as crisis management positions, at various companies with the goal of resolving conflicts, financial distress, and administrative disorganisation. She also worked on international projects with WHO and EU dealing with the spread of diseases and viruses.

Since 2014, Ms Sheppard has been a Personal Development Coach and Trainer in Germany.

### Professor David Sines

CBE BSc (Hons) RN RMN RNMH RNT PGCTHE PhD FRCN FRSA FHEA

Professor David Sines CBE was until recently Pro Vice Chancellor and Executive Dean and Professor of Community Health Care Nursing at the Faculty of Society and Health at Buckinghamshire New University and holds the position of Provost at the University.

He held previous roles as Executive Dean for the Faculty of Health & Social Care at London South Bank University and as Head of School of Health Sciences at the University of Ulster. David obtained his PhD in social policy from the University of Southampton in 1993 and has held four Secretary of State appointments, including appointments to the UKCC and NMC.

He has been a Governor of three NHS Foundation Trusts in London. He recently held an Honorary Appointment with Imperial College Healthcare NHS Trust as Associate Director of Nursing. He is a Fellow of the RCN and received a CBE in the 2010 Queen's Birthday Honours List for 'Services to Health Care'. David is a Non-Executive Director with the Central London NHS Community Healthcare Trust and an Associate Non-Executive Director with Buckinghamshire NHS Hospitals Trust. David is also an Emeritus Professor with Buckinghamshire New University and Strategic Advisor to the Vice Chancellor.

David is currently appointed as a professional advisor to Health Education England and works closely with primary and community care workforce strategy and transformation in North London. David is a Trustee with The Burdett Nursing Trust and is Patron with the Learning Disability Charity Choice Support and holds appointment as Honorary Vice President with the Northern Ireland Charity People and Professionals for Autism.

David has undertaken two previous periods of engagement with the HEE GP Deanery in both NWL and HENCEL and acted as a fully functioning Associate Director for the GP Deanery at the University of London for a twelve-month period as part of this role. David was Chair of the Health Education England Stakeholder Engagement Committee that produced the HEE (DHSC approved) Education and Training Framework for Non-Surgical Cosmetic interventions in 2015 and was subsequently appointed as Independent Chair of the Joint Council for Cosmetic Practitioners in January 2016.

### Dr Kathy Swanzy-Derben
Doctorate in Nursing, MBA, MSc, PG Dip, BSc(Hons), RMN, RGN.

Kathy is a Capital Nurse Foundation Programme Manager and Lead for International Healthcare Partnerships and BAME Mentoring at Central and North West London NHS Foundation Trust. Kathy has dual registration in Mental Health Nursing and Adult Nursing and has occupied a number of management and nurse leadership positions in a variety of clinical settings. She has a special interest in compassion and completed her doctoral thesis in Compassionate Care in Acute Mental Health'.

### Mike Waddington
Mike Waddington, 62, has been Communications Director at CNWL since 2014, with 17 years in the NHS and 38 years total experience in communication. Married to Jane, a language teacher with whom he goes in search of blue plaques. Struggles to play the, cello but the struggle is essential; he holds to the running adage that "pain is inevitable; suffering is optional".

### Dr Martin Weegmann

Martin Weegmann is a Clinical Psychologist and Group Analyst, with 30 years NHS experience, based on London. He has specialised in substance misuse, personality disorders and complex needs and has conducted workshops/lectured widely. Martin has published many papers and 6 books. His latest being the edited Psychodynamics of Writing (2018, Routledge). He is busy at work on a new, more popular book, Stories of an NHS Psychologist.

### Harvey Wells

Harvey Wells is a Senior Lecturer in Medical Education at Bart's and the London School of Medicine and Dentistry, Queen Mary University of London. By professional background, he is a psychotherapist with over 20 years of experience and has practised in the NHS, the charity sector and in private practice. He has specialised in working with patients with comorbid mental health and substance misuse.

### Nikki Yun

Nikki Yun is a Senior Staff Nurse in General Intensive Care at St George's University Hospitals NHS Foundation Trust. She is an Honorary Senior Lecturer at Kingston University and teaches medical students at Queen Mary University of London. Nikki qualified in 2015 and has since won two prestigious awards through The Nursing Times and a Cavell Star Award. In 2018 she was shortlisted for the Nursing Times Rising Star Award.

# References

AAP COUNCIL ON COMMUNITY PEDIATRICS. (2016). Poverty and Child Health in the United States. Pediatrics, 137(4): e20160339.

Abe, J.A.A. (2016) A longitudinal follow up study of happiness and meaning making, Journal of Positive Psychology, 11(5) 489-498.

Abramowitz, S. A. (2005). The poor have become rich, and the rich have become poor: Collective trauma in the Guinean Languette. Social Science & Medicine, 61(10), 2106-2118.

Ackroyd, K., Fortune, D. G., Price, S., Howell, S., Sharrack, B., & Isaac, C. L. (2011). Adversarial growth in patients with multiple sclerosis and their partners: relationships with illness perceptions, disability and distress. Journal of Clinical Psychology and Medicine, 18, 372–379.

Adams, R.E. & Boscarino, J.A. (2006). Predictors of PTSD and Delayed PTSD After Disaster. The Journal of Nervous and Mental Disease, 194(7) p.485-493. Doi: 10.1097/01.nmd.0000228503.95503.e9.

Age UK (2020) Loneliness, [Online] Age UK Retrieved from: https://www.ageuk.org.uk/information-advice/health-wellbeing/loneliness/, Accessed on 7th June, 2020.

Age UK. (2016) The Internet And Older People in The UK: Key Statistics. Age UK. Available at: https://www.ageuk.org.uk/globalassets/age-uk/documents/reports-and-publications/reports-and-briefings/active-communities/rb_july16_older_people_and_internet_use_stats.pdf (accessed 03 May 2020).

Ahorsu, D.K., Lin, C., Imani, V., Saffari, M., Griffiths, M.D. & Pakpour, A.H. (2020) The Fear of COVID-19 Scale: Development and Initial Validation. International Journal of Mental Health and Addiction, pp.1-9.

Akhtar, M. (2018) Positive Psychology for Overcoming Depression: Self help strategies to build strength, resilience and happiness, Watkins Publishing Limited.

Alegria, M., Atkins, M., Farmer, E., Slaton, E., & Stelk, W. (2010). One Size Does Not Fit All: Taking Diversity, Culture and Context Seriously. Administration and Policy in Mental Health and Mental Health Services Research, 37(1–2), 48–60. https://doi.org/10.1007/s10488-010-0283-2

Alkema, K., Linton, J.M. & Davies, R.A. (2008) Study of the relationship between self-care, compassion satisfaction, compassion fatigue, and burnout among hospice professionals. Journal of Social Work in End of Life Palliative Care, 4(2): 101–119.

Allen, A. cited by R. Pemblebury. (2020) 'Like the band on the Titanic, we keep on playing. But this ship will not sink: after 23 years in critical care, nothing prepared Anthea Allen for the war zone at her London hospital. Her diary from the coronavirus front like will horrify and inspire you.' Daily Mail Online. 28 April 2020. Available at: www.dailymail.co.uk/health/article-8262511/After-23-years-critical-care-prepared-ANTHEA-ALLEN-war-zone-London-hospital.html (Accessed 28 April 2020)

Allen, A.B. & Leary, M.R. (2010) Self-compassion, stress and coping, Social Personal Psychology Compass, 4(2), p.107-118.

Altman, D. (2011) Positively mindful: Skills, concepts and research, Positive Acorn.

American Psychiatric Association (APA) (2013) Diagnostic and Statisitical Manual – 5th Edition (DSM-5), New York, APA.

American Psychiatric Association, (2001). The principles of medical ethics: With annotations especially applicable to psychiatry. American Psychiatric Publication Incorporated.

Amin, A.A., Vankar, J.R., Nimbalkar, S.M., & Phatak, A.G. (2015) Perceived stress and professional quality of life in neonatal intensive care unit nurses in Gujarat, India. Indian Journal of Pediatrics, 82(11) p.1001–1005.

Amsruda, K.E., Lybergb, A. and Severinsson, E. (2019) Development of resilience in nursing students: A systematic qualitative review and thematic synthesis. Nurse education in Practice, 41, 102621.

Anderson, K., Delic, A., Komproe, I., Avdibegovic, E., van Ee, E. & Glaesmer, H. (2019) Predictors of posttraumatic growth among conflict-related sexual violence survivors from Bosnia and Herzegovina, Conflict and Health, 13(23) 1-11

Anderson, R.M., Heesterbeek, H., Klinkenberg, D. & Hollingsworth, T.D. (2020). How will country-based mitigation measures influence the course of the COVID-19 epidemic? Lancet. 395, pp. 31-34.

Andrews, K. (2016): The problem of political blackness: lessons from the Black Supplementary School Movement, Ethnic and Racial Studies. Online Available at: http:www.openaccess.bcu.ac.uk. [Accessed: 05/05/20]

Ansell-Pearson, K (2013) 'Attachment To Life, Understanding Death: Nietzsche and D.H. Lawrence'. Parrhesia, 18, pp.22-35

Arendt, H (1998i) Love and St Augustine. Chicago: University Of Chicago Press

Arendt, H (1998ii) The Human Condition, 2nd ed. Chicago: University Of Chicago Press

Ariapooran S. (2014) Compassion Fatigue and burnout in Iranian nurses: the role of perceived social support. Iran Journal of Nursing and Midwifery Research, 19(3) p. 279–284.

Arimitsu, K. (2016) The effects of a program to enhance self compassion in Japanese individuals: A randomized controlled pilot study, Journal of Positive Psychology. 11(6) p.559-571.

Aristotle. (1999) Nicomachean Ethics. (Trans. M. Ostwald). Upper Saddle river, NJ: Prentice-Hall (Original work published ca. 350 BCE).

Arnold-Forster, A. (2020) Has covid put practitioners back in touch with their reasons for becoming healthcare professionals? BMJ Blogs. Available at: https://blogs.bmj.com/bmj/2020/04/23/agnes-arnold-forster-has-covid-put-practitioners-back-in-touch-with-their-reasons-for-becoming-healthcare-professionals/ (Accessed 30 April 2020)

Ashir, M., & Marlowe, K. (2008). Traffic Lights: A practical clinical risk management system for community Early Intervention in Psychosis teams PO184. Early Intervention in Psychiatry, 2.

Asok, A., Kandal., E.R., & Rayman, J.B. (2019). The neurobiology of Fear Generalization. Frontiers in Behavioral Neuroscience. 12(329). p.1 – 15.

Austin, W., Goble, E., Leier, B. & Byrne, P. (2009) Compassion fatigue: The experience of nurses. Ethics and Social Welfare, 3(2), p.195-214.

AutisticPb (2020) My Positive about lockdown, [Online] Retrieved from: https://autisticpb.wordpress.com/my-positives-about-lockdown/, Accessed on 7th June, 2020.

Baddeley, A.D. (1986) Working Memory, Oxford, Oxford University Press.

Baddeley, A.D. and Logic, E.H. (1992) Auditory imagery and working memory IN Nickerson, R.G. (Editor) Attention and Performance VIII, Hillsdale, N.J., Lawrence Erlbaum.

Badger, K. & Royse, D. (2012) Describing compassionate care: The burn survivor's perspective. Journal of Burn Care & Research, 33(6), p.772-780.

Bai, Y; Lin, C. C; Lin, C. Y; Chen, J. Y; Chue, C. M; Chou, P. (2004) Survey of stress reactions among health care workers involved with the SARS outbreak. Psychiatr Serv; 55, pp. 1055–57.

Bali, S., Stewart, K.A. & Pate, M.A. (2016) Long shadow of fear in an epidemic: fearonomic effects of Ebola on the private sector in Nigeria. British Medical Journal Global Health. 1(3) p.2-13.

Bannink, F. (2014) Post Traumatic Success: Positive Psychology & Solution-Focused Strategies to Help Clients Survive & Thrive, W.W. Norton and Company.

Bar-Dayan, Y., Boldor, N., Kremer, I., London, M., Levy, R., Barak, M.I., and Bar-Dayan, Y. (2011) Who is willing to risk his life for a patient with a potentially fatal, communicable disease during the peak of A/H1N1 pandemic in Israel? Journal of Emergencies, Trauma and Shock, 4(2): 184–187.

Barnes, P.W. & Lightsey Jr., O.R. (2005) Perceived racist discrimination, coping, stress and life satisfaction, Journal of Multi-Cultural Counselling and Development, 33(1) p.48-61 (January)

Bataille, G. (2001) Theory of religion Translated by Robert Hurley original title:Th´eoriede la religion. New York. Zone Books

Bate, S. P., Bevan, H., & Robert, G. (2004). Towards a million change agents. A review of the social movements literature: Implications for large scale change in the NHS.

Baumeister, R.F., Vobs, K.D., Aaker, J.L. & Garbinsky, E.N. (2013) Some key differences between a happy life and a meaningful life, Journal of Positive Psychology, 8(6) p.505-516.

BBC, viewed May 2020, https://www.bbc.co.uk/news/localnews/2641673-Newcastle%20upon%20Tyne/0

Becker, E. (1971). The Birth and Death of Meaning: An Interdisciplinary Perspective on the Problem of Man (2nd ed.). New York: Free Press.

Bell, C.M., Davis, D.E., Griffin, B.J., Ashby, J.S. & Rice, K.G. (2017) The promotion of self-forgiveness, responsibility and willingness to make reparations through a workbook interventions, Journal of Positive Psychology, 12(6) 571-578.

Benson, G., Ploeg, J. and Brown, B. (2010) A cross-sectional study of emotional intelligence in baccalaureate nursing students. Nurse Education Today, 30, 49-53

Berge, M. S. (2017). Telecare – where, when, why and for whom does it work? A realist evaluation of a Norwegian project: Journal of Rehabilitation and Assistive Technologies Engineering. https://doi.org/10.1177/2055668317693737

Bergmann, I. (2017) Reflections on loneliness, limitation and liberation, Introduction in

Bergmann, I. and Hippler, S. (Eds) (2017)

Bergmann, I. and Hippler, S. (Eds) (2017) Cultures of Solitude: Loneliness, Limitation, Liberation. Frankfurt/New York, Peter Lang

Berry-Smith, S (2012) Death, Freedom, Isolation and Meaninglessness, And The Existential Psychotherapy of Irvin D. Yalom: A Literature Review. Available at: https://openrepository.aut.ac.nz/handle/10292/4611 (Accessed: 30 April 2020)

Billings, J., Kember, T., Greene, T., Grey, N., EL-LEithy, S., Lee, D., Kennerley, H., Robertson, M., Brewin, C., & Bloomfield, M. (2020). COVID Trauma Response Working Group Rapid Guidance. Guidance for Planners of the psychological response by hospital staff associated with COVID: Early Interventions.

Bion, W R (1957) Differentiation of the psychotic from the non-psychotic personalities.Int J Psychoanal. 1957 May-Aug;38(3-4): 266-75.

Bion, W R (1979) Making the Best of a Bad Job. In Clinical Seminars and Other Works London: Karnac Books, 2000. (Reprinted London: Karnac Books, 1994)

Blackmore, S. and Troscianko, E.T. (2015) Consciousness: an introduction, London, Routledge (Taylor and Francis Group).

Blanchard, D.C. & Blanchard, R.J. (2008) Defensive Behaviours, fear and anxiety handbook. Handbook of Behaviour Neuroscience, 17. p.63 – 79.

Blanchard, D.C. and Blanchard, R.J. (2008) Defensive behaviours, fear, and anxiety. Handbook of anxiety and fear. Academic Press, Amsterdam, The Netherlands.

Bleich, A., Gelkopf, M., & Solomon, Z (2003). Exposure to terrorism, stress-related mental health symptoms, and coping behaviours among a nationally representative simple in Israel. Journal of the American Medical Association. 290(5), 612-620.

Blows, W.T. (2010) The biological basis of nursing: mental health, London, Routledge

Bluth, K. (2017) The self compassion workbook for teens: Mindfulness and compassion skills to overcome self criticism and embrace who you are, Oakland CA, New Harbinger Publications Limited.

Bong, M. & Clark, R. E. (1999) Comparison between self-concept and self-efficacy in academic motivation research. Educational Psychology, 34: p.139–154.

Bong, M. & Skaalvik, E.M. (2003) Academic self concept and self efficacy: How different are they really? Educational Psychology Review, 15(10), p. 1-41.

Borges LM. Acceptance and Commitment Therapy for Moral Injury (ACT-MI): Moving with Moral Pain towards a meaningful life. HSR&D Cyberseminar May 2019.
https://www.hsrd.research.va.gov/for_researchers/cyber_seminars/archives/3592-notes.pdf

Bostock, L., Sheikh, A. I., & Barton, S. (2009). Posttraumatic growth and optimism in health-related trauma: A systematic review. Journal of Clinical Psychology in Medical Settings, 16, 281–296.

Botanaki, E. (1999) Seventeenth-Century Englishwomen's spiritual diaries: self-examination, covenanting, and account keeping', Sixteenth Century Journal, 30/1, p. 3–21

Bowlby, J. (1969). Attachment. Attachment and loss. Volume 1. Loss. New York: Basic Books.

Bradberry Travis & Lencioni Patrick,2009, Emotional Intelligence 2.0

Bradbury-Jones, C & Isham, L. (2020) The pandemic paradox: The consequences of COVID-19 on domestic violence. (Online). Available at: https://onlinelibrary.wiley.com/doi/pdf/10.1111/jocn.15296 (accessed on 01 May 2020).

Bramley, L. and Matiti, M. (2014) How does it really feel to be in my shoes? patients' experiences of compassion within nursing care and their perceptions of developing compassionate nurses. Journal of Clinical Nursing. 23, (19-20) pp.2790-2799.

Brand, C., Barry, L., & Gallagher, S. (2016). Social support mediates the association between benefit finding and quality of life in caregivers. Journal of Health Psychology, 21(6) 1126-1136.

Braunack-Mayer, A; Tooher, R; Collins, J; Street, J; Marshall, H. (2013) Understanding the school community's response to school closures during the H1N1 2009 influenza pandemic. Biomedical Central Public Health. 13, pp. 344.

Bray, L., O'Brien, M.R., Kirton, J., Zubairu, K. and Christiansen, A. (2014) The role of professional education in developing compassionate practitioners: A mixed methods study exploring the perceptions of health professionals and pre-registration students. Nurse Education Today. 34 (3), pp.480–486.

Brendtro, L. K., Brokenleg, M., & Van Bockern, S. (2005). The Circle of Courage and Positive Psychology. Reclaiming Children and Youth, 14(3), 130–136. Retrieved from http://graingered.pbworks.com/f/Circle+of+Courage-Positive+Psychology.pdf ?Accessed

Breslau, J., Kendler, KS., Su, M., Gaxiola-Aguilar, S., Kessler, R.C (2005). Lifetime risk and persistence of psychiatric disorders across ethnic groups in the United States. Psychological Medicine 35: 317-327.

Breslin, N., Baptiste, C., Gyamfi-Bannerman, C., Miller, R., Martinex, R., Bernstein, K., Ring, L., et al. (2020) COVID-19 infection among asymptomatic and symptomatic pregnant women: Two weeks of confirmed presentations to an affiliated pair of New York City hospitals. American Journal of Obstetrics & Gynecology MFM, 9;2(2):100118 doi: 10.1016/j.ajogmf.2020.100118.

Brewin, C.R. (2014) Episodic memory, perceptual memory, and their interactions: foundations for a theory of posttraumatic stress disorder, Psychological Bulletin, 140, 69-97

Brindley, P. (2020) Covid-19-Healthcare workers are scared but, in some ways, also lucky. BMJ Blogs. Available at: https://blogs.bmj.com/bmj/2020/03/31/peter-brindley-covid-19-healthcare-workers-are-scared-but-in-some-ways-also-lucky/ (Accessed 30 April 2020)

British Broadcasting Corporation (2020a) Coronavirus: Domestic Abuse Calls up 25% Since Lockdown, Charity Says. (Online). Available at: https://www.bbc.co.uk/news/uk-52157620  (accessed 01 May 2020).

British Broadcasting Corporation (2020b) Coronavirus: Remembering the NHS workers who have died. (Online). Available at: https://www.bbc.co.uk/news/health-52242856 (accessed 02 May 2020).

British Broadcasting Corportation (2012) BBC News: Met arrests in London domestic violence crackdown, [Online] London, BBC. (28th November) Retrieved from : https://www.bbc.co.uk/news/uk-england-london-20524486, Accessed on 8thy June, 2020.

British Medical Association. COVID-19 – Ethical Issues. A Guidance Note. 2020. https://www.bma.org.uk/media/2360/bma-covid-19-ethics-guidance-april-2020.pdf

British Medical Journal (BMJ) (2020) COVID-19 GUIDELINE WATCH Covid-19 and pregnancy, [Online] BMJ, 369:m1672 doi: 10.1136/bmj.m1672 (Published 4 May 2020) Retrieved from : https://www.bmj.com/content/bmj/369/bmj.m1672.full.pdf, Accessed on 7th June, 2020.

British Psychological Society (2020) The psychological needs of healthcare staff as a result of the Coronavirus outbreak. Available at https://www.bps.org.uk/sites/www.bps.org.uk/files/News/News%20-%20Files/Psychological%20needs%20of%20healthcare%20staff.pdf [Accessed 30/04/20].

British Psychological Society. Coronavirus resources. https://www.bps.org.uk/coronavirus-resources 2020

Brondolo, E., Gallo, L.C., & Myers, H.F. (2009). Race, racism and health: Disparities, mechanisms, and interventions. Journal of Behavioral Medicine, 32(1), p.1–8.

Brondolo, E., Ver Halen, N. B., Pencille, M., Beatty, D., & Contrada, R. J. (2009). Coping with racism: A selective review of the literature and a theoretical and methodological critique. Journal of Behavioral Medicine, 32(1), p.64–88.

Bronfenbrenner, U. (1979).The Ecology of Human Development. Cambridge, MA: Harvard University Press.

Bronk, K. C. (2011) The role of purpose in life in healthy identity formation: A grounded model. New Directions for Youth Development, 132, p.31–44.

Brooks, S. K; Webster, R.K; Smith, L. E; Woodland, L; Wessely, S; Greenberg, N; et al. (2020) The psychological impact of quarantine and how to reduce it: rapid review of the evidence. Lancet.395, pp. 912–20.

Brooks, S., Webster, R., Smith, L., Woodland, L., Wesley, S., Greenberg, N. Rubin, G. (2020) The Psychological impact of quarantine and how to reduce it: rapid review of the evidence. Lancet, 395, p. 912-920

Brown, G. (2020) Coronavirus: Rest pods for frontline staff in new Ninewells relaxation area. The Courier. May 10th 2020. Available at: https://www.thecourier.co.uk/fp/news/local/dundee/1311859/coronavirus-rest-pods-for-frontline-staff-in-new-ninewells-relaxation-area/ (Accessed 30 April 2020)

Brown, K.W., Ryan, R.M. & Cresswell, J.D. (2007) Mindfulness: Theoretical foundations and evidence for its salutary effects, Psychological Inquiry, 18(4) 211-237.

Bryant, R.A. (2006) Cognitive-behavior therapy: Implications from advances in neuroscience. In N.Kato, M. KAwata, & Pitman, R. K (Eds), PTSD: Brain Mechanisms and Clinical Implications (pp 255-270) Tokyo: Springer-Verlag.

Brzycki, H.G. (2009) Teacher Beliefs and Practices that Impart Self-System and Positive Psychology Attributes: A Dissertation in Educational Theory and Policy, Ann Arbor, MI, Pennsylvania State University (ProQuest LLC).

Burgess, R. (2020). COVID_19 mental health responses neglect social realities. Nature. 4th May 2020. Doi: 10.1038/d41586-020-01313-9.

Burki, T. K. (2020) Cancer guidelines during the COVID-19 pandemic. (Online). Available at: https://www.thelancet.com/journals/lanonc/article/PIIS1470-2045(20)30217-5/fulltext (accessed 03 May 2020).

Burns, J. K. (2015). Poverty, inequality and a political economy of mental health. Epidemiology and psychiatric sciences, 24(2), 107-113.

Byrne, E., Elliott, E., Saltus, R., & Angharad, J. (2018). The creative turn in evidence for public health: Community and arts-based methodologies. Journal of Public Health, 40(suppl_1), i24–i30.

Cacioppo, J. T. & Hawkley, L. C. (2009) Perceived social isolation and cognition. Trends Cogn Sci. 13, pp. 447–54.

Cacioppo, J. T., Hughes, M. E., Waite, L. J., Hawkley, L. C., & Thisted, R. A. (2006). Loneliness as a specific risk factor for depressive symptoms: Cross-sectional and longitudinal analyses. Psychology and Aging. 21(1), pp. 140–151.

Cambridge English Dictionary online (2020). Meaning of Fear and Anxiety. https://dictionary.cambridge.org/dictionary/english/fear [Accessed: 25/05/20]

Campaign to End Loneliness : Connections in Older Adults (2020) Coronavirus and Social Isolation, [Online], London, Campaign to End Loneliness, Retrieved from : https://www.campaigntoendloneliness.org/blog/coronavirus-and-social-isolation/, Accessed on 7th June, 2020.

Campbell, D. & Mason, R. (2020) Nurses sent to London as capital faces 'tsunami' of virus patients. The Guardian. 26 March 2020. Available at: https://www.theguardian.com/world/2020/mar/26/nhs-to-move-nurses-to-london-to-help-with-coronavirus-tsunami (Accessed 09 May 2020)

Care Quality Commission (2020a) Understanding the impact of coronavirus on autistic people and people with a learning disability, [Online] London, CQC. Retrieved from : https://www.cqc.org.uk/news/stories/understanding-impact-coronavirus-autistic-people-people-learning-disability, Accessed on 7th June, 2020.

Care Quality Commission (CQC) (2020b) Monitoring the Mental Health Act in 2018/19, [Online] Newcastle-Upon-Tyne, Retrieved from: https://www.cqc.org.uk/sites/default/files/20200206_mhareport1819_report.pdf, Accessed on : 7th June, 2020.

Carleton, N (2016) Fear of the unknown: One fear to rule them all? Journal of Anxiety Disorders. 41 (1), pp. 5–21.

Carleton, N. (2016) Fear of the unknown: One fear to rule them all? Journal of Anxiety Disorders. 41. p.5–21

Centers for Disease Control and Prevention (U.S.) (Ed.). (2005). Disaster mental health primer: Key principles, issues and questions. Drop of News ..., 2012(1). https://stacks.cdc.gov/view/cdc/29151

Chadwick, H. (1993) The Early Church. London, Penguin

Chen, N.; Zhou, M.; Dong, X.; Qu, J.; Gong, F.; Han, Y.; Qiu, Y.; Wang, J.; Liu, Y.; Wei, Y.; et al. (2020) Epidemiological and clinical characteristics of 99 cases of 2019 novel coronavirus pneumonia in Wuhan, China: A descriptive study. Lancet. 395, pp.507–513.

Cherniss C, Extein M, Goleman D, Weissberg RP (2006). Emotional intelligence: What does the research really indicate? Educ Psychol.41:239–45.

Chipps, J., Brysiewicz, P., & Mars, M. (2012). A systematic review of the effectiveness of videoconference-based tele-education for medical and nursing education. Worldviews on Evidence-Based Nursing, 9(2), 78–87.

Chochinov, H.M. (2007) Dignity and the essence of medicine: the A, B, C and D of dignity conserving care. British Medical Journal, 335, 184–187.

Chodron, P (2007) When Things Fall Apart: Heart Advice For Difficult Times. Rockport, MA: Element Books

Chyi, H.P. & McCombs, M. (2004) Media salience and the process of framing: coverage of the Columbine School shootings, Journalism & Mass Communication Quarterly, 81(1) p.22–35.

Circenis, K. & Millere, E. (2011) Compassion Fatigue, burnout and contributory factors among nurses in Latvia, Procedia: Social and Behavioral Sciences, 30, p.2042-2046.

Clare, S. & Reed, J. (2020) BBC News: Health : Coronavirius : The struggle of living with autism, [Online] London, British Broadcasting Corporation, Retrieved from: https://www.bbc.co.uk/news/health-52398144, Accessed on 6th June, 2020.

Cobb, S. (1976). Social support as a moderator of life stress. Psychosomatic Medicine. 38, pp. 300–314.

Cocker, F. & Joss, N. (2016) Compassion Fatigue among healthcare, emergency and community service workers: a systematic review, International Journal of Environmental Research and Public Health, 13(5) p.618.

Cohen, I. (2017) Tree types of deep solitude: religious quests, aesthetic retreats, and withdrawals due to personal distress. Chapter 7 in Bergmann, I. and Hippler, S. (Eds)

Cohen, J.A., Mannarino, A.P., & Deblinger, E. (2017) Treating Trauma and Traumatic Grief in Children and Adolescents – Second Edition. Guilford Press

Coltart, C.E.M., Lindsay, B., Ghinal, I., Johnson, A.M. & Heymann, D.L. (2017) The Ebola outbreak 2013-2016: Old lessons for new epidemics, Philosophical Transactions Royal Society, 372, 201602797. https://doi.org/10.1098/rstb.2016.0297

Conick, H. (2017) Social media, smartphones and other drugs. Marketing News, April/May, p.40-47.

Conklin, A. I., Forouhi, N. G., Surtees, P., Khaw, K. T., Wareham, N. J., & Monsivais, P. (2014). Social relationships and healthful dietary behaviour: evidence from over-50s in the EPIC cohort, UK. Social science & medicine, 100, 167-175.

Cordis, D (2016) 'Reflections On Israel.' Tikkun, 22 February. Available at: https://www.tikkun.org/major-american-jewish-leader-changes-his-mind-about-israel (Accessed: 16 April 2020)

Cornelia Funke, 2020, Inkheart, viewed 18 May 2020, <http://www.corneliafunke.com>

Covert, M.D. & Reeder, G.D. (1990) Negativity effects in impression formation: The role of unit information and schematic expectancies, Journal of Experimental Social Psychology, 26, p.49-62.

Cowen, K.J., Hubbard, L.J. and Hancock, D.C. (2018) Expectations and experiences of nursing students in clinical courses: A descriptive study. Nurse Education Today. 67:15-20

Craske, M.G. & Hazlett-Stevens, H. (2002) Facilitating symptom reduction and behavior change in GAD: the issue of control. Clinical Psychology: Science and Practice, 9, p.69-75.

Crawford, M. J., & Patterson, S. (2007). Arts therapies for people with schizophrenia: An emerging evidence base. Evidence Based Mental Health, 10(3), 69–70. https://doi.org/10.1136/ebmh.10.3.69

Crawford, P, Gilbert, P, Gilbert, J, Gale, C, Harvey, K (2013) The language of compassion in acute mental health care. Qualitative health research, 23(6), p.719-727.

Cumbie, S. A., & Rutherfoord, S. R. (1994). Weaving aesthetics into practice: The use of aesthetic techniques in group psychotherapy with clients remembering repressed traumatic memories. NLN Publications, 14–2611, 223–245.

Cunningham, C, O, Diaz, C, Slawek, D, E (2020) COVID-19: the worst days of our careers. Annals of Internal Medicine, pp.1-2.

Curtis, K. (2014) Compassion is an essential component of good nursing care and can be conveyed through the smallest actions. British Journal of Nursing. 18 (3), pp.95.

Cutter, V. (2020) Covid-19—the corona cohort of soon-to-be doctors. BMJ Blogs. Available at:  https://blogs.bmj.com/bmj/2020/03/31/vanessa-cutter-covid-19-the-corona-cohort-of-soon-to-be-doctors/ (Accessed 30 April 2020)

Czekierda, K., Banik, A., Park, C. L., & Luszczynska, A. (2017). Meaning in life and physical health: systematic review and meta-analysis. Health Psychology Review, 11(4), 387-418.

Dalton, L., Rapa, E. & Stein, A. (2020) Protecting the psychological health of children through effective communication about COVID-19, Lancet, V4.5, P346-347, May 2020

Danon, L., Brooks-Pollock, E., Bailey, M. & Keeling, M. (2020) A spatial model of CoVID-19 transmission in England and Wales: early spread and peak timing. medRxiv preprint; doi: doi:10 .1101/2020.02.12.20022566. Accessed 5 March 2020

Dashraath, P., Lin, J., Wong, J.,  Xian, M.,  Lim., K.,  Lim, L.M., Li, S., Biswas, A., Choolani, M., Mattar, C. & Su, L.L.  (2020) Coronavirus Disease 2019 (COVID-19) Pandemic and Pregnancy, [Online] American Journal of Obstetrics and Gynecology, (June) 222(6) p.521-531.  doi: 10.1016/j.ajog.2020.03.021.

De Paula Gebara, C.F., Ferri, C.P., Lourenço, L.M., de Toledo Vieira, M. de Castro Bhona, F.M., and Noto, A.R. (2015) Patterns of domestic violence and alcohol consumption among women and the effectiveness of a brief intervention in a household setting: a protocol study, BMC Women's Health (2015) 15(78) 1-8

Dean W, & Talbot SG. Hard Hits of Distress.  Journal of Pediatric Rehabilitation Medicine: an Interdisciplinary Approach, 2020, 13, 3-5.

Dean W, Talbot S & Dean A. Reframing Clinician Distress: Moral Injury not Burnout. Fed Prac, 2019 Sep; 36 (9): 400-402

Dean, E. (2020) COVID-19 pandemic presents new challenges for learning disability nurses. Learning Disability Practice, 23(3) p.8-9

Deci, E.L. & Ryan, R.M. (1985) Intrinsic motivation and self determination in human behaviour, New York, Plenium Press.

Dekel, S., Ein-Dor, T. & Solomon, Z. (2012) Posttraumatic growth and posttraumatic distress: a longitudinal study, Psychological trauma, theory, research, practice and policy, 4(1) pp. 94-101.

Delobelle P; Rawlison, L; Ntuli, S; Malatsi, I; Decock, R. & Deporter, A. (2009) HIV/AIDS knowledge, attitudes, practices and perceptions of rural nurses in South Africa. Journal of Advanced Nursing. 65 (5), pp. 1061–1073.

Department for Education (2020a) Guidance: Actions for early years and childcare providers during the coronavirus outbreak, London, Department for Education.

Department for Education (2020b) Guidance: Coronavirus (COVID-19): implementing protective measures in education and childcare settings, London, Department for Education

Department of Health (2008) High quality care for all: NHS next stage review final report. London: Department Health

Department of Health (2009) The Handbook of NHS Constitution the NHS belongs to us all. First edition. London: Department of Health

Department of Health (2012) Compassion in Practice Our Vision and Strategy: Nursing, Midwifery and Care Staff Our Vision and Strategy. The Stationery Office London.

Department of Health (2012) Compassion in practice, nursing, midwifery and care staff: our vision, our strategy. London: Department of Health.

Department of Health and Social Care (DHSC) (2018) Modernising the Mental Health Act: Increasing choice, reducing compulsion. Final report of the Independent Review of the Mental Health Act 1983, December 2018, London, DHSC.

Deutsch, M. (1961). Courage as a Concept in Social Psychology. The Journal of Social Psychology, 55(1), pp.49-58.

Devmukar, D., Shannon, G., Bhopal, S., Abubakar, I. (2020) Racism and discrimination in COVID-19 responses. Lancet. 395(10231) p.1194. Published online 2020 Apr 1. doi: 10.1016/S0140-6736(20)30792-3

Dewey, J. (1991). How we think. Lexington, MA:D. C. Heath and Company

Dickinson, E. (1994) The Selected Poems of Emily Dickinson. Ware, Hertfordshire, Wordsworth Publications

Dillon, A. (2020) Maya Angelo Inspirational Quotes and insights of a phenomenal woman, Andrea Dillon Publishing.

Dimmond, B. (2015) Legal Aspects of Nursing, Harlow, Pearson Publishing.

Diversity and inclusion in the NHS. Available on line: https://www.kingsfund.org.uk/sites/default/files/field/field_publication_file/Maki ng-the-difference-summary. [Accessed :11/05/20]

Dixon, H. (2020) Government's Stay At Home Message Too Successful, leaving people over-anxious and scared to go out. The Telegraph, 1st May 2020. Available on-line: https://www.telegraph.co.uk/news/2020/05/01/governments-stay-home-message-successful-leaving-people-anxious/ (accessed 3rd May 2020).

Driscoll, J. (2007) Practising Clinical Supervision. London. Elsevier.

Duckworth, A. L., Peterson, C., Matthews, M. and Kelly D. (2007) 'Grit: Perseverance and Passion for Long-Term Goals', Journal of Personality and Social Psychology, 92(6), pp. 1087–1101.

Dweck, C.S. (2017) Mindsets: Updated edition: Changing the way you think to fulfil your potential, Robinson.

Dworznik, G. (2006) Journalism and Trauma: How reporters and photographers make sense of what they see, Journalism Studies, 7(4) p.534-553.

Dyas, D., Edden, V. and Ellis, R. (eds.) (2005) Approaching Medieval English Anchoritic and Mystical Texts. Cambridge, D.S Brewer

Eckersley, R.M. (2007) Culture, spirituality, religion, and health: looking at the big picture. Medical Journal of Australia.186(10) p.S54.

Edmondson, A. (2003) Managing the risk of learning: Psychological safety in work teams. In: West, M.A., Tjosvold D. and Smith, K.G., (Editors) International Handbook of Organizational Teamwork and Cooperative Working. London: Blackwell.

Edwards, A., & Elwyn, G. (2009). Shared decision-making in health care: Achieving evidence-based patient choice. Oxford University Press.

Egnew, T.R. (2009) Suffering, Meaning, and Healing: Challenges of Contemporary Medicine, Annals of Family Medicine; 7(2) p.170-175. (MARCH/APRIL)

Ehlers, A. & Clark, D.M. (2008) Posttraumatic stress disorder: the development of effective psychological treatments, Nordic Journal of Psychiatry, 62(Suppl 47) pp.11-18.

Elderton, A., Berry, A. & Chan, C. (2017) A systematic review of posttraumatic growth in survivors of interpersonal violence in adulthood. Trauma Violence Abuse. 18(2):223–36.

Eleanor Roosevelt, 2020, Good Reads, viewed 21 June 2020, www.goodreads.com

Elliot, H.D. & Richardson, R. (2018) The effect of early life stress on context fear generalisation in adult rats. Behavioral. Neuroscience. 133(1) p.50

Emerson, RW (2018) 'Self-Reliance' in Selected Writings Of Ralph Waldo Emerson Broadview Press: Peterborough, ON

Emmons, R.A. & Stern, R. (2013) Gratitude as a psychotherapeutic intervention, Journal of Clinical Psychology, 69(8) 846-855.

Enenkel, K. and Göttler, C. (Eds.) (2018) Solitudo: Spaces and Places of Solitude in Late medieval and Early Modern Cultures. Leiden, Netherlands, Brill

England, N. H. S. (2014). Choice in Mental Health Care: Guidance on implementing patients' legal rights to choose the provider and team for their mental health care. NHS England, London.

Equality Act (2010), London, T.S.O.

Erikson, K. T. (1976). Trauma at Buffalo Creek. Society, 13(6), 58-65.

European Centre for Disease Prevention (2020b) Covid-19 Situation update worldwide, as of 6 June, 2020, [Online] ECDPC, Retrieved from https://www.ecdc.europa.eu/en/covid-19-pandemic, Accessed on 6th June, 2020.

European Centre for Disease Prevention and Control (ECDPC) (2020) Covid-19 Situation update worldwide, as of 27 May, 2020, [Online] ECDPC, Retrieved from https://www.ecdc.europa.eu/en/geographical-distribution-2019-ncov-cases, Accessed on 27th May, 2020.

European Centre for Disease Prevention and Control (ECDPC) (2020a) Covid-19 Situation update worldwide, as of 27 May, 2020, [Online] ECDPC, Retrieved from https://www.ecdc.europa.eu/en/geographical-distribution-2019-ncov-cases, Accessed on 27th May, 2020.

Evans, H. M. (2008). The Action in Therapeutic Action: Nonverbal Interventions. J. Amer. Psychoanal. Assn., 56, 565–572.

Fardin, M. A. (2020). COVID-19 and Anxiety: A Review of Psychological Impacts of Infectious Disease Outbreaks. Archives of Clinical Infectious Diseases, In Press.

Farnsworth JK, Drescher KD, Evans W, Walser RD. A Functional Approach To Understanding And Treating Military-Related Moral Injury. J Context Behav Sci 2017; 6: 391-397

Feely M. (2007) Depression: what's in a name? A psychiatric nursing theory of connectivity, (unpublished PhD thesis), Faculty of Health and Life Sciences, Jordanstown, University of Ulster.

Feeney, A. & Everett, S. (2019) Understanding supervision in nursing practice, Oxford, Sage Publishing,

Feldman, C, Kuyken, W (2011) Compassion in the landscape of suffering. Contemporary Buddhism, 12(1), pp.143-155.

Festinger, L. (1954) A theory of social comparison processes, Human Relations, 7(2) p.116-140.

Figley, C. R. (Ed.). (1995). Brunner/Mazel psychological stress series, No. 23. Compassion fatigue: Coping with secondary traumatic stress disorder in those who treat the traumatized. Brunner/Mazel.

Fiorillo & Gorwood (2020) The consequences of the COVID-19 pandemic on mental health and implications for clinical practice. European Psychiatry. 63 (1), pp.1-4.

Fiscella, K., & Williams, D. R. (2004). Health disparities based on socioeconomic inequities: implications for urban health care. Academic Medicine, 79(12), 1139-1147.

Fisher, M.L. & Exline, J.J. (2010) Moving towards self-forgiveness: Removing barriers related to shame, guilt and regret, Social and Personality Psychology Compass, 4, 548-558.

Foa, E.B. and McNally, R.J. (1996) Mechanisms of change in exposure therapy. Current controversies in the anxiety disorders. The Guilford Press, New York.

Fonagy, P & Allison, E (2014) The role of mentalizing and epistemic trust in the therapeutic relationship Psychotherapy, 51, 372-380.

Ford, M. (2020, April, 17). Exclusive: BME nurses 'feel targeted' to work on Covid-19 wards. Online: http//www.NursingTimes. [Accessed: 12/05/20]

Fosha, D., Siegel, D.J. & Solomon, M.F. (Editors) The healing power of emotion: Affective neuroscience, development and clinical practice, New York, NY. Norton. p.86-111.

Fotopoulou, A., & Tsakiris, M. (2017). Mentalizing homeostasis: The social origins of interoceptive inference. Neuropsychoanalysis, 19(1), 3–28.

Foucault, M. (1986) Of other spaces. Diacritics, 16/1, p. 22-27

Foulkes, S H (1948). Introduction to Group Analytic Psychotherapy London: Karnac.

Francati, V., Vermetten, E. & Bremner, J.D. (2007) Functional neuroimaging studies in posttraumatic stress disorder: reviewing current methods and findings, Depression and Anxiety, 24, 202-218.

Frankl, V. (1988) The will to meaning: foundations and applications of logotherapy, London, Penguin Books.

Frankl, V. (2011) Man's Search for Ultimate Meaning, London, Rider.

Frankl, V. E. (1959). Man's search for meaning: An introduction to logotherapy .(I. Lasch, Trans.) Boston.

Frankl, V. E. (1977). The Unconscious God – Psychotherapy And Theology. London: Hodder and Stoughton.

Frankl, V. E. (2006). Man's Search For Meaning. Boston, Ma: Beacon Press.

Frankl, V.E. (1979) The unheard cry for meaning: psychotherapy and humanism, New York, Touchstone.

Fredricks, J.A. (2014) Eight myths of student disengagement: Creating classrooms of deep learning, London, Corwin / Sage.

Fredrickson, B. (2001) Positivity: Groundbreaking research to release your inner optimist and thrive, Oneworld.

Fredrickson, B.L. (2012) Positivity: Groundbreaking research to release your inner optimism and thrive, Oxford, Oneworld Inc.

Fredrickson, B.L., Cohn, M., Coffey, K.A., Pek, J., & Finkel, S.A. (2008). Open hearts build lives: Positive emotions, induced through loving-kindness meditation, build consequential personal resources. Journal of Personality and Social Psychology, 95, 1045–1062.

French, M & Monahan, T. (2020) Disease Surveillance: How Might Surveillance Studies Address COVID-19? Surveillance & Society. 18 (1), pp. 1-11.

Fromm, E (1941) The Fear of Freedom, Farrar and Rinehart, USA.

Fuss, D. (1998) Interior chambers: the Emily Dickinson homestead. Differences: A Journal of Feminist Cultural Studies, 10/3, p. 1- 46

Gallicchio, M. (2013). World War II in historical memory. In T. W. Zeiler & D. M. DuBois (Eds.) A Companion to World War II, (pp.978-998): Oxford: Wiley-Blackwell.

Gee, W. (1931). Rural-Urban Heroism in Military Action. Social Forces, 10(1), p.102.

Gelb, A. and Gelb, B. (1960) O'Neill. New York, Harpers and brothers

General Medical Council (2013) Good medical practice. (Online). Available at: https://www.gmc-uk.org/ethical-guidance/ethical-guidance-for-doctors/good-medical-practice (accessed on 26 April 2020).

Gerbner, G. (1998). "Cultivation Analysis: An Overview". Mass Communication and Society. 1 (3–4): 175–194

Germer, C.K. (2009) The mindful path to self-compassion: freeing yourself from destructive thoughts and emotions, New York, NY., Guildford Press.

Giddens, A. (1990) Central problems in social theory: action, structure and contradiction in social analysis. Berkeley, CA: University of California Press

Gilbert, P. (2005) Compassion: Conceptualisations, research and use in psychotherapy, London: Routledge.

Gilbert, P. (2010). An introduction to compassion focused therapy in cognitive behavior therapy. International Journal of Cognitive Therapy. 3 (2): 97–112.

Gilbert, P. (2013) The Compassionate Mind, London, Robinson.

Gilbert, P. & Miles, J.N.V. (2000) Sensitivity to social putdown: its relationship to perceptions of social rank, shame, social anxiety, depression, anger and self-other blame, Personality and Individual Differences, 29, 757-774.

Gilbert, P., & Irons, C. (2004). A pilot exploration of the use of compassionate images in a group of self-critical people. Memory, 12(4), 507–516.

Gilbert, P., Clarke, M., Hempel, S., Miles, J. N. V., & Irons, C. (2004) Criticizing and reassuring oneself: An exploration of forms, styles and reasons in female students. British Journal of Clinical Psychology, 43, 31–50.

Gilligan C. & Attanucci, J. Two Moral Orientations: Gender Differences And Similarities. Merrill Palmer Quarterly, 1988; 34, 3, 223-237

Gilligan C. In a different voice. Psychological Theory and Women's Development. 1993. Cambridge, Massachusetts. Harvard University press

Goldman-Rakic, P.S. (1992) Topography of cognition, parallel distributed network in primate association cortex, Annual Review of Neuroscience, 11, 137-156.

Gopee, N. (2018) Supervision and Mentoring in Healthcare, Oxford, Sage Publishing.

Gottman, J.M. (1994) What predicts divorce? The relationship between marital processes and marital outcomes, Hillsdale N.J., Lawrence Erlbaum Associates.

Gracey, F., Kinsell, E.L., Muldoon, O.T. & Fortune, D.G. (2015) Post-Traumatic Growth following acquired brain injury: a systematic review aa meta-analysis, Frontiers in Psychology, 68(1162) 1-16.

Gracey, F., Palmer, S., Rous, B., Psaila, K., Shaw, K., O'Dell, J., Cope, J. & Mohamed, S.. (2008). "Feeling part of things": personal construction of self after brain injury. Neuropsychological Rehabilitation. 18, 627–650.

Greenberg, N., Docherty, M., Gnanapragasam, S., & Wessely, S. (2020). Managing mental health challenges faced by healthcare workers during covid-19 pandemic. BMJ, 368.

Greenburg N, Docherty M, Gnanapragasam S, Wessely S. Managing Mental Health Challenges Faced By Healthcare Workers During Covid-19 Pandemic BMJ 2020; 368:m1211

Greenstone, M. & Nigam (2020) Does Social Distancing Matter? (Online). Available at: http://iepecdg.com.br/wp-content/uploads/2020/04/SSRN-id3561244.pdf (accessed on 1 May 2020).

Griegson, J. (2020) Half of British drinkers starting earlier in the day during Covid-19 crisis, [Online] London, The Guardian, Retrieved from : https://www.theguardian.com/society/2020/jun/02/half-of-british-drinkers-starting-earlier-in-the-day-during-covid-19-crisis, Accessed on 7th June, 2020.

Grieve, W.E. & Staudinger, U. (2006) Resilience in adulthood and old age: resources and potentials for successful ageing, IN Cicchetti, D. & Cohen, D.J.

(Editors) Developmental Psychopathology: risk, disorders and adaptation (Volume 3), Hobeken, N.J., John Wiley, p.796-840.

Griffin, J. (2010) The Lonely Society? London, The Mental Health Foundation

Gross, R. & Kinnison, N. (2014) Psychology for Nurses and Health Professionals. London, CRC Press (Taylor & Francis).

Guardian (2019). Available at https://www.theguardian.com/society/2019/apr/04/nearly-one-in-seven-britons-could-live-alone-2039-study-shows

Guardian (2020) Zoom Booms As Demand For Video Conferencing Tech Grows. The Guardian Newspaper on-line (accessed 03 May 2020).

Guardian, 2020 available at https://www.theguardian.com/world/2020/mar/17/france-at-war-how-parisians-are-coping-with-life-under-lockdown.

Guile, A. (2020). Are we ready to give effective help to traumatised NHS staff and public following COVID 19?

Haffower, H. (2020). A certain horrible subset of the internet is calling the coronavirus 'boomer remover', Business Insider Australia. (Online). Available at: https://www.businessinsider.com/millennials-gen-z-calling-coronavirusboomer-remover-reddit-2020-3?r=US&IR=T (accessed 29 April 2020).

Hagelskamp, C., & Hughes, D. (2014). Workplace discrimination predicting racial/ethnic socialization across African American, Latino, and Chinese families. Cultural Diversity And Ethnic Minority Psychology, 20(4), p.550-560.

Hakala, S. (2009) Koulusurmat verkostoyhteiskunnassa. Analyysi Jokelan ja

Hall, J. H. & Fincham, F. D. (2008) The temporal course of self-forgiveness. Journal of Social and Clinical Psychology, 27, 174–202. doi.10.1521/jscp.2008.27.2.174.

Hammen, C. (1991) The generation of stress in the course of unipolar depression. Journal of abnormal psychology. 100(4) p.555-561

Hammen, C. (2016) Depression and stressful environments: identifying gaps I conceptualization and measurement. Anxiety, stress and coping. 29(2), p.335 – 351

Hannah, S. T., Sweeney, P. J., & Lester, P. B. (2007). The Courageous Mind-Set: A Dynamic Personality System Approach to Courage. In The Psychology of Courage: Modern Research on an Ancient Virtue. Share on Email Pury, Cynthia L. S. (Ed); Lopez, Shane J. (Ed) Washington, DC, US: American

Psychological Association, 125–148. https://doi.org/10.1016/S0969-4765(04)00066-9 Accessed?

Harris, R. (2019). ACT Made Simple: An Easy-To-Read Primer on Acceptance and Commitment Therapy – Second Edition. Harbinger Press.

Harris, R. (2020). FACE COVID: How to respond effectively to the Corona crisis. [Online] Coronado, Retrieved from: https://e-tmf.org/app/uploads/2020/03/FACE-COVID-How-to-respond-effectively-to-the-Corona-crisis-by-Russ-Harris.pdf. Accessed 17 May, 2020.

Harvey, M. R. (1996). An ecological view of psychological trauma and trauma recovery. Journal of traumatic stress, 9(1), 3-23.

Havsteen-Franklin, D. (2016). Mentalization-Based Art Psychotherapy. In J. Rubin (Ed.), Approaches to Art Therapy Theory and Techniques (pp. 144–164). Brunner/Mazel.

Havsteen-Franklin, D. (2019). Creative Arts Therapies. In A. W. Bateman & P. Fonagy (Eds.), Handbook of mentalizing in mental health practice (2nd ed., pp. 181–197). American Psychiatric Pub.

Hawker, L. (2020) Coronavirus second wave panic as scientists admit they're 'flying blind' over immunity. The Express, 29th April 2020. Available at: https://www.express.co.uk/news/uk/1275232/Coronavirus-second-wave-news-covid19-latest-testing-vaccine-Danny-Altmann (accessed 02 May 2020).

Hayes, S.C., Luoma, J.B., Bond, F.W., Masuda, A. & Lillis, J. (2006). "Acceptance and Commitment Therapy: Model, processes and outcomes". Behaviour Research and Therapy. 44 (1): 1–25. doi:10.1016/j.brat.2005.06.006. PMID 1630072

Hayes, S.C., Strosahl. K.D. & Wilson, K.G. (2011) Acceptance and Commitment Therapy: the process and practice of mindful change, New York, N.Y., Guilford Press.

Health & Care Professions Council (HCPC) (2020) Communicating during the COVID-19 pandemic. Available at: https://www.hcpc-uk.org/covid-19/advice/applying-our-standards/communicating-during-the-covid-19-pandemic/ (Accessed 09 May 2020)

Health and Safety Executive (HSE) (2020) RIDDOR Reporting of Covid-19, [Online] London, HSE. Retrieved from : https://www.hse.gov.uk/news/riddor-reporting-coronavirus.htm. Accessed on 7th June, 2020.

Health Education England (HEE) and the Nursing and Midwifery Council (NMC) (2015) Raising the bar: the shape of caring: a review of the future education and training of registered nurses, London, HEE & NMC.

Hearn, J. & Whitehead, A. (2006) Collateral damage: Men's 'domestic' violence to women seen through men's relations with men. The Journal of Community and Criminal Justice. 53 (1), pp. 55–74.

Hefferon, K. (2013) Positive Psychology and the Body: The somatopsychic side of flourishing, Maidenhead. Oxford University Press.

Hegney, D.G., Craigie, M., Hemsworth, D., Osseuran-Moisson, R., Aoun, S., Francis, K. & Drury, V. (2014). Compassion satisfaction, compassion fatigue, anxiety, depression and stress in registered nurses in Australia: study 1 results. Journal of Nurse Management, 22(4): 506–518.

Her Majesties Government / National Health Service (2020) COVID-19 Hospital Discharge Service Requirements  [Online] HMG/NHS (19th March) Retrieved from:  https://www.gov.uk/government/publications/coronavirus-covid-19-hospital-discharge-service-requirements, Accessed on 7th June, 2020.

Herbert, F. (2005). Dune (40th anniversary ed.). New York: Ace Books

Herman, J (1997). Trauma and Recovery: The aftermath of political violence-form domestic abuse to political terror. Basic Books.

Herron, JBT., Hay-David, AGC., Gilliam, AD., Brennan, PA (2020) Personal protective equipment and Covid 19- a risk to healthcare staff?  British Journal of Oral and Maxillofacial Surgery. online: April 13, 2020.

Hill, C. (1993) The English Bible in the Seventeenth-Century Revolution. London, Penguin

Hirschberger, G. (2018). Collective trauma and the social construction of meaning. Frontiers in Psychology, 9, 1441.

Ho, C. S., Chee, C. Y., & Ho, R. C. (2020). Mental Health Strategies to Combat the Psychological Impact of COVID-19 Beyond Paranoia and Panic. Annals of the Academy of Medicine, Singapore, 49(1), 1.

Hobfoll., S.E., Watson, P., Bell., C. et al. (2007). Five Essential Elements of Immediate and Mid-Term Mass Trauma Intervention: Empirical Evidence. Psychiatry 70 (4), pp283-315.

Hoffman, S.G., Grossman, P., & Hinton, D.E. (2011) Loving-Kindness and Compassion Meditation; Potential for Psychosis Intervention, Clinical Psychology Review, 41(7) 1126-1132.

Holm, J. and Bowker, J. (1994) Rites of Passage. London, Pinter publishers

Holmes EA, O'Connor RC, Perry VH, et al. (2020) Multidisciplinary research priorities for the COVID-19 pandemic: a call for action for mental health science. Lancet Psychiatry 2020; published online April 15. https://doi.org/10.1016/S2215-0366 (20)30168-1. Available at: https://www.thelancet.com/pdfs/journals/lanpsy/PIIS2215-0366(20)30168-1.pdf (Accessed 09 May 2020)

Holston, E. and Taylor, J. (2016) Emotional intelligence in nursing students. International Journal of Advanced Psychology, 5, 11-22.

Home Office (2020) Guidance: Coronavirus (COVID-19) and domestic abuse [Online] Retrieved from: https://www.gov.uk/government/publications/coronavirus-covid-19-and-domestic-abuse, Accessed on 7th June, 2020.

Hooper, C., Craig, J., Janvrin, D.R., Wetsel, M.A. & Reimels, E. (2010) Compassion Satisfaction, Burnout, and Compassion Fatigue among emergency nurses compared with nurses in other selected inpatient specialities, Journal of Emergency Nursing, 36(5) p.520-427.

Hopper, E (2003) The Social Unconscious: Selected Papers Jessica Kingsley: London

Horesh, D., & Brown, A.D. (2020). Traumatic Stress in the Age of COVID-19: A Call to Close Critical Gaps and Adapt to New Realities. Unpublished Manuscript, APA.

Horowitz, M. J. (1986). Stress Response Syndromes. Northville, NJ: Jason Aronson.

Howe, N and Strauss, W. (2000). Millennials Rising: The Next Great Generation. New York: Random House.

Hsu, L.M. & Langer, E.J. (2013) Chapter 76: Mindfullness and cultivating well being in older adults, IN David, S.E., Boniwell, I. & Ayers, A.C. (Editors) The Oxford Handbook of Happiness, Oxford, Oxford University Press, p.1026-1036.

HTA, C. (2016, January 28). Telehealth services for the treatment of psychiatric issues: Clinical effectiveness, safety, and guidelines. Centre for Reviews and Dissemination. http://www.crd.york.ac.uk/crdweb/Showrecord.asp?LinkFrom

Hughes, D.A. (2007). Attachment-Focused Family Therapy. Norton

Independent Television Network (2020) NHS Staff Fear PPE will run out this weekend. Available on-line at: https://www.itv.com/news/2020-04-18/coronavirus-nhs-staff-fear-ppe-will-run-out-this-weekend/ (accessed 03 May 2020).

Inspirational Quotations, 2020, Right Attitudes, viewed 29 May, http://www.inspiration.rightattitudes.com/authors/queen-victoria/

Intensive Care National Audit & Research Centre (ICNARC) (2020). Report on COVID-19 in critical care. [Online] ICNARC, (Updated 27 May). Retrieved from: https://www. icnarc.org/Our-Audit/Latest-News/2020/04/10/Report-On-5578-Patients-Critically-Ill-With-Covid-19] accessed 7 June 2020.

Ivtzan, I., Lomas, T., Hefferon, K. & Worth, P. (2016) Second wave positive psychology: embracing the dark side of life, Abingdon, Routledge.

Ivtzan, I., Lomas, T., Hefferon, K., & Worth, P. (2016). Second wave positive psychology: Embracing the dark side of life. Routledge. Abingdon.Oxon.

Jack Welch, 2020, General Electric, viewed 20 June 2020, www.ge.com

James.C, Green. J, Rodriquez, J. (2008) addressing disproposionality. wiley online, pp. 77-88.

Janoff-Bulman, R. (1992). Shattered Assumptions: Toward a new psychology of trauma. New York: Free Press.

Janoff-Bulman, R. (2004). Posttraumatic growth: three explanatory models. Psychol. Inq. 15, 30–34.

Janoff-Bulman, R. (2004). Posttraumatic growth: Three explanatory models. Psychological Inquiry, 15(1), 30-34.

Janoff-Bulman, R., & McPherson Frantz, C. (1997). The impact of trauma on meaning: From meaningless world to meaningful life. In M. J. Power & C. R. Brewin (Eds.), The transformation of meaning in psychological therapies: Integrating theory and practice (p. 91–106). John Wiley & Sons.

Jasinskaja-Lahti, I., Liebkind, K., & Perhoniemi, R. (2006). Perceived discrimination and well-being: A victim study of different immigrant groups. Journal of Community and Applied Social Psychology, 16(4), p.267–284

Jazaieri, H., Lee, I.A., McGonigal, K., Jinpa, T., Doty, J.T., Gross, J.J. & Goldin, P.R. (2016) A wandering mind is a less caring mind: Daily experience sampling during compassion meditation training, The Journal of Positive Psychology, 11(1), p.37-50.

Jenkins, B. and Warren, N.A. (2012) Concept analysis: Compassion fatigue and effects upon critical care nurses. Critical Care Nurse Quarterly, 35: p.388–395.

Jenkins, R. and Elliot, P. (2004). Stressors, burnout and social support: nurses in acute mental health settings. Journal of Advanced Nursing, 48(6), 622 - 631.

Jenner, S. (1997) The Parent-Child Game, London, Bloomsbury.

Johnstone, L. & Boyle, M. with Cromby, J., Dillon, J., Harper, D., Kinderman, P., Longden E., Pilgrim, D. & Read, J. (2018). The Power Threat Meaning Framework: Overview. Leicester: British Psychological Society.

Jonas-Simpson, C; Mitchell, G; Fisher, A. et al. (2006) The experience of being listened to: a qualitative study of older adults in long-term settings. Journal of Gerontology Nursing. 32 (1), pp. 46-54.

Jordan, R; Adab, P. & Cheng, K. (2020) Covid-19: risk factors for severe disease and death. (Online). Available at: https://www.bmj.com/content/368/bmj.m1198.long (accessed 10 May 2020).

Joseph, S. (2012) What doesn't kill; A guide to overcoming adversity and moving forward. London, Piakus

Joseph, S. (2012) What Doesn't Kill: A guide to overcoming adversity and moving forward, Piatkus.

Joseph, S. (2015) Positive Psychology in Practice: Promoting Human Flourishing in Work, Health, Education, and Everyday Life, John Wiley and Sons.

Joseph, S. (2016) Authentic: How to be yourself and why it matters, London, Pitkus.

Julian of Norwich (2015) Revelations of Divine Love.  Transl. B Windeatt. Oxford, Oxford University Press

JWT Intelligence (2012, March). JWT Marketing Communications : Fear of Missing Out (FOMO) Retrieved from:  http://www.jwtintelligence.com/wp-ontent/uploads/2012/03/F_JWT_FOMOupdate_3.21.12.pdf

Kabit-Zinn, J. (1994) Full catastrophic living: the program of the stress reduction clinic at the university of Massachusetts Medical Centre, New York, Delta Press.

Kabit-Zinn, J. (2014) Full catastrophic living: how to cope with stress, pain and illness using mindfulness practice, London, Piatkus.

Kang, L; Li, Y; Hu, S; Chen, M; Yang, C; Yang, B. et al. (2019) The mental health of medical workers in Wuhan, China dealing with the 2019 novel coronavirus. (Online). Available at: https://www.thelancet.com/journals/lanpsy/article/PIIS2215-0366(20)30047-X/fulltext (accessed 01 May 2020).

Kangas, M., Williams, J. R. & Smee, R. I. (2011). Benefit finding in adults treated for benign mengingioma brain tumours: relations with psychosocial wellbeing. Brain Impairment 12, 105–116.

Kanov, J, M, Maitlis, S, Worline, M, C, Dutton, J, E, Frost, P, J, Lilius, J, M (2004) Compassion in organizational life. American Behavioral Scientist, 47(6), 808-827.

Kanten, A.B. & Tiegen, K.H. (2008) Better than average and better with time: relative evaluation of self and others on the past, present and future, European Journal of Social Psychology, 38, 343-353.

Karafillakis, E., Jalloh, M.F., Nuriddin, A., Larson, H.J., Whitworth, J., Lees, S., Hageman, K.M., Sengeh, P., Jalloh, M.B., Bunnell, R., Carroll, D.D. & Morgan, O. (2016) Once there is life, there is hope' Ebola survivors' experiences, behaviours and attitudes in Sierra Leone, 2015. British Medical Journal Glob Health.1(3) e000108

Kashdan, T.B. & Kane, J.Q. (2011) Post-traumatic distress and the presence of post-traumatic growth and meaning of life: experiential avoidance as a moderator, Personality and Individual differences, 50(1) p.84-89.

Kauhajoen kriisien viestinn"ast" a. Helsingin yliopisto. Viestinn"an laitoksen tutkimusraportteja 2/2009. Viestinn"an tutkimuskeskus CRC.

Keats, J (1817) Private letter to his brothers. Available at http://mason.gmu.edu/~rnanian/Keats-NegativeCapability.html (Accessed: 23 April 2020)

Keeley, G. (2020). Corpses of the elderly found abandoned in Spanish care homes, https://www.aljazeera.com/news/2020/03/corpses-elderly-abandoned-spanish-care-homes200324141255435.html (accessed 01 May 2020).

Kellner, D. (2008) Guys and guns amok: domestic Terrorism and school shootings from the Oklahoma City bombings to the Virginia Tech massacre. London: Paradigm Publishers.

Kemp, R. (2020) The rhetoric of fear.

Kendi, I.X (2020, April 6). Ideas: What the Racial Data Show: The Pandemic seems to be hotting people of color the hardest. The Atlantic. On line: http://www.theatlantic.com/ideas. [Accessed: 14/04/2020]

Khan, O. (2020) u The Guardian, (20 April, 2020).

Kilburg, R. R. (2012). Wisdom, courage, temperance, justice, and reverence: Platonic virtues and leadership competence. Virtuous Leaders: Strategy, Character, and Influence in the 21st Century. BT - Virtuous Leaders: Strategy,

Character, and Influence in the 21st Century., 73–101.
https://doi.org/http://dx.doi.org/10.1037/13494-004

Kinchin, D. (2005) Post Traumatic Stress Disorder: The Invisible Injury, Success Unlimited.

Kinchin, D. (2007) A guide to psychological debriefing: managing emotional decompression and Post-Traumatic Stress Disorder, London, Jessica Kingsley Publishers, pp. 21.

King, L. A., Hicks, J. A., Krull, J. L., & Del Gaiso, A. K. (2006). Positive affect and the experience of meaning in life. Journal of Personality and Social Psychology, 90, 179–196.

King's Fund (2019) Public satisfaction with the NHS and social care in 2018: Results from the British Social Attitudes survey. The King's Fund. Available at: https://www.kingsfund.org.uk/publications/public-satisfaction-nhs-social-care-2018 (Accessed 09 May 2020)

King's Fund (2020) Public satisfaction with the NHS and social care in 2019: Results from the British Social Attitudes survey. The King's Fund. Available at: https://www.kingsfund.org.uk/publications/public-satisfaction-nhs-social-care-2019 (Accessed 09 May 2020)

Kissler, S. M., Tedijanto, C., Goldstein, E., Grad, Y. H., & Lipsitch, M. (2020). Projecting the transmission dynamics of SARS-CoV-2 through the postpandemic period. (Online). Available at: https://science.sciencemag.org/content/early/2020/04/24/science.abb5793 (accessed on 02 May 2020).

Klaidman, S. & Beauchamp, T.L. (1987) The virtuous journalist. Oxford. Oxford University Press.

Kline, R. (2015). The "snowy white peaks" of the NHS: a survey of discrimination in governance and leadership and the potential impact on patient care in London and England. Middlesex University Research Repository.

Knight, M, Bunch, K., Vousden, N., Morris, E., Simpson, N., Gale, C., O'Brien, P., Quigley, M., Brocklehurst, P. & Kurinczuk, J.J. (2020). Characteristics and outcomes of pregnant women hospitalised with confirmed SARS-CoV-2 infection in the UK: a national cohort study using the UK Obstetric Surveillance System (UKOSS). [Online] Retrieved from: https://www.npeu.ox.ac.uk/downloads/files/ukoss/ annual-repor ts/UKOSS%20COVID-19%20Paper%20pre-print%20draft%2011-05-20.pdf, , Accessed on 7th June, 2020.

Koh, D. (2020) Occupational risks for COVID-19 infection. (Online). Available at: https://www.ncbi.nlm.nih.gov/pmc/articles/PMC7107962/ (accessed 03 May 2020).

Kohlberg L. Discussion: Developmental Gains in Moral Judgement. American Journal of Mental Deficiency 1974, 79, 3, 142-146.

Kohut, H. (1981) Introspection, empathy and semi-circle of mental health, IN P. Omstein (Editor) The search for the self: selected writings of Heinz Kohut 1978-1981 (Volume 4), New York, N.Y., International University Press. p.537-566.

Kolakowski, L (2005) Main Currents Of Marxism. London: WW Norton

Korakidou, V., & Charitos, D. (2012). The spatial context of the aesthetic experience in interactive art: An inter-subjective relationship. Technoetic Arts, 9(2–3), 2–3.

Krout, R. E., Baker, F. A., & Muhlberger, R. (2010). Designing, piloting, and evaluating an on-line collaborative songwriting environment and protocol using Skype telecommunication technology: Perceptions of music therapy student participants. Music Therapy Perspectives, 28(1), 79–85.

Kutikov, A; Weinberg, D; Edelman, M; Horwitz, E; Uzzo, R. & Fisher, I. (2020) A War on Two Fronts: Cancer Care in the Time of COVID-19. (Online). Available at: https://annals.org/aim/fullarticle/2764022 (accessed 03 May 2020).

Kuyken, W. and Feldman, C. (2019) Mindfulness: Ancient Wisdom meets Modern Psychology. New York, Guildford Press

Lahad, M, & Leykin, D. (2010). Ongoing exposure versus intense periodic exposure to military conflict and terror attacks in Israel. Journal of Traumatic Stress, 23, 691-698. Doi:10.1002/jts.20583

LaMotte, S. (2020) Covid-19 appears to attack placenta during pregnancy, study says, [Online] CNN Retrieved from: https://edition.cnn.com/2020/05/22/health/placenta-covid-19-wellness/index.html, Accessed on 7th June, 2020.

Lamouroux A, Attie-Bitach T, Martinovic J, Leruez-Ville, M. & Ville, Y. (2020) Evidence for and against vertical transmission for SARS-CoV-2 (COVID-19). [Online] American Journal of Obstetrics & Gynecology, (4 May, In ress) https://www.sciencedirect.com/science/article/pii/S000293782030524X, Accessed on 7th June, 2020.

Lavietes, M. (2020) J.K. Rowling donates to coronavirus victims of domestic violence, homeless, [Online] Thomson Reuters Foundation (3 May), Retrieved from: https://news.trust.org/item/20200503164018-bhurd, Accessed on 8th June, 2020.

Layard, R. & Clark, D.M. (2015) Thrive: the power of psychological therapy, London, Penguin.

LeDoux, J. (2015) Anxious: Using the Brain to Understand and Treat Fear and Anxiety. Viking

Lee, B. & LiPuma, E. (2002) Cultures of circulation: the imagination of modernity, Public Culture, 14(1) p191–214.

Lehto RH, Stein KF. (2009) Death anxiety: an analysis of an evolving concept. Res Theory Nurs Pract.;23(1):23-41.

Lester, P. B., Vogelgesang, G. R., Hannah, S. T., & Kimmey, T. (2010). Developing Courage in Followers: Theoretical and Applied Perspectives. In Pury, Cynthia L. S. (Ed); Lopez, Shane J. (Ed). The Psychology of Courage: Modern Research on an   Ancient Virtue. Washington, DC, US: American Psychological Association. (2010). Xvi 247 Pp. Doi: 10.1037/12168-000, 187–207. https://doi.org/10.1037/12168-010

Levine, P. A (2008). Healing Trauma: A Pioneering Programme for Restoring the Wisdom of Your Body. Sounds True: Boulder, Colorado

Levy, C. E., Spooner, H., Lee, J. B., Sonke, J., Myers, K., & Snow, E. (2018a). Telehealth-based creative arts psychotherapy: Transforming mental health and rehabilitation care for rural veterans. The Arts in Psychotherapy, 57, 20–26.

Levy, C. E., Spooner, H., Lee, J. B., Sonke, J., Myers, K., & Snow, E. (2018b). Telehealth-based creative arts psychotherapy: Transforming mental health and rehabilitation care for rural veterans. The Arts in Psychotherapy, 57, 20–26.

Lewis, CS (1961) A Grief Observed. London: Faber and Faber

Li, Z-S. and Hasson, F. (2020) Resilience, stress, and psychological well-being in nursing students: A systematic review. Nurse Education Today, 90, 104440.

Liang, C.T.H., Nathwani, A., Ahmad, S., & Prince, J.K. (2010). Coping with discrimination: The subjective well-being of South Asian American women. Journal of Multicultural Counseling and Development, 38(2), p.77–87.

Lindsey, E.W. (2013) Emotional Development, IN Lopez, S.J. (Editor) The encyclopedia of Positive Psychology, Chicester, Wiley-Blackwell, p.307-315

Linehan, M (2016) DBT Skills Training Manual. New York: Guilford Press

Linehan, M (2019) 'Walking A Tightrope', Psychology Today. December 2020 Available at: https://www.psychologytoday.com/us/articles/201912/how-marsha-linehan-developed-the-central-feature-dialectical-behavior-therapy (Accessed: 16 April 2020)

Linley, A., Willars, J. & Biswas-Diener, R. (2010) The strengths book, Coventry, CAPP.

Linley, P. A. & Joseph, S. (2004). Positive change following trauma and adversity: a review. Journal of Trauma. Stress, 17, 11–21.

Lintern, S. (2020). World will face a mental health crisis after coronavirus pandemic, experts warn. The Independent Available at: https://www.independent.co.uk/news/health/coronavirus-mental-health-research-anxiety-a9466466.html (Accessed 09 May 2020)

Litz B.T., Stein N. Delaney E, Leibowitz L,Nash WP, Silva C Maguen, S. Moral Injury and Moral Repair in War Veterans: A Preliminary Model And Intervention Strategy.  Clin Psychol Rev 2009; 29; 695 - 206

Liu, X., Kaplan, H. B., & Risser, W. (1992) Decomposing the reciprocal relationship between academic achievement and general self-esteem. Youth and Society, 24, p.123–148.

Lomas, T., Hefferon, K. & Itzan, I. (2014) Applied Positive Psychology: integrated positive practice, Oxford, Sage Publishing.

Lopez, S. J., O'Byrne, K. K., Petersen, S., & Snyder, C. R. (2003). Profiling courage. Positive Psychological Assessment: A Handbook of Models and Measures., 185–197. https://doi.org/10.1037/10612-012 Lopez, S. J., Rasmussen, H. N., Skorupski, W. P., Koetting, K., Petersen, S. E., & Yang, Y. (2010). Folk Conceptualizations of Courage. In The Psychology of Courage: Modern Research on an Ancient Virtue. Share on Email Pury, Cynthia L. S. (Ed); Lopez, Shane J. (Ed) Washington, DC, US: American Psychological Association, 23–45. https://doi.org/10.1037/12168-002

Lopez, S. J., Rasmussen, H.N., Skorupski, W.P., Koetting, K. Petersen, S.E. and Yang, Y. (2010) 'Folk Conceptualizations of Courage', In The Psychology of Courage: Modern research on an ancient virtue.

Losada, M. & Heaphy, E. (2004) The role of positivity and connectivity in the performance of business teams: a nonlinear dynamic model. American Behavioral Scientists, 47: p.740-765.

Lovell, M. (2017) Thoreau and the landscapes of solitude: painted epiphanies of undomesticated nature. Chapter 3 in Bergmann, I. and Hippler, S. (Eds)

Lowe, S. M., Okubo, Y., & Reilly, M. F. (2012). A qualitative inquiry into racism, trauma, and coping: Implications for supporting victims of racism. Professional Psychology: Research and Practice, 43(3), 190–198.

Lyubomirsky, S. (2010) The How of Happiness: a practical guide to getting the life you want, London, Piatkus.

Lyubomirsky, S. (2012) The How of Happiness, New York: Penguin Books.

Maben, J. & Griffiths, P (2008) Nurses in society: starting the debate. London: Kings College London.

Macedo, M., Wilheim, L., Goncalves, R., Cantinho, E., Vilete, L., Figueira, I., Ventura, P. (2014) Building resilience for future adversity: a systematic review of interventions in non-clinical samples of adults. BSC Psychiatry.

Maddux, J.E. & Kleiman, E.M. (2016) Chapter 7: Self efficacy: a foundational concept for positive clinical psychology, IN Wood, A.M. & Johnson, J. (Editors) The Wiley Handbook of Positive Clinical Psychology, Oxford, Wiley Blackwell.

Maital, S. & Barzani, E. (2020) -The Global Economic Impact of COVID-19: A Summary of Research. Samuel Neaman Institute for National Policy Research.

Malott, K.M. & Schaefle, S. (2015). Addressing Clients' Experiences of Racism: A Model for Clinical Practice. Journal of Counseling & Development, 93, 361–369.

Mancini, C., Mears, D.P., Stewart, E.A., Beaver, K.M., & Pickett, J.T. (2015).Whites' Perceptions About Black Criminality. Crime & Delinquency, 61(7), p.996–1022.

Manstead, A.S.R. (2018) The psychology of social class: How socioeconomic status impacts thought, feelings, and behaviour British Journal of Social Psychology, 57(2) p,267-291. McLellan A. (2020) Please stay home too: an open letter to NHS managers and other admin staff [Online] Health Service Journal 30 March 2020 Retrieved from; https://www.hsj.co.uk/comment/please-stay-home-too-an-open-letter-to-nhs-managers-and-other-admin-staff/7027257.article

Marieb, E.N. & Hoehn, K. (2016) Human anatomy and physiology, Oxford, Pearson

Marsh, H.W. & Parker, J.W. (1984) Determinants of student self concept: is it better to be a relatively large fish in a small pond even if you don't learn to swim well? Journal of Personality and Social Psychology, 41(1) 213-231.

Martel, Y. (2001). Life of Pi: A novel. New York: Harcourt.

Martin, G. R. R. (2011). A Game of Thrones. New York: Bantam Books

Martin, G.N. (2006) Human Neuropsychology, Pearson / Prentice Hall.

Marx Memorial Library (2019) 'Why Is Marxism A Better Kind Of Philosophy?' Morning Star, 29 July 2019.

Maslow, A.H. (2013) A theory of human motivation, Wilder Publications.

Mason, B. (1993) Towards positions of safe uncertainty, Human Systems: The Journal of Systemic Consultation and Management, 4, 189-200.

Mason, H. & Birch, K. (Eds). (2018) Yoga for Mental Health Handspring Publishing. National Institute for Health and Care Excellence (2018). Post-Traumatic Stress Disorder. NG116 https://www.nice.org.uk/guidance/ng116

Mason, R, & Campbell, D. (2020) Pressure on Johnson A UK's daily coronavirus testing to get missed again, The Guardian, 7th May, 2020.

Mason, R. and Stewart, H. (2020). UK government has no exit plan for Covid-19 lockdown, say sources. (Online). Available at: https://www.theguardian.com/world/2020/apr/15/uk-governmenthas-no-exit-plan-for-covid-19-lockdown-say-sources (accessed 02 May 2020).

Matsui, M. and Braun, K. (2014) Nurses' and care workers' attitudes toward death and caring for dying older adults. International Journal of Palliative Nursing. 16(12), p.593–8

Matthews, M., Eid, J., Kelly, D., Bailey, J. and Peterson, C. (2006). 'Character Strengths and Virtues of Developing Military Leaders: An International Comparison'. Military Psychology, 18(sup1), pp.S57-S68. doi: 10.1207/s15327876mp1803s_5.

May, R. & Powis, S. (2020) Letter from Chief Nursing Officer and National medical Director, [Online] London, NHS England and NHS Improvement, Retrieved at : https://www.england.nhs.uk/coronavirus/wp-content/uploads/sites/52/2020/04/maintaining-standards-quality-of-care-pressurised-circumstances-7-april-2020.pdf, Accessed on 7th June, 2020.

McCaully, M., Ministry, S. & Viswanath, K (2013) The H1N1 Pandemic: Media frames, stigmatisation and coping. Bio Medical Cente Public Health. 13(1116) p.1-16.

McInerney, D. & Putwain, D. (2017) Developmental and Educational Psychology for Teachers: an applied approach, Abingdon, Routledge (Taylor & Francis Group)

McIntosh, D. N., Poulin, M. J., Silver, R. C., & Holman, E. A. (2011). The distinct roles of spirituality and religiosity in physical and mental health after collective trauma: a national longitudinal study of responses to the 9/11 attacks. Journal of Behavioral Medicine, 34(6), 497-507.

McNamer, S. (2010) Affective Meditation and the invention of Medieval Compassion. Pennsylvania, University of Pennsylvania Press

Mehta, P; McAuley, D; Brown, M & Sanchez, E; Tattersall, R; Manson, J. et al. (2020) COVID-19: consider cytokine storm syndromes and immunosuppression. (Online). Available at: https://www.thelancet.com/journals/lancet/article/PIIS0140-6736(20)30628-0/fulltext#%20 (accessed on 02 May 2020).

Mencap (2020) Press Release: Emergency measures must have the interests and safety of the most vulnerable in our society at it's heart. [Online] Mencap, Retrieved from : https://www.mencap.org.uk/press-release/emergency-measures-must-have-interests-and-safety-most-vulnerable-our-society-its, Accessed on 7th June, 2020.

Merleau-Ponty, M. (1982). Phenomenology of perception. London: Routledge.

Michel, G., Taylor, N., Absolom, K., & Eiser, C. (2010). Benefit finding in survivors of childhood cancer and their parents: Further empirical support for the Benefit Finding Scale for Children. Child: Care, Health and Development, 36(1), 123–129.

Middleton, A. (2019). Post 9/11 Rural Veterans with PTSD: A Meta-narrative Analysis on How the Use of Telehealth Can Improve Access to Creative Art Therapy and Decrease Physician Burnout [PhD Thesis]. Northcentral University.

Miller, W.R. & Seligman, M.E.P. (1975) Depression and learned helplessness in man, Journal of Abnormal Psychology, 84, 228-238.

Mills, R. (2020) Prince Charles opens up on missing his family during coronavirus lockdown, [Online] Sky News, Retrieved from: https://news.sky.com/story/prince-charles-opens-up-on-missing-his-family-during-coronavirus-lockdown-12000638. Accessed on 7th June, 2020.

MIND (2020) Loneliness, [Online] London, MIND. Retrieved from: https://www.mind.org.uk/information-support/tips-for-everyday-living/loneliness/about-loneliness/, Accessed on 7th June, 2020.

Ministry for Housing, Communities & Local Government and Public Health England (2020) COVID-19: guidance on isolation for domestic abuse safe-accommodation settings, [Online] London, Ministry for Housing, Communities & Local Government and Public Health England (March) Retrieved from: https://assets.publishing.service.gov.uk/government/uploads/system/uploads/attachment_data/file/874568/COVID-19_-

_guidance_on_isolation_for_domestic_abuse_safe-accommodation_settings.pdf, Accessed on 7th June, 2020.

Miscall Brown, K., & Sorter, D. (2008). Voice and Cure: The Significance of Voice in Repairing Early Patterns of Disregulation. Clinical Social Work Journal, 36(1), 31–39. SocINDEX with Full Text.

Mitchell, G. (2020) Suicide among health workforce rising warns shadow minister, Nursing Times, (May 4)

Molendijk T, Kramer E-H, & Verweij D.  Moral Aspects of "Moral Injury": Analyzing Conceptualizations on the Role of Morality In Military Trauma. Journal of Military Ethics, 2018, 17:1, 36-53, DOI: 10.1080/15027570.2018.1483173

Mor, G. & Cardenas, I. (2010) The immune system in pregnancy: a unique complexity. American Journal of Reproductive Immunology, 63(6):425-33.

Morganstein, J. & Ursano, R. (2020) Ecological disasters and mental health: causes, consequences, and interventions. Frontiers in Psychiatry, 11 p.1-15 (accessed 01 May 2020).

Morse, J, Bottorff, J, Anderson, G (2006) Beyond empathy: expanding expressions of caring. Journal of Advanced Nursing, 53(1), 75-87.

Mosoeunyane, N.M (2015). My Life in England. Dorrance Pub Co. Pittsburg.Pennysylavia.USA

Moss, G. (2019). Inclusive Leadership. Routledge.

Moss, R.H. (1993) Coping responses inventory: Professional manual.

Mouse, A, E. (1919) Funny Stories From The Great War As Told By The Soldiers. Chicago: Shrewsbury Publishing Company.

Msiska, G., Smith, P., Fawcett, T. and Nyasulu, B. M. (2014) Emotional labour and compassionate care: What's the relationship? Nurse Education Today. (34), pp. 1246–1252.

Muschert, G.W. (2007a) Research in school shootings, Sociology on Compass, 1: p. 60–80.

Muschert, G.W. (2007b) The Columbine victims and the juvenile super predator, Youth Violence and Juvenile Justice, 5: p 351–366.

Muschert, G.W. & Carr, D. (2006) Media salience and frame changing across events: coverage of nine school shootings, Journalism & Mass Communication Quarterly, 83: p.747–766.

Nathoo, B. A. S. (2017) An Exploration of the Concepts of Compassion in the Care of Older People amongst Key Stakeholders in Nursing Education: Pre-Qualifying Nursing Students, Nurse Educators and Clinical Mentors—a Qualitative Study. Unpublished Doctorate Thesis. Portsmouth. University, Portsmouth.

National Autistic Society (NAS) (2020) Coronavirus: Your stories, [Online] Nottingham. NAS. Retrieved from: https://www.autism.org.uk/services/helplines/coronavirus/resources/stories-from-the-spectrum.aspx, Accessed on 7th June, 2020.

National Health Service (2020b) Legal guidance for mental health, learning disability and autism, and specialised commissioning services supporting people of all ages during the coronavirus pandemic, [Online] London, NHS. Retrieved from: https://www.england.nhs.uk/coronavirus/wp-content/uploads/sites/52/2020/03/C0454-mhlda-spec-comm-legal-guidance-v2-19-may.pdf, Accessed on 7th June, 2020.

National Health Service (NHS) (2020a) Covid-19 deaths of patients with a learning disability notified to LeDeR [Online] Learning Disability Mortality Review (LeDeR), University of Bristol. Retrieved from: https://www.england.nhs.uk/publication/covid-19-deaths-of-patients-with-a-learning-disability-notified-to-leder/ Accessed on 7th June, 2020.

National Health Service (NHS) (2020c) Who's at higher risk from coronavirus, [Online] London, NHS. Retrieved from: https://www.nhs.uk/conditions/coronavirus-covid-19/people-at-higher-risk/whos-at-higher-risk-from-coronavirus/, Accessed on 7th June, 2020.

National Health Service England (2020) NHS warning to seek help for cancer symptoms, as half of public report concerns with getting checked. (Online). Available at: https://www.england.nhs.uk/news/?filter-category=uec (accessed 01 May 2020).

National Health Service, (2020). Your NHS Needs You - NHS callf or volunteer army. [online]. Available from: https://www.england.nhs.uk/2020/03/your-nhs-needs-you-nhs-call-for-volunteer-army/ [accessed 20.04.20].

National Institute for Health and Care Excellence (2005) Post-Traumatic stress disorder (PTSD): The management of PTSD in adults and children in primary and secondary care (CG26), London, NICE.

National Institute for Health and Care Excellence (NICE) (2019) Guidance (NG28) Type 2 Diabetes in Adult managers, London, NICE.

National Institute of Health and Care Excellence (2020) COVID-19 Rapid Guideline: Critical Care, London. NICE.

NCBI (2018, November 21). Application and Effectiveness of Telehealth to Support Severe Mental Illness Management: Systematic Review. JMIR mental health. http://www.ncbi.nlm.nih.gov/pubmed/30463836

Neely, M.E., Schallert, D.L., Mohammed, S.S., Roberts, R.M. & Chen, Y-J (2009) Self-kindness when facing stress: The role of self-compassion, goal regulation, and support in college students' well-being. Motivational Emotion, 33, p.88–97.

Neff, K. D. (2003a) Self-compassion: an alternative conceptualization of a healthy attitude toward oneself. Self and Identity, 2, 85–102.

Neff, K. D. (2003a) The development and validation of a scale to measure self-compassion. Self and Identity, 2, 223–250.

Neff, K. D. (2003b) Self-compassion: an alternative conceptualization of a healthy attitude toward oneself. Self and Identity, 2, 85–102.

Neff, K. D., Hseih, Y., & Dejitthirat, K. (2005) Self-compassion, achievement goals, and coping with academic failure. Self and Identity, 4, p.263–287.

Neff, K. D., Kirkpatrick, K. L., & Rude, S. S. (2007a) Self compassion and adaptive psychological functioning. Journal of Research in Personality, 41, p.139–154.

Neff, K. D., Kirkpatrick, K. L., & Rude, S. S. (2007a) Self compassion and adaptive psychological functioning. Journal of Research in Personality, 41, p.139–154. doi:10.1016/j.jrp.2006.03.004.

Neff, K. D., Kirkpatrick, K., & Rude, S. S. (2007b) Self-compassion and its link to adaptive psychological functioning. Journal of Research in Personality, 41, p.908–916.

Neff, K. D., Rude, S. S., & Kirkpatrick, K. L. (2007) An examination of self-compassion in relation to positive psychological functioning and personality traits. Journal of Research in Personality, 41, p.908–916. doi:10.1016/j.jrp.2006.08.002.

Neff, K.D. (2003b) Self-compassion: stop beating yourself up and leave insecurity behind, New York, Harper Collins.

Neff, K.D. (2003c) Self-compassion: stop beating yourself up and leave insecurity behind, New York, Harper Collins.

Neff, K.D. (2011) Self-compassion: stop beating yourself up and leave insecurity behind, New York, NY. Harper Collins.

Neff, K.D. (2017) Introduction, IN Bluth, K. (Author) The self compassion workbook for teens: Mindfulness and compassion skills to overcome self criticism and embrace who you are, Oakland CA, New Harbinger Publications Limited.

Neff, K.D. (2020) Self compassion, Retrieved , http://self-compassion.org

Neff, K.D. & Germer, C. (2018) The Mindful Self-Compassion Workbook: A proven way to accept yourself, build inner strengths and thrive, New York, NY, Guilford Press.

Neff, K.D. & Vonk, R. (2009) Self-Compassion Versus Global Self Esteem: Two different ways of relating to oneself, Journal of Personality, 77(1) p.1-50.

Neibuhr, R. (circa. 1932- 1933) The Serenity Prayer

Neil. (2020) Neil's Experience of COVID-19 Emergency, [Online] Scottish Commission on Learning Disabilities, Retrieved from: https://www.scld.org.uk/neils-experience-of-covid-19-emergency/, Accessed on 7th June, 2020.

Neimeyer, R. A. (2004). Fostering posttraumatic growth: A narrative elaboration. Psychological inquiry, 15(1), 53-59.

Neimeyer, R. A., Burke, L. A., Mackay, M. M., & van Dyke Stringer, J. G. (2010). Grief therapy and the reconstruction of meaning: From principles to practice. Journal of Contemporary Psychotherapy, 40(2), 73-83.

Neria, Y. & Rechkemmer, A. (2016) The role of fear-related behaviors in the 2013-2016 West Africa Ebola Virus Disease Outbreak. Current Psychiatry Report, 18(11) p.104.

New Economics Foundation (2006) Five ways to well being. (online) London, New Economics Foundation, Retrieved from http:// www.nef-consulting.co.uk/our-services/strategy-culture/five-ways-to-wellbeing/ Accessed on 15th May, 2020

Newman, K.S., Cybelle, F., David, J.H., Mehta, J. & Rota, W. (2004) Rampage. The social roots of school shootings. New York: Basic Books

Newman, M. (2020) Covid-19: doctors' leaders warn that staff could quit and may die over lack of protective equipment. (Online). Available at: https://www.bmj.com/content/368/bmj.m1257?casa_token=rU0VsQPDbn8AA AAA:vdNLMrPpGBrYtpk9xqp8GZoX4G8ZGuQPRAFbQMA_jzBxt5Mnz1s-KiTWniuvByAtxY2yZrJpEA (accessed 03 May 2020).

Newman, M. & Zainal, N. (2020) The value of maintaining social connections for mental health in older people. (Online). Available at: https://www.thelancet.com/pdfs/journals/lanpub/PIIS2468-2667(19)30253-1.pdf (accessed 01 May 2020).

NHS (2020) 10 tips to help if you are worried about coronavirus. NHS Website. Available at: https://www.nhs.uk/oneyou/every-mind-matters/coronavirus-covid-19-anxiety-tips/ (Accessed 09 May 2020)

NHS England (2019) NHS Staff experiencing discrimination at work by ethnicity and area, [Online] London, NHS England, Retrieved from: https://www.ethnicity-facts-figures.service.gov.uk/workforce-and-business/nhs-staff-experience/nhs-staff-experiencing-discrimination-at-work/latest, Accessed on 27th May, 2020.

NHS England (2020, April 4). Total number of COVID-19 deaths in England by date of death. Online: https://www.england.nhs.uk/2020/04/total-number-of-covid-19-deaths-in-england-by-date-of-death/. [Accessed: 12/05/20].

NHS England (2020) Coronavirus: principles for increasing the nursing workforce in response to exceptional increased demand in adult critical care (25 March 2020) Version 1. Available at: https://www.england.nhs.uk/coronavirus/wp-content/uploads/sites/52/2020/03/specialty-guide-critical-care-workforce-v1-25-march-2020.pdf (Accessed 9 May 2020)

NHS, Scottish Government, Department of Health, Welsh Government, Council of Deans of Health, NMC, RCN, Unison & Unity, (2020) Joint statement on expanding the nursing workforce in the Covid-19 outbreak, [Online] NHS, Scottish Government, Department of Health, Welsh Government, Council of Deans of Health, NMC, RCN, Unison & Unity, Retrieved from: https://www.nmc.org.uk/news/news-and-updates/joint-statement-on-expanding-the-nursing-workforce/, Accessed on 23/5/2020.

Nimmo, A., & Huggard, P. (2013) A Systematic Review of the Measurement of Compassion fatigue, Vicarious Trauma, and Secondary Traumatic Stress in Physicians. Australasian Journal of Disaster Trauma Studies, 1: 37– 44.

Nishi, D., Matsuoka, Y., & Kim, Y. (2010) Post traumatic growth: post traumatic stress disorder and resilience of motor vehicle accident survivors, BioPsychoSocial Medicine, 4(1) p.7.

NMC (2018) The Code: Professional standards of practice and behaviour for nurses, midwives and nursing associates, London, NMC.

NMC (2020) Joint statement on expanding the nursing workforce in the Covid-19 outbreak. Available at  https://www.nmc.org.uk/news/news-and-updates/joint-statement-on-expanding-the-nursing-workforce/ [Accessed 19 May 2020]

Nursing and Midwifery Council (2018) The Code: Professional standards of practice and behaviour for nurses and midwives. London: Nursing & Midwifery Council.

Nursing and Midwifery Council (NMC) (2008) The Code: Standards of conduct, performance and ethics for nurses and midwives, London, NMC.

Nursing and Midwifery Council, (2020). NMC Covid-19 emergency register goes live with more than 7,000 former nurses and midwives ready to support health and social care services across the UK [online]. Available from: https://www.nmc.org.uk/news/press-releases/nmc-covid-19-emergency-register-goes-live/. [accessed 20.04.20].

O'Brien, J. (2020) Emotional NHS nurse: We're exhausted and broken, please stay at home. LBC. 7 April 2020. Available: https://www.lbc.co.uk/radio/presenters/james-obrien/emotional-nhs-nurse-exhausted-broken-coronavirus/ (Accessed 28 April 2020)

O'Hanlon, B. & Bertolino, B. (2012) The therapist's notebook on Positive Psychology: Activities, exercises and handouts, Hove, Routledge.

O'Leary, K., Jalloh, M.F. & Neria, Y. (2018) Fear and culture: contextualising mental health impact of the 2014-2016 Ebola epidemic in West Africa, BMJ Global Health, 3(3) e0000924.

Odell-Miller, H., Hughes, P., & Westacott, M. (2006). An investigation into the effectiveness of the arts psychotherapies for adults with continuing mental health problems. Psychotherapy Research, 16(1), 122–139.

Odessa, FL, Psychological assessment Incorporation.

Office of National Statistics (2020a) Coronavirus (COVID-19) Infection Survey pilot: 5 June, 2020, [Online] London, ONS. (15th June) Retrieved from https://www.ons.gov.uk/peoplepopulationandcommunity/healthandsocialcare/conditionsanddiseases/bulletins/coronaviruscovid19infectionsurveypilot/5june2020, Accessed pm 6th June, 2020.

Office of National Statistics (2020b) Deaths involving Covid-19, England and Wales: deaths occurring in April 2020, [Online] London, ONS. (15th June) Retrieved from https://www.ons.gov.uk/peoplepopulationandcommunity/birthsdeathsandmarriages/deaths/bulletins/deathsinvolvingcovid19englandandwales/deathsoccurringinapril2020, Accessed on 6th June, 2020.

Office of National Statistics (ONS) (2020) Personal and economic well-being in Great Britain: May 2020. Available at: https://www.ons.gov.uk/peoplepopulationandcommunity/wellbeing/bulletins/personalandeconomicwellbeingintheuk/may2020 (Accessed 7 May 2020)

Öhman, A. (2000). "Fear and anxiety: Evolutionary, cognitive, and clinical perspectives". In M. Lewis & J.M. Haviland-Jones (Eds.). Handbook of emotions. pp. 573–93. New York: The Guilford Press.

Orsillo, S.M., Roemer, L., Blocklerner, J. & Tull, M.T. (2011) Chapter 4: Acceptance, Mindfulness and cognitive-Behavior Therapy: Comparisons, contrasts and application to anxiety, IN Hayes, S.C., Follette, V.M. & Lineham, M.M. (Editors) Mindfulness and acceptance: expanding the Cognitive-Behavioral Tradition, London, Guilford Press, p.66-95.

Overall, S. (2015). Walking against the current: Generating creative responses to place. Journal of Writing in Creative Practice, 8(1), 11–28.

Oxford University Press (1996) The Oxford English Reference Dictionary, Oxford, Oxford University Press.

Ozer, E.J., Best, S.R., Lipsey, T.L. & Weiss, D.S. (2003) Predictors of posttraumatic stress disorder and symptoms in adults: a meta analysis, Psychological Bulletin, 129, 52-73.

Panagioti, M; Geraghty, K; Johnson, J; Zhou, A; Panagopoulou, E; Chew-Graham, C. et al. (2018) Association Between Physician Burnout and Patient Safety, Professionalism, and Patient Satisfaction: A Systematic Review and Meta-analysis. JAMA Internal Medicine. 178 (10), pp. 1317-1330.

Park M., Cook, A., Lim, J., Sun J. and Dicken, B. (2020) A Systematic Review of COVID-19 Epidemiology Based on Current Evidence. Journal of Clinical Medicine. 9 (967), pp.1-13.

Park, V. (2020) COVID-19: what to expect if you are deployed to a critical care setting. Nursing Standard. Available at: https://rcni.com/nursing-standard/careers/career-advice/covid-19-what-to-expect-if-you-are-deployed-to-a-critical-care-setting-159646  Accessed 09 May 2020

Patel, P. (2020) Speech: Home Secretary's statement on domestic abuse and coronavirus (COVID-19), [Online] London, Home Office, (11 April) Retrieved from:   https://www.gov.uk/government/speeches/home-secretary-outlines-support-for-domestic-abuse-victims, Accessed on 7th June, 2020.

Patel, R., Spreng. R.N., Shin, L.M. & Girard, T.A. (2012) Neurocircuitry models of posttraumatic stress disorder and beyond: a meta analysis of functional neuroimaging studies, Neuroscience and Biobehavioral Review, 36(3) 2130-2142.

Paterson, R (2011) Can we mandate compassion? The Hastings Center Report, 41(2), 20-23.

Pavlicevic, M. (1997). Music therapy in context: Music, meaning and relationship. Jessica Kingsley Publishers.

Penman, J. & Ellis, B. (2015) Paliative care clients' and care givers' notion of fear and their strategies for over coming it. Journal of paliative and supportive care. 13(3), p.777-785.

Pennebaker, J.W. & Seagel, J.D. (1994) Forming a story the health benefits of narrative, Journal of Clinical Psychology, 55, 1243-1254.

Pennebaker, J.W., Kiecolt-Glaser, J.K. & Glaser, R. (1988) Disclosure of trauma and immune functions: health implications of psychotherapy, Journal of Consulting and Clinical Psychology, 56, 239-245.

Penner, L.A., Dovidio, J.F., West, T.V., Gaertner, S.L., Albrecht, T.L., Dailey, R.K., & Markova, T. (2010) Aversive racism and medical interactions with Black patients: A field study. Journal of Experimental Social Psychology, 46(2) p.436-440.

Perrin, A. (2017) 10 facts about Smart phones as the iPhone turns 10, [Online] Pew Research Centre, Retrieved from https://www.pewresearch.org/fact-tank/2017/06/28/10-facts-about-smartphones/ Accessed on 26th May, 2020.

Perry, B. (2008) Why exemplary oncology nurses seem to avoid compassion fatigue. Canadian Oncology Nursing Journal, 18(2), 87-92.

Peterson, C., Meier, S.F. & Seligman, M.E.P. (1995) Learned Helplessness: a theory for the age of personal control, Oxford University Press.

Piaget, J. (1929) The child's conception of the world, London, Routledge and Kegan Paul Limited.

Piaget, J. The Moral Judgment of the Child. 1965. New York, USA. First Free Press

Pidd, H., Barr, C., & Mohdin, A. (2020, May 1st). Calls for health funding to be prioritised as poor bear brunt of Covid-19. The Guardian (Online Edition).

Pines, E., Rauschhuber, M., Cook, J., Norgan, G,, Canchola, L., Richardson, C., and Jones, M. (2014) Enhancing resilience, empowerment and conflict management among baccalaureate students: outcomes of a pilot study. Nurse Educator, 39 (2) pp. 85-90

Porges, S.W. (2009). The Polyvagal Theory: new insights into adaptive reactions of the autonomic nervous system. Cleve. Clin. J. Med. 76, 86-90. Doi: 10.3949/ccjm.76.s2.17.

Potter, P., Deshields, R. & Rodriguez, S. (2013), Developing a systematic program for compassion fatigu", Nursing Administration Quarterly, 37(4) p.326-332.

Prem, K; Liu, Y; Russell, T; Kucharski, A; Eggo, R; Davies, N. et al. (2020) The effect of control strategies to reduce social mixing on outcomes of the COVID-19 epidemic in Wuhan, China: a modelling study. (Online). Available at: https://www.thelancet.com/journals/lanpub/article/PIIS2468-2667(20)30073-6/fulltext (accessed on 02 May 2020).

Pryce, J. (2020) TV Advert, Alzheimer's Disease Society.

Przybylski, A., Murayama, K., DeHaan, C. & Gladwell, V. (2013). Motivational, emotional, and behavioral correlates of fear of missing out. Computers in Human Behavior, 29(4), p.1841-1846.

Psychologytools.com/psychological-resources-for-coronavirus-covid-19. May 2020

Public Health Agency of Canada (2020) Coronavirus disease (covid-19) pregnancy, childbirth and caring for newborns: advice for mothers during COVID-19, [Online] Toronto, Public Health Agency of Canada, Retrieved from: https://www.canada.ca/content/dam/phac-aspc/documents/services/diseases-maladies/pregnancy-advise-mothers/pregnancy-advise-mothers-eng.pdf, Accessed on 7th June, 2020.

Public Health England (2020, April 1st): Corona virus (Covid-19). Guidance PHE data series on deaths in people with COVID-19: technical summary. Online: https://www.gov.uk/government/organisations/public-health-england: [Accessed: 09/05/20].

Public Health England (2020a). Guidance on social distancing for everyone in the UK. 2020. [Online] London, Public Health England, Retrieved from: www.gov.uk/government/publications/covid-19-guidance-on-social-distancing-and-forvulnerable-people/guidance-on-social-distancing-for-everyone-in-the-uk-and-protectingolder-people-and-vulnerable-adults, Accessed on 7th June, 2020.

Public Health England (2020b). Guidance on shielding and protecting people who are clinically extremely vulnerable from COVID19. [Online] Retrieved from: https://www.gov.uk/government/publications/ guidance-on-shielding-and-protecting-extremely-vulnerable-persons-from-covid-19/, Accessed on 7th June, 2020.

Pury, C. L. S. (2013). Courage: What makes an action courageous? Activities for Teaching Positive Psychology: A Guide for Instructors., 13–17. https://doi.org/10.1037/14042-002

Pury, Cynthia L. S. (Ed); Lopez, Shane J. (Ed) Washington, DC, US: American Psychological Association, pp. 23–45.

Putman, D. (2001). The emotions of courage. Journal of Social Philosophy, 32(4), 463–470. https://doi.org/10.1111/0047-2786.00107

Putman, D. (2010). Philosophical roots of the concept of courage. The Psychology of Courage: Modern Research on an Ancient Virtue, (1974), 9–22. https://doi.org/10.1037/12168-001

Pynoos, R., Steinberg, A., & Wraith, R. (1995). A Developmental Model of Childhood Traumatic Stress In D. Cicchetti & D. Cohen (Eds) Manual of Developmental Psychopathology Vol 2 Risk, Disorder & Adaptation. pp72-95. Wiley

Queen Mary University of London, (2020) The ClinComm Podcast, Episode 1. Queen Mary University of London. April 2020. Available at: https://media.qmplus.qmul.ac.uk/channel/The%2BClin%2BComm%2BPodcas t/162031521 (Accessed on: 30 April 2020)

Qun Li, M., Xuhua G., Peng W., Xiaoye W., Lei Z., Yeqing T., et al. (2020) Early Transmission Dynamics in Wuhan, China, of Novel Coronavirus–Infected Pneumonia. The New England Journal of Medicine. 382 (13), pp. 1199-1207.

Race Relations Act (1965) H.M.S.O.

Rachman, S. (1980) Emotional processing. Behaviour Research and Therapy, 18 (1) 51-60

Rachman, S. J. (2010). Courage: A Psychological Perspective. 91–107.

Raghubir, A. (2018). Emotional intelligence in professional nursing practice: A concept review using Rodgers's evolutionary analysis approach. International Journal of Nursing Sciences, 5, 126-130.

Raittila, P., Koljonen, K. & V¨aliverronen, J. (2010) Journalism and school shootings in Finland 2007–2008. Tampere: Tampere University Press.

Rajakaruna SJ, Liu WB, Ding YB & Cao, G.W. (2017) Strategy and technology to prevent hospital-acquired infections: Lessons from SARS, Ebola, and MERS in Asia and West Africa. Military and Medical Research; 4: 32.

Ramluggun, P. and Anjoyeb, M. (2017) Mental health nursing students' views on their readiness to address the physical health needs of service users on registration. International journal of mental health nursing, 26(6):570-579. doi: 10.1111/inm.12279.

Ramluggun, P., Lacy, M., Cadle, M. and Anjoyeb, M. (2018) Managing the demands of the preregistration mental health nursing programme: The views of students with mental health conditions. International journal of mental health nursing, 27, 6, 1793-1804

Randomised Control Trial of a Low-Intensity Cognitive-Behaviour Therapy Intervention to Improve Mental Health in University Students. Australian Psychologist, 51(2), 145–153. https://doi.org/10.1111/ap.12113

Ranney, M; Griffeth, V. & Jha, A. (2020) Critical Supply Shortages — The Need for Ventilators and Personal Protective Equipment during the Covid-19 Pandemic. (Online). Available at: https://www.nejm.org/doi/full/10.1056/NEJMp2006141 (accessed 03 May 2020).

Rashid, T. (2015) Chapter 31: Strength based assessment, IN Joseph, S. (Editor) Positive Psychology in Practice: Promoting human flourishing in work, health, education and everyday life, Hoboken NJ, John Wiley & Sons.

Rashid, T. & Seligman, M.E.P. (2018) Positive Psychotherapy: Clinicians Manual, Maidenhead, Oxford University Press.

Rashid, T. & Seligman, M.E.P. (2020) Positive Psychotherapy: Workbook, Maidenhead, Oxford University Press.

Rate, C. R. (2010). Defining the Features of Courage. The Psychology of Courage: Modern Research on an Ancient Virtue, 47–66.

Refuge (2020) Covid19 Response. Available at: https://www.refuge.org.uk/refuge-responds-to-covid-19/ (accessed 03 May 2020)

Renick, M.J. & Harter, S.J. (1989) Impact of social comparisons on the developing and perceptions of learning disabled students, Journal of Educational Psychology, 81(4) 631-638.

Reporting of Injuries, Diseases and Dangerous Occurrences Regulations (RIDDOR) (2013)

Rev, 2020, Queen Elizabeth II Coronovirus Speech Transcript, viewed 1 May 2020, https://www.rev.com/blog/transcripts/queen-elizabeth-ii-coronavirus-speech-transcript

Reynolds, R., Palmer, S. & Green, S. (2019) Chapter 8: Positive Psychology Coaching for Health and Well being, IN Green, S. & Palmer, S. (Editors) Positive Psychology Coaching in Practice, Abingdon, Routledge (Taylor & Francis).

Richards, D.P. (2020) Covid-19 is bringing unpredictability and fear to the rheumatology community. BMJ Blogs. Available at: https://blogs.bmj.com/bmj/2020/03/31/dawn-p-richards-covid-19-is-bringing-unpredictability-and-fear-in-the-rheumatology-community/ (Accessed 30 April 2020)

Rig, P. (2020) Member Blog: Support During Lockdown for people with Learning disability, [Online] Mencap, Retrieved on: https://healthunlocked.com/mencap/posts/143327056/support-during-lockdown-for-people-with-learning-disability., Accessed on: 7th June, 2020.

Rimmer, A. (2020) Covid-19: Disproportionate impact on ethnic minority healthcare workers will be explored by government.  BMJ 2020;369:m1562

Rimmer, A. (2020) Covid-19: Disproportionate impact on ethnic minority healthcare workers will be explored by government. (Online). Available at: https://www.bmj.com/content/369/bmj.m1562 (accessed 02 May 2020).

Robins, C.J., Schmidt III, H. & Lineham, M.M. (2011) Chapter 2: Dialectic behavior therapy: Synthesizing radical acceptance with skilful meaning, IN Hayes, S.C., Follette, V.M. & Lineham, M.M. (Editors) Mindfulness and Acceptance: Expanding the cognitive-behavioral tradition, London, Guilford Press. p.30-44.

Robinson, C & Rose, S. (2013) Locus of Control, IN Lopez, S.J. (Editor) The encyclopedia of Positive Psychology, Oxford, Wiley-Blackwell Publishing, pg. 585-589

Robinson, M., & Cottrell, D. (2005). Health professionals in multi-disciplinary and multi-agency teams: Changing professional practice. Journal of Interprofessional Care, 19(6), 547–560.

Rosenberg, M. (1979) Conceiving the Self, Basic Books, New York.

Rossi, A, Cetrano, G, Pertile, R, Rabbi, L, Donisi, V, Grigoletti, L, Curtolo, C, Tansella, M, Thornicroft, G, Amaddeo, F (2012) Burnout, compassion fatigue, and compassion satisfaction among staff in community-based mental health services. Psychiatry Research, 200(2), 933-938.

Rotter, J. B. (1966). Generalized expectancies for internal versus external control of reinforcement. Psychological Monographs, 80(1) 609.

Rowling, J.K. (1999) Harry Potter and The Prisoner of Azkaban. Pottermore Publishing.

Rowntree, G., Atayero, S., O'Connell, M.D., Hoffman, M., Jassi, A., Narusevicius, V. & Tsapekos, D. (2015) Resilience in Emergency Medical Responders: A pilot study of a reflective journal intervention using a mixed methods approach, Journal of European Psychology Students, 6(2), p79-84.

Royal College of Midwives (RCM) (2020) Domestic Abuse. [Online] London, RCM. Retrieved from: https://www.rcm.org.uk/ media/4067/identifying-caring-for-and-supporting-women-at-risk-of_victims-of-domestic-abuse-duringcovid-19-v1__13052020final.pdf] accessed 7th June, 2020.

Royal College of Midwives (RCM) and Royal College of Obstetricians & Gynaecologists (RCOG) (2020) Coronavirus (Covid-19) Infection in Pregnancy: Information for Healthcare Professionals, (Version 10) [Online] London, RCM & (RCOG), (4th June) Retrieved from: https://www.rcog.org.uk/globalassets/documents/guidelines/2020-06-04-coronavirus-covid-19-infection-in-pregnancy.pdf, Accessed on 7th June, 2020.

Royal College of Physicians. Ethical Dimensions of COVID-19 for frontline staff. 2020.

Royal College of Psychiatrists (2020) Impact of Covid-19 on Black, Asian and Minority Ethnic (BAME) staff in mental healthcare settings/assessment and management of risk. Available at http.//rcpsych.ac.uk. [Accessed: 18/05/20]

Rozin, P. & Royzman, E.B. (2001) Negativity bias, negativity dominance and contagion, Personality and Social Psychology Review, 5, p.296-320.

Rutter, M. (1997) Psychosocial resilience and protective mechanisms. American Journal of Orthopsychiatry, 57, 316-331.

Sajnani, N. (2012). The implicated witness: Towards a relational aesthetic in dramatherapy. Dramatherapy, 34(1), 6–21.

Salas, J. (1990). Aesthetic experience in music therapy. Music Therapy, 9(1), 1–15.

Salvatore, J., & Shelton, J.N. (2007). Cognitive costs of exposure to racial prejudice. Psychological Science, 18(9), p.810–815.

Sanghavi, D.M. (2006). What Makes for a Compassionate Patient-Caregiver Relationship? Journal on Quality and Patient Safety. 32 (5) pp.283-292.

Santini, Z; Jose, P; Cornwell, E; Koyanagi, A; Nielsen, L; Hinrichsen, C. et al. (2020) Social disconnectedness, perceived isolation, and symptoms of depression and anxiety among older Americans (NSHAP): a longitudinal mediation analysis. Lancet Public Health. 5, pp. 62–70.

Schaufeli W, Bakker A (2013) [The psychology of labor and health, 3th ed.] De psychologie van arbeid en gezondheid. Derde geheel herziene druk ed. Bohn Stafleu van Loghum, Houten. cited in van Mol, Kompanje, Benoit, Bakker & Nijkamp, 2015

Schavarien, J (2004) Boarding school: the trauma of the 'privileged' child' Journal of Analytical Psychology, 49(5) p.683-706

Scheier, M. F., Carver, C. S. & Bridges, M. W. (1994). Distinguishing optimism from neuroticism (and trait anxiety, self-mastery, and self-esteem): A re-evaluation of the Life Orientation Test. Journal of Personality and Social Psychology, 67, 1063–1078.

Schimmenti, A., Billieux, J, Starcevic, V (2020) The four horsemen of fear: An integrated model of understanding fear experiences during the COVID-19 pandemic. Clinical Neuropsychiatry, 17(2), 41-45.

Schubert, C. F., Schmidt, U., & Rosner, R. (2016). Posttraumatic growth in populations with posttraumatic stress disorder—A systematic review on growth-related psychological constructs and biological variables. Clinical psychology & psychotherapy, 23(6), 469-486.

SCOPE (2020) The disability report: Disabled people and the coronavirus crisis, [Online] SCOPE, (May) Retrieved from: https://www.scope.org.uk/campaigns/disabled-people-and-coronavirus/the-disability-report/, Accessed on: 7th June, 2020.

Scottish Commission for people with a Learning Disabilities (SCLD) (2020) Statement on Human Rights and COVID-19, [Online) Glasgow, SCLD, Retrieved from: https://www.scld.org.uk/wp-content/uploads/2020/03/SCLD-COVID-19-Human-Rights-Statement.pdf, Accessed on 7th June, 2020.

Sears, S. R., Stanton, A. L., & Danoff-Burg, S. (2003). The Yellow Brick Road and the Emerald City: Benefit-finding, positive reappraisal coping, and posttraumatic growth in women with early stage breast cancer. Health Psychology, 22, 487–497

Seery, M., Holman, A. & Silver, R. (2010) Whatever does not kill us: cumulative lifetime adversity, vulnerability and resilience, Journal of Personality and Social Psychology, 99(6) 1025-1041.

Seligman, M. E. P. and Peterson, C. (2006) 'Character strengths in fifty-four nations and the fifty US states', Journal of Positive Psychology, 1(3), pp. 118–129. doi: 10.1080/17439760600619567.

Seligman, M.E.P. (1995) Optimistic child: a proven program to safeguard children against depression and build lifelong resilience, Houghton Mifflin (Harper-Collins).

Seligman, M.E.P. (2001) Learned optimism: how to change your mind and your life, Simon and Schuster.

Seligman, M.E.P. (2011) Flourish; a new understanding of happiness and well – being and how to achieve them. London, Nicholas Brealey Publishing.

Seligman, M.E.P. (2011) Flourish: a new understanding of happiness and wellbeing and how to achieve them, London, Nicholas Brealey Publishing.

Seligman, M.E.P. (2011) Flourish: A New Understanding of Happiness and Wellbeing: The practical guide to using positive psychology to make you happier and healthier, Nicholas Brealey Publishing.

Semple, S. and Cherrie, J.W. (2020) Covid-19 protecting worker health, Annals of Work Exposure and Health, 1-4.

Seneca (2004) Letters From A Stoic. London: Penguin Classics

Shapin, S. (1991) 'The mind in its own place': science and solitude in seventeenth-century England. Science in Context, 4/1, 191-218

Shapiro, F. (1995). Eye Movement Desensitisation and Reprocesing: Basic Principles, Protocols and Procedures. The Guilford Press.

Shapiro, S., De Sousa, S. & Hauck, C. (2016) Chapter 25: Mindfulness in Positive Clinical Psychology, IN Wood, A.M. & Johnson, J. (Editors) IN Wood, A.M. & Johnson, J. (Editors) The Wiley Handbook of Positive Clinical Psychology, John Wiley & Sons, p.381-394.

Shay, J. Achilles in Vietnam: Combat Trauma and the Undoing of Character. 1994. New York. Simon and Schuster.

Sheryl Sanberg, 2020, Good Reads, viewed 21 June 2020, www.goodreads.com

Shigemura, J; Ursano, R;Morganstein, J; Kurosawa, M. & Benedek, D. (2020) Public responses to the novel 2019 coronavirus (2019-nCoV) in Japan: mental health consequences and target populations. Psychiatry Clin Neurosci. 74, pp. 277–283.

Shoshani, A. & Aviv, I. (2012) The pillars of strength for first grade adjustment – Parental and children's character strengths and the transition to elementary school, Journal of Positive Psychology, 7(4) p.315-326.

Shoshani, A. & Steinmetz, S. (2014) Positive Psychology at School: A School-Based Intervention to Promote Adolescents' Mental Health and Well-Being, Journal of Happiness Studies, 15, p.1289–1311.

Shultz, J.M., Cooper, J.L., Baingana, F., Pguendo, M.A., Espinel, Z., Althouse, B.M., Marcelin, L.H., Towers, S., Espinola, M., McCoy, C.B., Mazurik, L., Wainberg, M.L.,

Siddique, H (2020, May, 1st) BAME Covid-19 death rate 'more than that of whites'. The Guardian, Available at http//.www.theguardian.com. [Accessed:21/04/20]

Simpkin, A (2020). Embracing uncertainty: could there be a blueprint from COVID-19? BMJ Blog Post: https://blogs.bmj.com/bmj/2020/04/16/embracing-uncertainty-could-there-be-a-blueprint-from-covid-19/

Simpkin, A.L. & Schwartzstein, R.M. (2016) Tolerating Uncertainty – The Next Medical Revolution. New England Journal of Medicine, 375: p.1713-5

Sinclair, A., & Haines, F. (1993). Deaths in the workplace and the dynamics of response. Journal of Contingencies and Crisis Management, 1(3), 125–137.

Singh, R., & Adhikari, R. (2020). Age-structured impact of social distancing on the COVID-19 epidemic in India. (Online). Available at: https://arxiv.org/pdf/2003.12055.pdf (accessed on 02 May 2020).

Sky News (2020) Coronavirus: Stars and notable figures who have died after contracting COVID-19, [Online] Sky News, Retrieved from: https://news.sky.com/story/coronavirus-stars-and-notable-figures-who-have-died-after-contracting-covid-19-11969431, Accessed on 7th June, 2020.

Sky News (2020b) Report: TV Programme, Sky News (6th June).

Slatten, L., David Carson, K. & Carson, P. (2011), Compassion fatigue and burnout: what managers should know, The Health Care Manager, 30(4), p.325-333.

Smart, D., English, A., James, J., Wilson, M., Daratha, K., Childers, B. & Magera, C. (2014), Compassion fatigue and satisfaction: a cross-sectional survey among US healthcare workers, Nursing & Health Science, 16(1), pp. 3-10.

Smith, C.A, and Ellsworth, P.C. (1985) Patterns of cognitive appraisal in emotion. Journal of Personality and Social Psychology, 48 (4) (1985), pp. 813-838.

Smith, G.D., Ng, F., Li, W.H.C. (2020) COVID-19: Emerging compassion, courage and resilience in the face of misinformation and adversity. Journal of Clinical Nursing, 29(9-10), 1425.

Smithies, D. (2011) Attention in rational-access consciousness, IN Mole, D.,

Smithies, D. & Wu, W. (Editors) Attention: Philosophical and psychological essays, Oxford, Oxford University press, p.247-273.

Smoke Gets In Your Eyes (2017) Mad Men. Series 1, Episode 1. Lionsgate Television. Available at: Netflix (Accessed: 30 April 2020).

Snyder, C.R. (2002). Hope Theory: Rainbows in the Mind. Psychological Inquiry, 13(4), 249–275.

Social Care Institute for Excellence (SCIE) (2020) COVID-19 guide for carers and family supporting adults and children with learning disabilities or autistic adults and children [Online] London, SCIE, Retrieved from: https://www.scie.org.uk/care-providers/coronavirus-covid-19/learning-disabilities-autism/carers-family, Accessed on 7th June, 2020.

Sodeke-Gregson, E.A., Holttum, S. & Billings, J. (2013) Compassion satisfaction, burnout and secondary traumatic stress in UK therapists who work with adult trauma clients. European Journal of Psychotraumatology, 4, https://www-ncbi-nlm-nihgov.ezproxy.lib.ucalgary.ca/pmc/articles/PMC3877781/ (accessed 12 May 2017).

Solomon, Z., Mikulincer, M. & Benbenishty, R. (1989) Locus of control and combat related PTSD: The intervening role of battle intensity, threat appraisal and coping, British Journal of Psychology, 28(3) p133-144.

Somasundaram, D. (2014). Addressing collective trauma: Conceptualisations and interventions. Intervention, 12(1), 43-60.

Sonis, J.D., Kennedy, M., Aaronson, E.L., Baugh, J.J., Raja, A.S., Yun, B.J. & White, B.A. (2020) Humanism in the Age of COVID-19: Renewing Focus on Communication and Compassion. Western Journal of Emergency Medicine: Integrating Emergency Care with Population Health, 21(3), 499-502.

Sorgaard, K. W., Ryan, P., & Dawson, I. (2010). Qualified and Unqualified (N-R C ) mental health nursing staff - minor differences in sources of stress and burnout. A European multi-centre study.

Spinoza (2017) Definitions Of The Emotions in The Ethics. Available at: https://www.gutenberg.org/files/3800/3800-h/3800-h.htm (Accessed: 15 April 2020)

Sprang, G., Clark, J.J. & Whitt-Woosley, A. (2007) Compassion fatigue, compassion satisfaction, and burnout: factors impacting a professional's quality of life. Journal of Loss and Trauma, 12(3), 259-280.

Stallman, H. M., Kavanagh, D. J., Arklay, A. R., & Bennett-Levy, J. (2016).

Steimer, T. (2002) The biology of fear- and anxiety-related behaviours. Dialogues in Clinical Neuroscience. 4 (3), pp. 231–249.

Steinbuch, Y. Italian nurse with coronavirus kills herself over fear of infecting others, New York Post, (March 25)

Stenger, J. (2018) 'Other' spaces in ancient civilisation- Christian ascetism as heterotopia. Journal for Ancient Studies, 7, p. 64-84

Stephenson, J (2020, April 12). Exclusive: Are we whitewashing coronavirus? Nursing Times, Available at https://www.nursingtimes.net/news/coronavirus/exclusive. [Accessed: 24/04/20]

Storr, A. (1988) Solitude. London, HarperCollins Publishers

Strawson, G (2008) 'Against Narrativity' in Real Materialism and Other Essays. Oxford: Clarendon Press

Streeter, C.C., Gerbarg, P., Saper, R., Ciraulo, D. & Brown, R. (2012) Effects of yoga on the autonomic nervous system, gamma-aminobutyric-acid, and allostasis in epilepsy, depression, and post-traumatic stress disorder. Med Hypotheses, May 78 (5): p.571-9.

Strengthscope (2019) Strengthscope Accreditation (Sample Report), Strengthscope.

Struyf, D., Zaman, J., Hermans, D. & Vervliet, B. (2017) Gradients of fear: How perception influences fear generalization. Behaviour Research and Therapy. 93 p. 116–122.

Sumiala, J. & Tikka, M. (2011) Imagining globalised fears: school shooting videos and circulation of violence on You-tube. Social Anthropology. 19(3) p.254-266.

Talbot SG & Dean W. Beyond Burnout: The Real Problem Facing Doctors is Moral Injury. Medical Economics 2019; 96: 10

Taylor Buck, E., & Havsteen-Franklin, D. (2013). Connecting with the image: How art psychotherapy can help to re-establish a sense of epistemic trust. ATOL: Art Therapy OnLine, 4(1), 1–24.

Taylor, S. E. (1983). Adjustment to threatening events: A theory of cognitive adaptation. American Psychologist, 38, 1161–1173

Teasdale, J.D., Segal, Z.V., Williams, J., Ridgeway V.A., Soulsby, J. & Lau M.A., (2000) Prevention of relapse/recurrence in major depression by Mindfulness-Based Cognitive Therapy, Journal of Consulting and Clinical Psychology, 68 (4): 615-23. (740 citations in ISI Web of Knowledge, October 2013). DOI: 10.1037//0022-006X.68.4.615

Tedeschi, R. & Calhoun, L. (2004). Posttraumatic growth: conceptual foundations and empirical evidence. Psychological Inquiry. 9, 405–412.

Tedeschi, R. G. & Calhoun, L. G. (1996) The posttraumatic growth inventory. Measuring the positive legacy of trauma. Journal of Trauma and Stress 9, 455–471.

Tedeschi, R.G., Shakespeare-Finch, J., Taku, K. & Calhoun, L.G. (2018) Posttraumatic Growth: theory, research and application, Routledge (Taylor and Francis

Tempesta, E. (2020) 'We're walking biological weapons': Healthcare workers candidly share their fears about COVID-19 and the devastating toll it has taken on them and their loved ones. (Online). Available at: https://www.dailymail.co.uk/femail/article-8278331/Coronavirus-Healthcare-workers-share-fears-COVID-19.html (accessed 01 May 2020).

Terry, M.L. & Leary, M.R. (2011) Self-compassion, self-regulation, and health, Self Identity, 10(3) 352-362.

The Critical Care National Network Nurse Leads (CC3N). (2020) Non-Critical Care Staff in Critical Care - Emergency Induction. CC3N. Available at: www.cc3n.org.uk/covid-19-resources-- guidance.html  (Accessed 09 May 2020)

The Moral Injury Project, Syracuse University.  What is Moral Injury?  2020. https://moralinjuryproject.syr.edu/about-moral-injury/

Thomas, H. (2020) Hancock setting a bad example on social distancing, say NHS leaders. [Online]  Health Service Journal, 10 April 2020,  Retrieved from https://www.hsj.co.uk/coronavirus/updated-hancock-setting-a-bad-example-on-social-distancing-say-nhs-leaders/7027385.article, Accessed on 14th May, 2020.

Thomas, K. (1984) Man and the Natural World. London, Penguin Books

Thomas, R. (2020) 'Unprecedented' number of Do Not Resuscitate Orders for Learning Disability Patients, [Online] Health Service Journal,  (24 April). Retrieved from: https://www.hsj.co.uk/coronavirus/unprecedented-number-of-dnr-orders-for-learning-disabilities-patients/7027480.article, Accessed on 7th June, 2020.

Thompson, G. (2019) Trauma and Meaning, Positive Living in Difficult Times, [Online] Accessed at: https://www.mwaning.ca/article/trauma-and-memory, Retrieved at: 24th April, 2020.

Thoreau, H. (2017) Walden. London, Vintage Classics

Togashi, K. & Kottler, A. (2015) Kohut's Twinship across cultures: The psychology of being human, Routledge.

Town&Country, 2020, viewed 20 May 20202, https://www.townandcountrymag.com

Townsend, M. (2020) Domestic abuse cases soar as lockdown takes its toll. (Online). Available at:

https://www.theguardian.com/world/2020/apr/04/domestic-abuse-cases-soar-as-lockdown-takes-its-toll (accessed on 02 May 2020).

Tranel, D., Nikolas, M.A. & Markin, J. (2020) Chapter 2L Psychopathology: a neurobiological perspective, IN Maddux, J.E. & Winstead, B.A. (Editors) Psychopathology: Foundations for a contemporary understanding, London, Routledge (Taylor and Francis Group).

Traynor M (2017) Critical Resilience for Nurses: An Evidence-Based Guide to Survival and Change in the Modern NHS. Routledge, Abingdon.

Triplett, K. N., Tedeschi, R. G., Cann, A., Calhoun, L. G., & Reeve, C. L. (2012). Post-traumatic growth, meaning in life, and life satisfaction in response to trauma. Psychological Trauma: Theory, Research, Practice, and Policy, 4, 400–410..

Tronick, E. (2009) Multilevel meaning making and dyadic, expansion of consciousness theory: the emotional and polymorphic polysemic flow of meaning, IN

Turner, K. and McCarthy, V.L. (2017) Stress and anxiety among nursing students: A review of intervention strategies in literature between 2009 and 2015. Nurse Education in Practice, 22:21-29.

Turner, V. (1969) The Ritual Process: Structure and Anti-Structure. Ithaca, New York, Cornell University Press

Uduak, A., and Aliya, D. (2010) The Involvement of Black and Minority Ethnic Staff in NHS Disciplinary Proceedings. Available on line at: https://www.nhsemployers.org/~/media/Employers/Documents/SiteCollection Documents/Disciplinary. [Accessed on 25/05/20]


United Kingdom Home Office. (2020). Coronavirus (COVID-19): Support for Victims of Domestic Abuse. (Online). Available at: https://www.gov.uk/guidance/domestic-abuse-how-to-get-help#coronavirus-covid-19-and-domestic-abuse (accessed on 01 May 2020).

United Nations (2020) UN working to ensure vulnerable groups not left behind in Covid-19 response, [Online] New York, Department of Global Communication, United Nations, Retrieved from: https://www.un.org/en/un-coronavirus-communications-team/un-working-ensure-vulnerable-groups-not-left-behind-covid-19, Accessed on 9th June, 2020.

Updegraff, J. A., Silver, R. C., & Holman, E. A. (2008). Searching for and finding meaning in collective trauma: results from a national longitudinal study of the 9/11 terrorist attacks. Journal of personality and social psychology, 95(3), 709.

Usherwood, T. (2020) I gasped for life from the coronavirus. At 38, I might never see my son again. The Sunday Times, March 29 2020. Available at: https://www.thetimes.co.uk/article/theo-usherwood-on-coronavirus-i-gasped-for-life-at-38-i-might-never-see-my-son-again-fgr5lr8z0 (Accessed 09 May 2020)

Van Der Kolk, B (2014). The Body Keeps the Score: Mind, Brain and Body in the Transformation of Trauma. Penguin.

Van der Kolk, B. (2014) The body keeps the score: Mind, brain and body in the transformation of trauma, London, Penguin (Random House)

Van Deurzen-Smith, E. (1997). Everyday Mysteries – Existential Dimensions of Psychotherapy. London: Routledge.

Van Gennet, A. (1960) The Rites of Passage. London, Routledge and Kegan Paul

Van Lith, T., Schofield, M. J., & Fenner, P. (2013). Identifying the evidence-base for art-based practices and their potential benefit for mental health recovery: A critical review. Disability and Rehabilitation, 35(16), 1309–1323.

Van Mol, M.M.C., Kompanje, E.J.O., Benoit, D.D., Bakker, J. & Nijkamp, M.D. (2015) The Prevalence of Compassion Fatigue and Burnout among Healthcare Professionals in Intensive Care Units: A Systematic Review. PLoS ONE, 10(8): e0136955. doi:10.1371/ journal.pone.0136955

Voltaire Quotes. Quotes.net. STANDS4 LLC, 2020. Web. 17 May 2020. https://www.quotes.net/quote/6751; https://dakebyhuferowybo.benjaminpohle.com/dalai-lama-critical-thinking-quote-15921cl.html

Walker, C. (2020) NEWS: COVID-19: critical care guide updated amid fears for people with learning disabilities. Learning Disability Practice, (25th March) [Online] Retrieved from:   https://rcni.com/learning-disability-practice/newsroom/news/covid-19-critical-care-guide-updated-amid-fears-people-learning-disabilities-159221, Accessed on 7th June, 2020.

Walker, C. & Gerada, C. (2020) Extraordinary times: coping psychologically through the impact of covid-19. BMJ Blogs. Available at: https://blogs.bmj.com/bmj/2020/03/31/extraordinary-times-coping-psychologically-through-the-impact-of-covid-19/ (Accessed 30 April 2020)

Walters, E.T., Carew, T. J., & Kandel, E.R. (1981). Associative learning in aplysia: evidence for conditioned fear in an invertebrate. Science, 211, p 504–506. doi:10.1126/science.7192881.

Wang, C; Pan, R; Wan, X; Tan, Y; Xu, L; Cyrus, S. et al. (2020) Immediate Psychological Responses and Associated Factors during the Initial Stage of the 2019 Coronavirus Disease (COVID-19) Epidemic among the General Population in China. (Online). Available at: https://www.mdpi.com/1660-4601/17/5/1729 (accessed 02 May 2020).

Warren, R., Smeets, E. & Neff, K. (2016) Self-criticism and self-compassion: risk and resilience, Current Psychiatry, 15(12), p.18-32.

Watkins, A., Rothfeldm M., Rashbaum. W.K. & Rosenthal, B.M. (2020) Top E.R. Doctor who treated virus patient dies by suicide, The New York Times, (April 27)

Weber, M. (1963). The Sociology of Religion. Boston: Beacon Press

Welch, S. E., & Bunin, J. (2010). Glove use and the HIV positive massage therapy client. Journal of Bodywork and Movement Therapies. 14(1), pp.35–39.

Wenzell, M., Woodyatt, L. & Hedrick, K. (2012) No genuine self-forgiveness without accepting responsibility: value reaffirmation as a key to maintaining positive self regard, European Journal of Social Psychology, 42(5), 617-627.

Werdel, M.B. & Wicks, R.J. (2012) Primer on Post Traumatic growth: an introduction and guide, Hove, John Wiley and Sons.

West, M., Dawson, J., & Kaur, M. (2015) The Kings Fund: Making the difference

Wheaton, M.G., Abramowitz, J.S., Berman, N.C., Fabricant, L.E., & Olatunji, B.O (2011). Psychological Predictors of Anxiety in Response to the H1N1: (Swine Flu) Pandemic. Available online: Springer Science+Business Media.[Accessed:12/05/20].

White, E., Hille K., Stefanie, P. Liu, N. (2020). Asia struggles to find coronavirus exit strategies. (Online). Available at: https://www.ft.com/content/04e9c5fe-52b1-4eb8-bf9c-793d71a0524d (accessed on 2 May 2020).

WHO, 2020, Munich Security Conference, viewed 21 June 2020, https://www.who.int/dg/speeches/detail/munich-security-conference

WHO. (2020). Mental health and psychosocial considerations during the COVID-19 outbreak, 18 March 2020. World Health Organization.

Williams R, Murray E, Neal A & Kemp V. Top ten Messages for Supporting Healthcare staff During the COVID-19 Pandemic. A discussion Document. Royal College of Psychiatry 2020

Williamson V, Murphy M & Greenburg N. COVID-19 And Experiences Of Moral Injury In Front-Line Key Workers. Occupational Medicine, 2020, Apr. Published online: https://doi.org/10.1093/occmed/kqaa052

Williamson V, Stevelink SAM, Greenberg N. Occupational Moral Injury and Mental Health: Systematic Review and Meta-Analysis. Br J Psychiatry 2018; 12: 339-346

Willis Commission (2012) Quality with compassion: the future of nurse education, Royal College of Nursing.

Windeatt, B. (2016) Medieval life-writing: types, encomia, exemplars, patterns. Chapter 2 in A. Smyth (Ed) A History of English Autobiography. Cambridge, Cambridge University Press

Windeatt, B. (2015) Introduction. In Julian of Norwich (2015) Revelations of Divine Love. Transl. B Windeatt. Oxford, Oxford University Press

Winnicott, D. (2018) The capacity to be alone. Chapter 2 in The Maturational Process and the Facilitating Environment. London, Routledge

Wohl, M.A., DeShea, L. & Wahkinney, R.L. (2008) Looking within: measuring state self-forgiveness and its relationship to psychological well being, Canadian Journal of Behavioural Science/Revue Canadienee Des Sciences Du Comportement, 40, 1-10.

Wolters, C. A. & Pintrich, P. R. (1998) Contextual differences in student motivation and self-regulated learning in mathematics, English, and social studies classrooms. Instructional Science, 26: p.27–47.

Woodward, C. (2004). 'Hardiness and the concept of courage'. Unpublished manuscript, The Groden Centre, providence, RI.

World Bank (2020) Population density (people per square kilometer of land area), [Online] World Bank, Retrieved from https://data.worldbank.org/indicator/EN.POP.DNST?view=map, Accessed on 27/5/2020.

World Health Organisation (2014) Ebola response roadmap. (Online). Available at: https://www.who.int/csr/resources/publications/ebola/response-roadmap/en/ (accessed 30 April 2020).

World Health Organisation (2020, April 27). WHO Timeline - COVID-19. Online: https://www.who.int/news-room/detail/27-04-2020-who-timeline---covid-19 [Accessed: 06/05/20]

World Health Organisation (2020a) Disability considerations during the COVID-19 outbreak. (Online). Available at: https://www.who.int/who-documents-detail/disability-considerations-during-the-covid-19-outbreak (accessed 26 April 2020).

World Health Organisation (2020b) Considerations for quarantine of individuals in the context of containment for coronavirus disease (COVID-19). (Online). Available at: https://apps.who.int/iris/bitstream/handle/10665/331497/WHO-2019-nCoV-IHR_Quarantine-2020.2-eng.pdf (accessed on 30 April 2020)

World Health Organisation (2020c) Staying at home and away from others (social distancing). (Online). Available at: https://www.gov.uk/government/publications/full-guidance-on-staying-at-home-and-away-from-others (accessed 26 April 2020).

World Health Organisation (2020d) Rational use of personal protective equipment for coronavirus disease 2019 (COVID-19). (Online). Available at: https://apps.who.int/iris/bitstream/handle/10665/331215/WHO-2019-nCov-IPCPPE_use-2020.1-eng.pdf (accessed on 30 April 2020).

World Health Organisation (2020e) Mental health and psychosocial considerations during the COVID-19 outbreak. (Online). https://apps.who.int/iris/bitstream/handle/10665/331490/WHO-2019-nCoV-MentalHealth-2020.1-eng.pdf (accessed 02 May 2020).

World Health Organisation (2020f) Shortage of personal protective equipment endangering health workers worldwide. 3rd March 2020. Available on-line at: https://www.who.int/news-room/detail/03-03-2020-shortage-of-personal-protective-equipment-endangering-health-workers-worldwide (accessed 03 May 2020).

World Health Organisation (WHO) (2013) International Classification of Disease 10th Edition (ICD-10) Geneiva, WHO.

World Health Organisation (WHO) (2018) International Classification of Disease 11th Edition (ICD-11). Geneiva, WHO.

World Health Organisation. (2020) Basic protective measures against the new coronavirus. https://www.who.int/emergencies/diseases/novel-coronavirus-2019/advice-for-public. Accessed 5 March 2020.

World Health Organization (2007) Practical Guidelines for Infection Control in Health Care Facilities. WPRO Regional Publication, Manila.

World Health Organization (2015) WHO Statement on Caesarean Section Rates, Geneva, Switzerland. Human Reproduction Programme World Health Organization.

World Health Organization (2019) Report of the WHO-China Joint Mission on Coronavirus Disease (COVID-19). (Online).  Available at:

https://www.who.int/docs/default-source/coronaviruse/who-china-joint-mission-on-covid-19-final-report.pdf (accessed 29 April 2020).

World Health Organization (2020b) Pregnancy, Childbirth, breastfeeding and COVID-19, [Online], Geneva, WHO, Retrieved at : https://www.who.int/reproductivehealth/publications/emergencies/COVID-19-pregnancy-ipc-breastfeeding-infographics/en/ Accessed on 7th June, 2020.

World Health Organization (WHO) (2006) Intimate partner violence and alcohol, [Online] Geneva, WHO, Retrieved from : https://www.who.int/violence_injury_prevention/violence/world_report/factsheets/fs_intimate.pdf, Accessed on 7th June, 2020.

World Health Organization (WHO) (2020a). WHO Timeline – Worldwide (Regional) COVID-19 Staistics. [Online] Geneva, WHO. April 27 Retrieved from : https://www.who.int/news-room/detail/27-04-2020-who-timeline---covid-19, Accessed: 5th June, 2020

Wu, S., Singh-Carlson, S., Odell, A., Reynolds, G, & Su, Y. (2016) Compassion fatigue, burnout, and compassion satisfaction among oncology nurses in the United States and Canada. Oncology Nurse Forum; 43(4): E161–E169.

Yackle, K., Schwartz, L.A., Kam, K., Sorokin, J., Huguenard, J., Feldman, J., Luo, L. & Krasnow, M. (2017) Breathing control center neurons that promote arousal in mice. Science, 355(6332): 1411-1415ty

Yalom, I. D. (1980). Existential Psychotherapy. New York, NY: Basic Books.

Yalom, I. D. (2013). Love's Executioner And Other Tales Of Psychotherapy. New York, NY: Basic Books.

Yalom, L.D. (1980) Existential Psychotherapy, New York, Basic Books.

Yoder, E.A. (2010) Compassion fatigue in nurses. Applied Nursing Research, 23: p.191–197.

Young, J.L., Derr, D.M., Cicchillo, V.J. & Bressler, S. (2011) Compassion satisfaction, burnout, and secondary traumatic stress in heart and vascular nurses. Critical Care Nursing Quarterly, 34(3), p.227-234.

Youngson, R (2008) Compassion in healthcare: the missing dimension of healthcare reform. London, NHS Confederation

Zeng, K., Chiu, C.P.K., Wang, R., Oei, T.P.S. & Leung, F.Y.K. (2015) The effects of Loving Kindness meditation on positive emotions: a meta analytical review, Frontiers in Psychiatry, p.1-14.

Zhang, Y-Y., Zhang, C., Xiao Rong Han, M.D., Wei, I.J. & Ying-Lei Weung, M.D. (2018) Determinants of compassion satisfaction, compassion fatigue and burnout in nursing a correlation meta-analysis, Medicine (Baltimore), 97(26) e11086.

Zimmerman, B. J. (1995) Self-efficacy and educational development. IN: Bandura, A. (Editor), Self-Efficacy in Changing Societies, New York, Cambridge University Press, p.202–231.

Zimmerman, P.B., Pojul, H., Rohoe, A., Roser, K., Powell, G., Lin=vingston, G. & Hagman, G. (2019) Chapter 1: An introduction to Intersubject Self Psychology, IN Hagman, G., Paul, H. & Zimmerman, P.B. (Editors) Intersubject Self Psychology: a primer, Routledge (Taylor and Francis Group).

Zoellner, L.A., Graham, B.& Bedard-Gillingan, M.A. (2020) Trauma and Stressor Related Disorders, IN Maddux, J.E. & Winstead, B.A. (Editors) Psychopathology Foundations for a contemporary understanding, London, Routledge (Taylor and Francos Group)

Printed in Great Britain
by Amazon

50070327R00219